T0259162

Models of Protection Against HIV/SIV

Avoiding AIDS in humans and monkeys

Models of Protection Against HIV/SIV

Avoiding AIDS in humans and monkeys

Edited by
Gianfranco Pancino
Guido Silvestri
Keith R. Fowke

AMSTERDAM • BOSTON • HEIDELBERG • LONDON
NEW YORK • OXFORD • PARIS • SAN DIEGO
SAN FRANCISCO • SINGAPORE • SYDNEY • TOKYO

Academic Press is an imprint of Elsevier

ELSEVIER

Academic Press is an imprint of Elsevier
32 Jamestown Road, London NW1 7BY, UK
225 Wyman Street, Waltham, MA 02451, USA
525 B Street, Suite 1800, San Diego, CA 92101-4495, USA

First edition 2012

Notice
No responsibility is assumed by the publisher for any injury and/or damage to persons or
property as a matter of products liability, negligence or otherwise, or from any use or
operation of any methods, products, instructions or ideas contained in the material
herein. Because of rapid advances in the medical sciences, in particular, independent
verification of diagnoses and drug dosages should be made

British Library Cataloguing-in-Publication Data
A catalogue record for this book is available from the British Library

Library of Congress Cataloging-in-Publication Data
A catalog record for this book is available from the Library of Congress

ISBN : 978-0-12-387715-4

For information on all Academic Press publications
visit our website at elsevierdirect.com

Typeset by TNQ Books and Journals Pvt Ltd.
www.tnq.co.in

Contents

Section I
Simian Models of Non-Pathogenic SIV Infection

1. Natural SIV Infection: Virological Aspects
Jan Münch and Frank Kirchhoff

2. Natural SIV Infection: Immunological Aspects
Béatrice Jacquelin, Roland C. Zahn, Françoise Barré-Sinoussi,
Jörn E. Schmitz, Amitinder Kaur and Michaela C. Müller-Trutwin

Section II
HIV-1-Exposed Seronegative Individuals

6. Host Genetics and Resistance to HIV-1 Infection

Ma Luo, Paul J. McLaren and Francis A. Plummer

7. The Immune System and Resisting HIV Infection

Keith R. Fowke, Catherine M. Card and Rupert Kaul

Section III
HIV-1 Controllers

8. Definition, Natural History and Heterogeneity of HIV Controllers

Asier Sáez-Cirión, Gianfranco Pancino and Olivier Lambotte,
for the ANRS CO18 Cohort

Section IV
Genetic Basis of Protection Against HIV

Contributors

T. Blake Ball, National Laboratory for HIV Immunology, National HIV & Retrovirology Laboratories, Public Health Agency of Canada, Winnipeg, Manitoba, Canada; and Department of Medical Microbiology, University of Manitoba, Winnipeg, Manitoba, Canada

Françoise Barré-Sinoussi, Institut Pasteur, Unité Régulation des Infections Rétrovirales, Paris, France

Mara Biasin, Universita degli Studi di Milano, Milan, Italy

Joel N. Blankson, Johns Hopkins University School of Medicine, Baltimore, Maryland, USA

Kristina Broliden, Karolinska Institutet, Department of Medicine Solna, Center for Molecular Medicine, Stockholm, Sweden

Robert W. Buckheit III, Johns Hopkins University School of Medicine, Baltimore, Maryland, USA

Catherine M. Card, Laboratory of Viral Immunology, Department of Medical Microbiology, University of Manitoba, Winnipeg, Manitoba, Canada

Mario Clerici, Universita degli Studi di Milano, Milan, Italy; and Fondazione Don Gnocchi, ONLUS, Milano, Italy

Thushan de Silva, Nuffield Department of Medicine, Weatherall Institute of Molecular Medicine, John Radcliffe Hospital, Oxford, UK

Jacques Fellay, Global Health Institute, School of Life Sciences, Federal Institute of Technology—EPFL, Lausanne, Switzerland; and Institute of Medical Microbiology, University Hospital, University of Lausanne, Lausanne, Switzerland

Keith R. Fowke, Laboratory of Viral Immunology, Department of Medical Microbiology, and Department of Community Health Sciences, University of Manitoba, Winnipeg, Manitoba, Canada

Béatrice Jacquelin, Institut Pasteur, Unité Régulation des Infections Rétrovirales, Paris, France

Rupert Kaul, Departments of Medicine and Immunology, University of Toronto, Toronto, Canada

Amitinder Kaur, Division of Immunology, New England Primate Research Center, Southborough, Massachusetts, USA

Frank Kirchhoff, Institute of Molecular Virology, Ulm University Medical Center, Ulm, Germany

Olivier Lambotte, Inserm U1012, and Hôpital Bicêtre, Service de Médecine Interne et Maladies Infectieuses, Le Kremlin-Bicêtre, France

Alan L. Landay, Department of Immunology/Microbiology, Rush University Medical Center, Chicago, Illinois, USA

Ma Luo, Department of Medical Microbiology, University of Manitoba, Winnipeg, Manitoba, Canada; and National Microbiology Laboratory, Public Health Agency of Canada, Winnipeg, Manitoba, Canada

Paul J. McLaren, Department of Medicine, Division of Genetics, Brigham & Women's Hospital, Harvard Medical School, Boston, Massachusetts, USA

Eirini Moysi, Nuffield Department of Medicine, Weatherall Institute of Molecular Medicine, John Radcliffe Hospital, Oxford, UK

Michaela C. Müller-Trutwin, Institut Pasteur, Unité Régulation des Infections Rétrovirales, Paris, France

Jan Münch, Institute of Molecular Virology, Ulm University Medical Center, Ulm, Germany

Gianfranco Pancino, INSERM and Institut Pasteur, Unité de Régulation des Infections Rétrovirales, Paris, France

Ivona Pandrea, Department of Pathology, Center for Vaccine Research, University of Pittsburgh, Pittsburgh, Pennsylvania, USA

Florencia Pereyra, Ragon Institute of MGH, MIT & Harvard and Division of Infectious Diseases, Brigham and Women's Hospital, Boston, MA, USA

Francis A. Plummer, Department of Medical Microbiology, University of Manitoba, Winnipeg, Manitoba, Canada; and National Microbiology Laboratory, Public Health Agency of Canada, Winnipeg, Manitoba, Canada

Sarah Rowland-Jones, Nuffield Department of Medicine, Weatherall Institute of Molecular Medicine, John Radcliffe Hospital, Oxford, UK

Asier Sáez-Cirión, Institut Pasteur, Unité de Régulation des Infections Rétrovirales, Paris, France

Jörn E. Schmitz, Division of Viral Pathogenesis, Beth Israel Deaconess Medical Center, Harvard Medical School, Boston, Massachusetts, USA

Gene M. Shearer, Experimental Immunology Branch, Center for Cancer Research, NCI, NIH, Bethesda, Maryland, USA

Guido Silvestri, Department of Pathology and Laboratory Medicine, Emory University School of Medicine, and Division of Microbiology & Immunology, Yerkes National Primate Research Center, Emory University, Atlanta, Georgia

Amalio Telenti, Institute of Medical Microbiology, University Hospital, University of Lausanne, Lausanne, Switzerland

Bruce D Walker, Ragon Institute of MGH, MIT & Harvard, Massachusetts General Hospital—East Campus, Charlestown, Massachusetts, USA

Roland C. Zahn, Division of Viral Pathogenesis, Beth Israel Deaconess Medical Center, Harvard Medical School, Boston, Massachusetts, USA

MODELS OF PROTECTION AGAINST HIV/SIV

Over 30 years have passed since the acquired immune deficiency syndrome (AIDS) was recognized as a new disease entity. The notification in the *Mortality & Morbidity Weekly Report* in the summer of 1981 of a small number of young men in US cities with *Pneumocystis* pneumonia or Kaposi's sarcoma heralded the emergence to the medical world of the AIDS pandemic. The major routes of AIDS transmission—via sex and blood, as well as from mother to child—were already firmly established from epidemiological data during the 2 years before the causative agent, human immunodeficiency virus type 1 (HIV-1), was discovered in 1983 at the Institut Pasteur in Paris. The disastrous fall in the number of CD4+ T-helper lymphocytes in the peripheral circulation was already characterized in 1981, and the immune activation that precedes immune collapse was soon noted in the form of raised plasma levels of neopterin and beta-globulin.

Rapid progress on the cell and molecular biology of infection followed the discovery of HIV-1, including the sequencing of the viral genome, the identification of CD4 as the attachment receptor on the target cells (T-helper lymphocytes and macrophages), and the potent inhibition of HIV replication by the first antiretroviral drug, azidothymidine. There were high hopes for the early development of an HIV vaccine by those who did not realize that no efficacious vaccine had yet been developed for well-known veterinary lentiviral diseases such as Maedi-Visna of sheep and equine infectious anemia. The lentiviruses of non-human primates (SIV) and of cats (FIV) were only identified after the discovery of HIV-1 and shortly before that of HIV-2. Ironically, one could say that the pioneering and intensive study of HIV and AIDS in humans provided an excellent model for the investigation of SIV in monkeys!

It took a little longer to realize that simian AIDS in macaques represented an unusual pathogenic infection by a recently introduced virus, in parallel with the virulence of HIV-1 in humans, whereas most of the African non-human primates naturally infected with their own SIV strains can sustain high levels of virus infection without ill effect. Moreover, a small proportion of people with HIV-1 infection and a majority of people with HIV-2 infection do not progress to AIDS.

This volume of authoritative and up-to-date review chapters provides a synthesis of our emerging knowledge of human and simian infection by HIV and SIV, respectively. The main focus is on these intriguing examples of exposed or infected persons, and African non-human primates, who remain in relatively good health.

The study of those who do not become sick when exposed to a potentially lethal pathogen can be as informative as the study of pathogenesis itself. A greater understanding of the delicate balance between control of infection and progression to disease in host—pathogen interactions offers the hope of developing rational intervention to prevent disease, through immune modulation, and through prophylactic and therapeutic vaccines. That is why this book represents a major contribution to HIV/AIDS.

Robin A. Weiss

Division of Infection & Immunity, University College London

Simian Models of Non-Pathogenic SIV Infection

Natural SIV Infection: Virological Aspects

Jan Münch and Frank Kirchhoff

Institute of Molecular Virology, Ulm University Medical Center, Ulm, Germany

Chapter Outline

INTRODUCTION

Since the discovery almost 30 years ago that the acquired immune deficiency syndrome (AIDS) is caused by a lentivirus, detailed insights have been achieved about the origin of the viruses causing AIDS in humans [1−3]. It has become clear that a large number of African non-human primates (NHPs) are infected with simian immunodeficiency viruses (SIVs) that are genetically closely related to the human immunodeficiency viruses (HIVs) (reviewed in [1−5]). The original source of HIV-1 group M, the main form of the AIDS virus infecting humans, has been traced to SIVcpz infecting the central subspecies of

Models of Protection Against HIV/SIV. DOI: 10.1016/B978-0-12-387715-4.00001-0

chimpanzees (Cpz; *Pan troglodytes troglodytes*) [6]. Most likely, the virus was initially transmitted to humans early in the 20th century in south-eastern Cameroon [7]. Another NHP species, the sooty mangabey (SM, *Cercocebus atys*) has been identified as the original host of the second human immunodeficiency virus (HIV-2) [8,9]. Altogether, our current knowledge suggests that SIVs have been independently transmitted from chimpanzees, gorillas and sooty mangabeys (SMs) to humans at least a dozen times in the past two centuries [3], and that African NHPs have represented natural hosts for lentiviruses for many thousands or even millions of years [10−12]. Interestingly, well-adapted natural simian hosts of SIV do not develop AIDS despite high levels of virus replication. A variety of host and viral properties that most likely cooperate and synergize to allow a well-balanced and benign virus−host relationship have been identified (reviewed in [13−16]). Their relative contribution and importance, however, remain largely elusive and may differ between primate species, and even among individuals of the same species, as well as viral strains. This chapter aims to provide a brief overview of the distribution and biological properties of primate lentiviruses, and of the emergence of the human immunodeficiency viruses. Especially, we want to highlight some features of HIV-1 that distinguish it from HIV-2 and from SIVs that replicate efficiently in African NHPs without causing disease, and speculate on the development of these properties and their potential role in the pathogenesis of AIDS.

PRIMATE LENTIVIRAL INFECTIONS IN THE WILD

The discovery that HIV and AIDS are the result of relatively recent zoonotic transmissions of SIVs from African NHPs to humans [1−3,6] aroused a great deal of interest in natural primate lentiviral infections. Initially, studies on the prevalence, distribution and genetic diversity of SIVs in their natural habitats were complicated because wild monkeys are difficult to sample and blood or other tissues from endangered species hardly available. In the past decade, however, effective non-invasive methodologies for the detection and analysis of SIV-specific antibodies and of virion RNA in fecal and urine samples of wild NHPs have been developed. These methods have allowed large-scale sero-epidemiological and molecular studies of wild primate populations and yielded key insights into the genetic diversity and natural history of primate lentiviruses [17−20]. Meanwhile, these non-invasive approaches have been considerably improved. For example, they now allow the generation of full-length infectious molecular clones of SIV from fecal viral consensus sequences [21]. Such unpassaged representative SIV clones represent suitable tools to unravel the biological properties of the various primate lentiviruses, and their analysis will help to better assess the risk for further cross-species transmissions of SIVs to humans.

To date, SIVs or SIV-specific antibodies have been detected in more than 40 different African NHPs [4,22]. Thus, a large number of African monkey and ape species carry their own specific SIV. In contrast, SIVs have—thus far—not been detected in Asian or New World primates. The prevalence rates of SIV in different naturally infected primate species vary substantially, ranging from the apparent absence of SIV infection to prevalence rates greater than 50 percent (in adult animals) for SIVagm and SIVmnd infecting African green monkeys (AGM; *Chlorocebus species*) and mandrills (*Mandrillus sphinx*), respectively [23,24]. In the latter species SIV infection rates are generally high, irrespectively of the population examined. In contrast, SIVcpz is unevenly distributed, and forms foci of SIVcpz endemicity in some but not all wild chimpanzee communities [17—19]. The reasons for the wide variability in SIV infection rates in different primate species and the uneven distribution of SIVcpz in East African apes, as well as the routes of SIV transmission in the wild, are poorly understood. The high prevalence rates of SIV in adult members of some monkey species, such as AGMs, SMs and mandrills, suggest that transmission through sexual contact and/or biting is common. In contrast, vertical transmission in the natural host of SIV seems rare [25—27].

NATURAL HISTORY OF PRIMATE LENTIVIRUSES

HIV and SIV belong to the genus of lentiviruses, and are generally referred to as "immunodeficiency" viruses. Both designations are misleading, because "lenti" means slow whereas primate lentiviruses actually spread very rapidly and eliminate most memory CCR5+CD4+ helper T cells in lymphoid tissues within a few weeks after infection. Furthermore, it has become clear that some SIVs do not cause immunodeficiency in their natural simian hosts. Primate lentiviruses are highly diverse (Figure 1.1), and those for which full-length genomic sequences are available fall into six approximately equidistant major lineages, specifically (i) SIVcpz/SIVgor/HIV-1 infecting chimpanzees, gorillas and humans; (ii) SIVsmm/HIV-2 found in SMs and humans; (iii) SIVagm from various African green monkey species; (iv) SIVsyk infecting Sykes' monkeys; (v) the SIVlhoest lineage, which encompasses viruses from mandrills, l'Hoest and sun-tailed monkeys; and (vi) SIVcol from Colobus monkeys. Furthermore, various recombinant forms, such as SIVrcm or SIVgsn from red-capped mangabeys and greater spot-nosed monkeys, respectively, have been detected, and other SIVs remain to be fully characterized [1,28].

Some SIVs may have coevolved with their African NHPs for long time periods because they form host-specific clusters in phylogenetic tree analyses. Thus, closely related monkey species are infected with closely related viruses. The most prominent examples are the four species of African green monkeys (i.e., sabaeus, tantalus, vervet and grivet monkeys: *Chlorocebus sabaeus, tantalus, pygerythrus* and *aethiops*, respectively) which are all infected by SIVagm at high prevalence [29—31]. Viruses from each AGM species form a distinct monophyletic cluster, and these four SIVagm clusters are in turn more closely related to one another than to other SIVs [29—31]. One straightforward explanation for host-specific viral

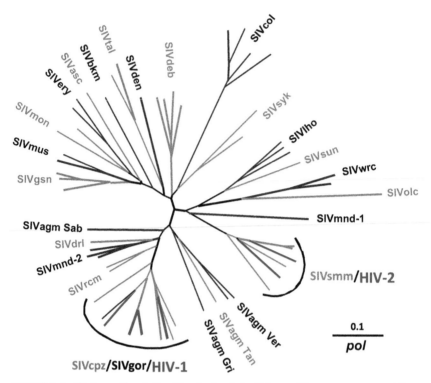

FIGURE 1.1 **Phylogenetic relationship of primate lentiviruses.** The tree was generated from fragments of the *pol* gene. Sequences derived from HIV-1 and HIV-2 are highlighted by red lines. SIVagm-Sab does not cluster with the remaining SIVagm Gri, Tan and Ver strains in the *pol* gene because it represents a recombinant [31]. *Tree reproduced courtesy of Martine Peeters.*

clustering is ancient SIV infection of the common precursor of the four AGM species followed by co-divergence and virus–host adaptation.

It is also evident, however, that not all primate lentiviral infections are the result of long-term virus–host co-evolution, and several cases of cross-species transmission of SIVs between different NHP species have been reported. One well-known example is the transmission of SIVsmm from captive SMs to macaques (*Macaca spec.*), which is associated with rapid disease progression in the non-natural host [32]. Thus, experimental infection of macaques with SIVsmm (named SIVmac after passage in macaques) represents one of the best animal models for AIDS in humans. Recent examples of simian–simian cross-species SIV transmission both in the wild and in captivity—for example, of SIVagm from AGMs to patas monkeys, baboons and the white-crowned mangabeys—have also been reported [33–35]. Furthermore, two distinct primate lineages infecting chimpanzees and gorillas or sooty mangabeys have been introduced into the human population at least 12 times, giving rise to HIV-1 and HIV-2 [1–3]. Notably, exposure of non-natural hosts to SIV or HIV can have very different outcomes. The AIDS pandemic gives a sobering example that in some cases the virus may spread and cause disease in the non-adapted host. Very likely, however, most cross-species transmission events went unnoticed because the virus was unable to replicate in the new species due to the non-functionality of essential virus-dependency factors (cellular factors that the virus needs to complete its life cycle), or due to its inability to antagonize or evade antiviral host factors. Thus, primate lentiviruses usually have a specific host range and can be more easily transmitted between closely related species. For example, HIV-1 infects humans and chimpanzees, but does not replicate in small monkey species.

The natural variation and genetic complexity of primate lentiviruses is further increased by their ability to recombine if a species becomes co-infected with two different viruses [36,37]. After experimental co-infection of a rhesus macaque monkey with two attenuated molecular clones of SIVmac that had either combined deletions in *vpx* and *vpr* or in the *nef* gene, only the virulent recombined wild-type virus containing intact *vpx*, *vpr* and *nef* genes was recovered at 2 weeks post-infection [38]. This example illustrates that genetic recombination can occur very rapidly and yield novel virus variants with increased fitness. Phylogenetic analyses strongly suggest that viruses infecting red-capped mangabeys (SIVrcm), sabaeus monkeys (SIVagm sab) and chimpanzees (SIVcpz) represent recombinants because parts of their genomes cluster with different viral lineages [31,39−41]. Obviously some of these chimeric viruses were pretty "fit" and successful, since SIVsab and SIVrcm are currently widespread in their natural hosts and SIVcpz was further transmitted to gorillas and to humans to cause the AIDS pandemic.

It has been estimated that the most recent common ancestor of AGMs existed approximately 3 million years ago [42]. In comparison, phylogenetic analyses of primate lentiviral sequences yielded much more recent estimates of diversification—for example, only hundreds or thousands of years for the SIVagm lineage [43]. As an alternative model to SIV infection of the common precursor of AGMs and subsequent virus/host co-diversification, it has been proposed that SIVs may have a more recent origin and that the apparent co-divergence between viruses and their hosts is due to the fact that viruses are more likely to be transmitted between closely related hosts [42]. This model is also plausible, and may apply in some cases. It is conceivable, however, that the exceedingly high mutation rates of primate lentiviruses do not allow accurate assessment of the distant evolutionary history of viruses based on contemporary sequence data. A phylo-geographic approach demonstrated that SIVs are at least 32,000 years old [10]. Furthermore, the recent discovery that lentiviruses repeatedly infiltrated the germline of prosimian species millions of years ago clearly suggests that primates have been exposed to lentiviruses for a very long time [11,12].

The evidence that primate lentiviruses are substantially more ancient than previously anticipated does not imply, however, that all naturally infected NHPs live in a well-adapted benign relationship with their SIVs. In fact, experimental evidence only comes from 3 of the 40 SIV-infected species: SM, AGMs and (to a lesser extent) mandrills [4−6]. Thus, virtually nothing is known about most natural SIV infections. Notably, recent data have demonstrated that SIVcpz causes disease in naturally infected chimpanzees [19], and thus changed the common view that natural SIV infections are generally non-pathogenic. One interesting question is how long it may take to achieve a benign well-balanced virus−host relationship. It has been established that only two of four distinct subspecies of common chimpanzees (*P. t. troglodytes* and *P. t. schweinfurthii*) are infected with SIVcpz [3,17]. If SIVcpz indeed already circulated in the most recent common ancestor of *P.t.t* and *P.t.s*, estimated to have existed about 380,000 years ago [44], chimpanzees did not achieve a non-pathogenic relationship with their virus for a long period of coexistence. A more recent origin of SIVcpz certainly cannot be excluded. Nonetheless, the results obtained from the natural hosts of SIV suggest that the development of a more benign relationship between HIV and humans should not be expected soon.

ORIGIN OF HIV-1 AND HIV-2

As described above, African NHPs represent a huge reservoir of lentiviruses that have the potential to cross species barriers. Zoonotic transmission to humans, however, has thus far "only" been reported for three of these viruses: SIVcpz from chimpanzees (*Pan troglodytes troglodytes*), SIVgor from gorillas (*Gorilla gorilla gorilla*), and SIVsmm from sooty mangabeys (*Cercocebus atys*) [1−3] (Figure 1.2). Soon after the discovery of HIV-2 in individuals from West Africa in 1986, a closely related virus (SIVsmm) was identified in SMs [8,9,45,46]. Sooty mangabeys are widespread in West Africa and have a high rate of infection with SIVsmm in the wild [46]. Furthermore, the natural habitat of these monkeys overlaps with the region where HIV-2 is endemic in humans, and where the animals are frequently hunted for food or kept as pets [46]. Thus, humans are frequently in contact with SIVsmm-infected animals, and exposure to blood or biting provides plausible routes of virus transmission. Notably, HIV-2 strains can be divided into no less than eight different groups that are interspersed among the SIVsmm lineages [9,46,47]. Thus, SIVsmm has crossed the species barrier from SMs to humans on several independent occasions (Figure 1.2B). Only HIV-2 groups A and B, however, have spread in the human population. The remaining six groups were usually only detected in single individuals [48].

Elucidating the origin of HIV-1 was more difficult. Initially, a virus closely related to HIV-1, named SIVcpz, was detected in two captive chimpanzees [49,50]. SIVcpz was a strong candidate for the origin of HIV-1, because both have the same genetic organization and contain a *vpu* gene that is absent in most other primate lentiviruses. For a long time, however, it remained a matter of debate whether chimpanzees represent the natural source of HIV-1, because the prevalence of SIVcpz in the wild seemed to be very low. One reason for this lack of knowledge was that studies of the distribution of SIVcpz in wild chimpanzee populations were initially hardly feasible, because they required testing of blood or tissues. The development of reliable non-invasive approaches to detecting SIV RNA and antibodies in fecal samples of wild primates was a major breakthrough in this area of research, and showed that SIVcpz infection is actually common and widespread in Central and Eastern chimpanzees (*P. t. troglodytes* and *P. t. schweinfurthii*) but absent in the remaining two subspecies (*P. t. verus* and *P. t. ellioti*) [17−19]. The finding that only two of the four subspecies of chimpanzees are infected suggests an evolutionarily "recent" origin of SIVcpz. Furthermore, it explained the apparent scarcity of SIVcpz in the wild, because initially mainly *P. t. verus* was tested for the presence of SIVcpz [51]. Meanwhile, SIVcpz strains that are closely related to two of the four groups of HIV-1 (M and N) have been identified in the *P. t. troglodytes* subspecies of chimpanzees [17−19]. Furthermore, chimpanzees living in the southeast corner of Cameroon have been identified as the probable source of pandemic HIV-1 group M strains [6]. Interestingly, the closest relatives of the remaining two groups of HIV-1 (O and P) have been detected in gorillas [20,52,53]. The prevalence of SIVgor in wild-living gorillas seems to be low, and is thus far limited to a few sites in Cameroon. Currently, it is unclear whether gorillas were the immediate source of HIV-1 O or whether gorillas and humans were both infected with a yet-to-be-identified SIVcpz strain [20,52]. HIV-1 group P is very closely related to SIVgor, and thus most likely the result of a gorilla−human transmission [53]. Altogether, it is evident that SIVs infecting chimpanzees or gorillas have been transmitted to humans at at least four independent times (Figure 1.2A), but only the event that led to the development of HIV-1 group M is responsible for the AIDS pandemic.

Lentiviruses have infected African NHPs since primeval times. Thus, humans must have been exposed to diverse SIVs many times, and it appears that at least a dozen independent transmissions of SIVs to humans have occurred in the past one or two centuries. Certainly, many more transmissions occurred in the past but did not spread significantly in the human populations. The reasons for this presumably high number of dead-end infections remain a matter of speculation. However, population densities, changes in social structures, migration and traveling, behavioral changes, wars, the presence of other sexually transmitted diseases, as well as the increasing use of intravenous injections, may all explain why successful zoonotic transmissions of SIVs to humans have occurred only recently. Other interesting questions are why only 3 of more than 40 non-human primate species and only one of two subspecies of chimpanzees have transmitted their virus to humans. As discussed below in more detail, accumulating evidence suggests that besides viral determinants, species-specific differences in virus dependency and host restriction factors play a key role in zoonotic lentiviral transmission. Thus, adaptation of SIVs to chimpanzees and gorillas—our closest non-human relatives—lowered the

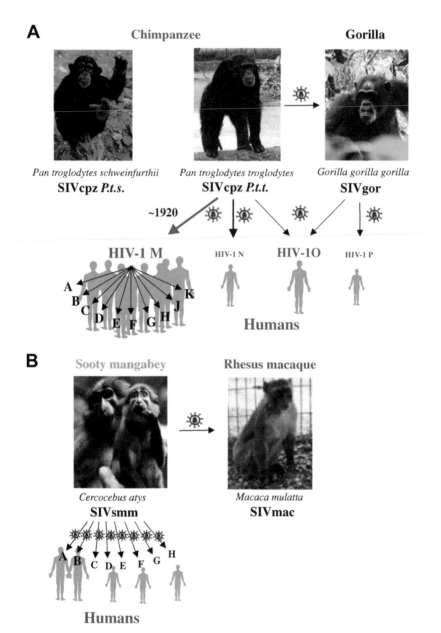

FIGURE 1.2 Schematic outline of the origin of HIV-1 and HIV-2. (A) SIVcpz was transmitted from the *P. t. troglodytes* (but not the *P. t. schweinfurthii*) subspecies of chimpanzees to humans and gorillas, evolving into HIV-1 groups M and N, and SIVgor, respectively. HIV-1 group P was most likely originally transmitted from gorillas. As indicated by the dashed line, it is unknown whether HIV-1 group O strains originated from chimpanzees or gorillas. (B) HIV-2 originated from several zoonotic transmissions of SIVsmm infecting sooty mangabeys to humans. Experimental infection

of rhesus macaques is an animal model for AIDS in humans and macaque-derived SIVsmm strains are named SIVmac. The recent human and non-adapted macaque hosts develop AIDS (red), whereas sooty mangabeys are well adapted to SIVsmm and do usually not develop disease (green). It is currently unknown whether or not SIVgor causes immunodeficiency in gorillas. *Photographs of non-human primates reproduced courtesy of M.L. Wilson, Beatrice H. Hahn, Cecile Neel and Martine Peeters.*

genetic barrier to zoonotic transmission of SIVs to humans. Finally, it must be considered that of all these independent introductions of SIVs into humans, only the one that resulted in the evolution of HIV-1 group M strains is responsible for the AIDS pandemic. Even today, AIDS would be a relatively rare and presumably poorly known tropical disease without the occurrence of pandemic HIV-1 group M strains.

STRUCTURAL AND GENETIC FEATURES OF PRIMATE LENTIVIRUSES

As outlined above, primate lentiviruses are highly divergent, and some viral proteins share less than 30 percent amino acid identity between the different strains of SIV and HIV. Nonetheless, many structural, molecular and biological features seem to be generally conserved. All primate lentiviral particles have a diameter of about 100–150 nm and are surrounded by a cell-derived lipid membrane containing the viral glycoproteins and some cellular factors. The HIV-1 and SIVmac Env glycoprotein is a trimer that generally interacts with CD4 as the primary receptor, and one or several chemokine receptors (most often CCR5) as the entry cofactor. The matrix protein forms a layer underneath the lipid membrane. The viral genome is surrounded by a cone-shaped capsid, composed of capsid proteins, and consists of two copies of positive single-stranded viral RNAs that are associated with the nucleocapsid protein, a tRNA primer, and enzymes required for reverse transcription and integration (http://visualscience. ru/en/illustrations/modelling/hiv/). Notably, the viral RNA genome has a highly ordered and complex structure [54].

Primate lentiviruses are complex retroviruses with a genome of about 10,000 nucleotides that contains 8–9 genes and encodes about 15 different proteins. In addition to the *gag, pol* and *env* genes that are present in all other retroviruses and encode structural (Env and Gag) and enzymatic proteins (reverse transcriptase, integrase and protease), all lentiviruses contain *tat* and *rev* genes encoding essential regulatory proteins. Furthermore, all present-day primate lentiviruses are equipped with at least three additional small genes, i.e., *vif, vpr* and *nef* (Figure 1.3). Lentiviruses acquired these accessory genes during co-evolution with their hosts, and the "prosimian" lentivirus pSIVgml that invaded the genome of a lemur several million years ago only contains the *vif* reading frame [11]. The finding that *vif* was the first accessory gene acquired during lentiviral evolution is in agreement with the fact that it is also present in the genomes of the ovine-caprine, bovine and feline (but not in the equine)

HIV-1, SIVcpz, SIVgor, SIVgsn, SIVmon, SIVmus, SIVden

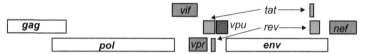

HIV-2, SIVsmm, SIVmac, SIVdrl, SIVmnd-2

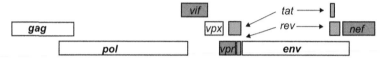

SIVagm, SIVsyk, SIVlhoest, SIVsun, SIVmnd-1, SIVasc, SIVcol

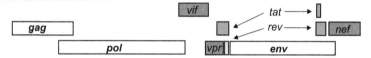

FIGURE 1.3   Genomic organization of primate lentiviruses. The *vpu* gene that is only found in HIV-1 and its closest SIV counterparts is indicated in red and the *vpx* gene that is encoded by HIV-2 and SIVs infecting the Papionini tribe of monkeys is highlighted in yellow. ORFs encoding regulatory proteins Tat and Rev are shown in blue, and the accessory genes *vif*, *vpr* and *nef* in orange.

groups of lentiviruses, whereas *vpr* and *nef* are characteristic for all SIV and HIV strains but absent in other lentiviruses [55]. Two other accessory genes are only found in some primate lentiviruses. A factor named viral protein X (Vpx) is only encoded by SIVs infecting the Papionini tribe of monkeys (SIVsmm, SIVrcm, SIVmnd-2 and SIVdrl) and in HIV-2. Most likely, *vpx* was originally acquired by a non-homologous recombination that resulted in a duplication of the *vpr* gene [56,57]. Finally, another accessory viral gene, named *vpu*, distinguishes HIV-1 and its most closely related SIVs (i.e., SIVcpz, SIVgor, SIVgsn, SIVmus, SIVmon and SIVden) from most other primate lentiviruses, such as SIVagm, SIVsmm and HIV-2 [40,58]. The acquisition of a *vpu* gene in the primate lentiviral lineage that ultimately led to the emergence of AIDS may have had an impact on their virulence [15], and is thus discussed below in more detail.

BARRIERS TO CROSS-SPECIES TRANSMISSION: VIRUS DEPENDENCY FACTORS

In order to replicate in a new host, the virus must be capable of using all cellular factors required for the completion of its life cycle and be able to evade or counteract the host defense mechanisms. It is well known that viruses have to exploit cellular factors to infect and replicate in their target cells. The recent application of advanced technological methods suggests that the interaction between HIV-1 and its host may be far more complex than previously anticipated. Several genome-wide RNA interference-based screens have evaluated the great majority of about 23,000 human genes and identified more than 1,000 that reduced HIV infection when knocked-down (reviewed in [59,60]). Most of the latter are involved in specific pathways, such as ubiquitination and proteasomal targeting, nuclear transport, transcription, cytoskeletal regulation, immune response, RNA binding/splicing and protein folding. These studies suggest that HIV and SIV may depend on cellular factors at essentially each step of their life cycle, such as attachment, fusion, reverse transcription, uncoating, nuclear import, integration, viral transcription, translation, post-translational modification of viral proteins, virion assembly and budding. It is noteworthy, however, that the overlap between the different studies was minimal, and a specific role of the vast majority of these potential "virus dependency" factors in the virus life cycle remains to be defined. Despite some limitations, these analyses provide first insights into the complexity of the virus—host interaction, and clearly suggest that primate lentiviruses depend on a large array of cellular cofactors. One way that the host can become resistant to a pathogen is thus to acquire changes in virus dependency factors that disrupt the interaction with and misuse by the pathogen. In fact, it has been demonstrated that cellular proteins that interact with pathogens are under positive selection pressure and evolve at an unusually fast rate [61—64]. Thus, these host proteins often show sequence variations between different primate species, and are used by primate lentiviruses in a species-specific manner. In many cases, virus exposure to a new host will therefore not result in productive infection. In other cases, the cellular factors may not work optimally for the virus, but allow some replication. Obviously, this is particularly likely if the pathogen is transmitted between closely related species. Primate lentiviruses are particularly well qualified for cross-species transmission because they are highly variable and thus capable of rapidly adapting to a new host environment. Furthermore, retroviruses integrate their genomes into that of the host cell. Thus, they have an opportunity for retreat and can be passively propagated by divisions of the host cells. Subsequently, the increased number of virally infected cells, together with the high error rate of the reverse transcriptase, may facilitate the selection of virus variants with increased fitness in the new host. A specific variation of M30R in the Gag protein may represent such an adaptation that increased the replication fitness of HIV-1 in humans [65].

BARRIERS TO CROSS-SPECIES TRANSMISSION: HOST RESTRICTION FACTORS

Although viruses are dependent on the support of many cellular factors, it has become clear that cells—particularly those of new hosts—are not a friendly environment for invading pathogens. Specifically, the innumerable encounters between our ancestors and pathogens have not only resulted in the development of innate and adaptive immune systems, but also driven the evolution of specific factors against viruses that were refractory to conventional immune mechanisms (reviewed in [66−72]). These intrinsic immunity or host restriction factors are constitutively expressed and active in some cell types, and can thus protect us and other mammals against invading pathogens without previous encounters. However, like innate immunity, they can also be strongly upregulated and induced by type I interferons (reviewed in [68,69]). Initially it was thought that they specifically target eukaryotic retroviruses, but it has become clear that some of them have broad activity and inhibit viruses belonging to different families. The three major antiretroviral factors known to date target different steps of the viral life cycle: TRIM5α proteins inactivate incoming viral capsids; cytidine deaminases (e.g., APOBEC3G) inhibit reverse transcription and induce lethal hypermutations of the viral genome; and tetherin (also known as CD317, BST2 or HM1.24) tethers budding virions to the cell surface [66−72] (Figure 1.4). All these host restriction factors have evolved under positive selection pressure due to past encounters with ancient viruses to evade viral antagonists or to gain activity against new invading pathogens [61−64]. Thus, the antiviral factors and their antagonists often act in a species-specific manner, and this actually facilitated their discovery.

TRIM5α (tripartite motif 5-alpha) was initially identified by a genetic screen of a cDNA library prepared from primary rhesus monkey lung fibroblasts [73]. The rhesus homologue inhibited HIV-1, as opposed to human TRIM5α [74]. TRIM5α is a member of the tripartite motif family of proteins (hence the name TRIM), and contains a RING, B-box 2, coiled-coil and a C-terminal PRY/SPRY domain. The latter is required for retroviral restriction, and determines viral specificity [75]. Notably, a single amino acid substitution of R332I in the SPRY domains of human TRIM5α is sufficient to render it active against HIV-1 [75]. The exact antiviral mechanism remains to be clarified, but it seems generally accepted that TRIM5α binds to the incoming capsids of sensitive retroviruses and rapidly recruits them to the proteasome to prevent reverse transcription and thus viral DNA synthesis [71].

APOBEC3G (apolipoprotein B mRNA-editing enzyme, catalytic polypeptide-like 3G) is a cytidine deaminase, and was the first host gene identified as an inhibitor of HIV-1 infection [76]. Most antiviral factors are constitutively expressed in some but not all cell types, and APOBEC3G was discovered by comparison of the mRNA expression profiles of cells that do or do not support efficient replication of *vif*-defective HIV-1 [76]. In the absence of Vif, APOBEC3G is incorporated into lentiviral virions and inhibits reverse transcription and induces the deamination of cytidine to uridine during negative strand DNA synthesis [76−81]. These changes lead to the degradation of the viral DNA or become fixed as G-to-A mutations.

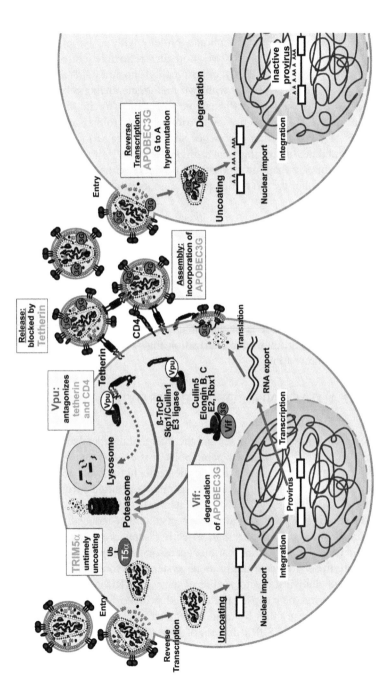

FIGURE 1.4 Host restriction factors and their viral antagonists. To date, three antiretroviral factors have been well characterized. TRIM5α interacts with incoming HIV-1 capsids and deregulates uncoating by proteasomal degradation. Vif binds to a cullin 5-based ubiquitin ligase complex and to APOBEC3G to induce the degradation of the restriction factor in proteasomes. In the absence of Vif, APOBEC3G is incorporated into progeny virions and inhibits reverse transcription and causes lethal G-to-A hypermutations of the retroviral genome in the next round of infection. Finally, tetherin inhibits the release of mature viral particles from the cell surface and is antagonized by the HIV-1 group M Vpu protein [82, 83]. Notably, many other primate lentiviruses use Nef to counteract tetherin [119–121]. *Reproduced from Kirchhoff (2010) [55], with permission.*

Tetherin (BST-2, CD317 or HM1.24) is a recently discovered restriction factor, that "tethers" nascent enveloped viral particles to the cell membrane [82,83]. Tetherin is a type II transmembrane protein with a cytoplasmic N-terminal region, a transmembrane (TM) domain, a flexible coiled-coil extracellular domain and a C-terminal glycophosphatidyl-inositol (GPI) anchor [84]. Tetherin has an unusual topology, with two membrane anchors; both of these, the cytoplasmic tail and the GPI anchor, are critical for its antiviral activity [82]. Thus, it seems to tether nascent virions directly to the surface of the producer cells, with one membrane anchor sticking in the virion and the other in the cell membrane. Interestingly, an artificial "tetherin" with a different amino acid sequence but comparable topology also inhibits virus release [85], suggesting that no cellular or viral cofactors are required for its antiviral activity.

It is noteworthy that treatment with type I interferons *in vivo* induces several hundred different factors, and the function of most of them is unknown. Recent elegant experiments examined about 400 interferon-stimulated genes for their capability to inhibit various viral pathogens, and identified several additional inhibitors of HIV and other viruses [86]. Furthermore, it has long been known that macrophages and dendritic cells express a yet to be identified restriction factor that is antagonized by the viral protein X (Vpx) [87–89] (see "Latest advances", this chapter). Thus, it is evident that additional antiviral factors remain to be discovered, and their characterization may provide new opportunities for therapy or prevention.

EVASION AND ANTAGONISM OF ANTIRETROVIRAL FACTORS

Despite the specific antiviral host defenses and the many viral dependencies of cellular factors discussed in the previous paragraphs, it is evident that primate lentiviruses can jump species barriers and replicate to high levels in their respective hosts. In fact, recent data have demonstrated a positive correlation between the induction of "antiviral" IFN-stimulated genes in HIV-1-infected individuals and viral loads [90]. This finding suggests that IFN-induced factors have become mere indicators rather than effective suppressors of HIV-1 replication. Their wide variability and various accessory viral gene functions allow primate lentiviruses to evade the immune system and to develop resistance against some antiviral factors. For example, TRIM5α interacts specifically with the viral p24 capsid protein, and primate lentiviruses can become resistant to this restriction by acquiring mutations in the capsid that abolish p24 binding to the PRY/SPRY domain of TRIM5 proteins (reviewed in [71]). Thus, although TRIM5α is most likely an important determinant of the species-specificity of primate lentiviruses, it does not seem to be very difficult for the virus to evade this restriction factor. In comparison, it is more challenging for SIV and HIV to evade antiviral factors targeting components in a relatively unspecific manner, such as the viral RNA (APOBEC3G) or membrane (tetherin), because they cannot just avoid them by escape mutations. Instead, primate lentiviruses have acquired specific tools, such as Vif, Vpu, Vpr, Vpx and Nef, to antagonize these antiviral defense mechanisms (Figures 1.3, 1.4). As a consequence, HIV and SIV are capable of replicating efficiently and continuously in the presence of apparently strong antiviral immune responses.

Vif (viral infectivity factor) specifically antagonizes APOBEC3G by linking a Cullin 5-based E3 ubiquitin ligase complex to the restriction factor, thereby inducing its poly-ubiquitination and proteasomal degradation (reviewed in [67,91]). As a consequence, APOBEC3G is not packaged into budding virions and fully infectious virions are produced. Initially it was thought that differential susceptibilities of APOBEC proteins to Vif proteins may play an important role in the host-specificity of primate lentiviruses, because SIV Vif proteins are often poorly effective against human APOBEC3G in transient transfection experiments. Subsequent experiments demonstrated, however, that several SIV strains replicate efficiently in human cells despite of this lack of Vif function [92]. Thus, the role of Vif-dependent APOBEC3G antagonism in the host range of primate lentiviruses seems complex and needs further study.

Vpr (viral protein R) is a virion-associated factor of about 14 kDa that is encoded by all primate lentiviruses. Its main function is not entirely clear, but multiple activities, such as cell cycle arrest in the G2 phase, activation of proviral transcription, induction of cell death and enhancement of the fidelity of reverse transcription, have been reported (reviewed in [68,93]). Vpr-mediated G2 cell-cycle arrest involves its interaction with the Cullin 4A−DDB1 complex via DCAF-1 (initially named VprBP) [94]. It is currently unknown whether Vpr increases the activity of the Cullin 4A−DDB1−DCAF-1 complex for its normal substrates, or allows it to recruit a new one for poly-ubiquitination and degradation [68,93]. Notably, HIV-1 Vpr also facilitates infection of macrophages [95,96], suggesting that it antagonizes an as yet unknown host restriction factor in this cell type.

Nef (negative factor) is the third accessory factor encoded by all HIV and SIV strains, and by far the one with the greatest number of reported interactions and functions. Nef is a myristoylated protein of about 24−27 kDa in HIV-1, and between 25 and 37 kDa in SIVs (reviewed in [97,98]). It can associate with cytoplasmic membranes, and is expressed at high levels throughout the viral life cycle. Nef is required for efficient viral replication *in vivo*, and accelerates disease progression in HIV-1-infected humans and in rhesus macaques experimentally infected with SIVmac [99−101]. Nef seems to be the "all purpose" tool of primate lentiviruses, and manipulates viral target cells in complex ways. In virally infected T cells, the HIV-1 Nef protein down-modulates CD4, MHC-I and (less efficiently) CD28 and CXCR4 from the surface by interacting with the cytoplasmic tails of these receptors and recruiting them to the endocytic machinery, and/or by rerouting them to lysosomes for degradation (reviewed in [97,98,102−104]). Altogether, these Nef functions may facilitate the release of fully infectious virions, prevent super-infection, protect the virally infected T cells against CTL lysis, and reduce their migration in response to the chemokine SDF-1 (CXCL12) as well as their responsiveness to stimulation. Furthermore, these Nef activities modulate the functionality of virally infected T cells and reduce their recognition and elimination by the immune system, thereby expanding the time period of virus production. Notably, Nef also affects MHC-II antigen presentation of antigen-presenting cells by up-modulation of the Invariant chain (Ii or CD74) at the cell surface [105,106], and may thus contribute to the impaired helper T cell responses observed in AIDS patients. The HIV-1 Nef protein also interacts with a variety of cellular kinases to modulate signal transduction pathways (reviewed in [102,104]) and to promote the induction of cellular transcription factors, such as NF-AT, NF-κB, and AP-1, that elevate the transcription of the viral LTR promoter and thus viral replication [107−113].

Notably, primate lentiviral Nef proteins differ fundamentally in their effect on the responsiveness to stimulation via the CD3−TCR complex. In stark contrast to *nef* alleles of HIV-1 and some (usually *vpu* containing) SIVs, the great majority of primate lentiviral Nefs effectively down-modulate TCR−CD3 from the surface of infected T cells and block their responsiveness to TCR-mediated activation [114]. The possible reasons for and consequences of the loss of Nef-mediated down-modulation of TCR−CD3 by the primate lentiviral lineage that gave rise to HIV-1 are discussed below in more detail. Recent data suggest that Nef may also affect the survival and function of bystander cells [115−117]. However, these results remain to be confirmed in independent studies. Altogether, it is evident that Nef induces complex changes in cellular trafficking, gene and receptor surface expression, antigen presentation, and signal transduction, and that these effects cooperate to suppress the elimination of virally infected cells by the immune system and to turn them into more effective producers of fully infectious virions. Nef is commonly considered to be an early viral gene product. It is noteworthy, however, that it also performs important functions during the late stage of the viral life cycle. For example, the great majority of primate lentiviral Nefs enhance virion infectivity by a poorly defined mechanism that likely involves the interaction of Nef with the GTPase Dynamin-2, a regulator of clathrin-mediated endocytosis [118]. Finally, as discussed below, some SIV strains use their Nef proteins to antagonize tetherin [119−121].

Vpx (viral protein X) is only encoded by HIV-2, SIVsmm and SIVs infecting drills or mandrills, and most likely arose from *vpr* [55,56]. Interestingly, the two main functions of Vpr seem to be segregated in *vpx* containing primate lentiviruses: Vpr induces cell cycle arrest, and Vpx facilitates infection of macrophages [89,122,123]. Just like Vpr, Vpx binds DCAF-1 to interact with the Cullin 4A−DDB1 complex, and this interaction seems to be required for its ability to promote macrophage infection [89,124]. Thus, Vpx and Vpr may both induce the ubiquitination and degradation of an as yet unknown restriction factor expressed in macrophages and dendritic cells, although Vpx is substantially more effective than Vpr [125]. In fact, both accessory proteins may compensate for one another, because an individual defect in each gene had little if any effect on virus replication or pathogenicity in the SIV/macaque model, whereas combined deletions in both accessory genes resulted in a severely attenuated viral phenotype [126]. Further studies to clarify whether macrophage infection is particularly common in infections with *vpx* containing viruses, such as SIVsmm or HIV-2, and whether the presence of this accessory gene affects the viral coreceptor tropism, will be interesting.

Vpu (viral protein U) is a small 16 kDa integral membrane protein that is only present in HIV-1 and its closest SIV counterparts. Vpu is expressed during the late stage of the viral life cycle from a bicistronic RNA that also encodes the viral envelope glycoprotein (reviewed in [127–130]). The Vpu proteins of pandemic HIV-1 M strains have two well-documented functions. First, they interact with CD4 and recruit a ubiquitin ligase complex to its cytoplasmic tail to mediate poly-ubiquitinylation and proteasomal degradation [131,132]. Vpu-mediated CD4 degradation may facilitate virion release and prevent super-infection as well as the formation of inactive gp120/CD4 complexes in virally infected cells, but most of these effects have only been observed under artificially high levels of CD4 expression. Secondly, the HIV-1 group M Vpu antagonizes the interferon-induced host restriction factor "tetherin" (BST-2) to promote virion release [82,83]. Vpu interacts specifically with the trans-membrane domain of tetherin and seems to target it to the trans-Golgi network or to early endosomes for proteasomal or lysosomal degradation by a mechanism that may involve β-TrCP [61,133–138]. While the exact mechanism of Vpu-mediated tetherin antagonism is a matter of debate, it is clear that Vpu sequesters tetherin away from the sites of virus assembly to enhance virion budding. Notably, the Vpu proteins of pandemic and non-pandemic HIV-1 strains and SIV show major differences in their capability to antagonize tetherin, and different primate lentiviruses use different proteins to antagonize tetherin [120,139]. Recently, it has been reported that HIV-1 Vpus also affect the function of Natural Killer (NK) and NKT cells by down-modulation of NTB-A and CD1d, respectively [140,141]. However, these effects are relatively modest compared to tetherin antagonism and CD4 degradation, and their relevance needs further study.

Altogether, accumulating evidence suggests that the major function of the viral accessory proteins is to antagonize specific host restriction factors and to modulate adaptive immune responses. A common scheme for many of them is that they recruit ubiquitin complexes to the cellular factors to mediate their proteasomal degradation (reviewed in [68]). Another interesting feature is that most accessory viral proteins are multifunctional. Thus, even if some specific activities are lost after cross-species transmission, the selective advantage of the remaining functions will help the virus to maintain intact accessory genes. Some key functions seem conserved between most or all primate lentiviruses, but the bulk of knowledge comes from studies of pandemic HIV-1 M strains, and we are only beginning to gain a more comprehensive picture of primate lentiviral accessory gene function.

DEVELOPMENT OF HIV-1

As outlined above and shown in Figure 1.3, all primate lentiviruses have a "standard" repertoire of accessory genes (i.e., *vif, vpr* and *nef*), and many functions and properties are conserved. It has also become clear, however, that HIV-1 differs in several ways from SIVsmm and SIVagm, which replicate to high levels in their natural hosts without causing disease. Distinctive features of HIV-1 are the presence of a *vpu* gene, lack of Nef-mediated down-modulation of TCR−CD3, and the frequent utilization of CXCR4 as entry cofactor during late stages of infection (Table 1.1). Meanwhile, we have a pretty detailed picture about the acquisition of these properties that may contribute to the virulence of HIV-1 in humans.

One of the first important events for the latter emergence of HIV-1 was the acquisition of a *vpu* gene by a distant SIV precursor of HIV-1, most likely a common ancestor of SIVs infecting *Cercopithecus* monkeys (SIVgsn/mus/mon) (Figure 1.5) [15,40]. The emergence of a *vpu*-containing subset of primate lentiviruses is actually somewhat surprising, because some SIVs without a *vpu* gene, such as SIVsmm and SIVagm, have apparently achieved an ideally balanced relationship with their primate hosts since they maintain high viral loads and spread efficiently without causing disease. This does not seem to be the case for the *vpu*-containing SIVs, because the prevalence in greater spot-nosed and mustached monkeys is surprisingly low (about 2−3 percent) and SIVcpz causes disease in its natural chimpanzee host [18,22,23].

TABLE 1.1 Differences between HIV-1 and SIVagm or SIVsmm

HIV-1	SIVsmm, SIVagm
Vpu: CD4, tetherin, CD1d, NTB-A	No Vpu
Nef: no CD3 modulation; weak effects on CD28 and CXCR4	Nef: effective CD3, CD28 and CXCR4 modulation; tetherin antagonism
Frequently CXCR4-tropic	Rarely CXCR4-tropic
→ **Deregulates T cell activation**	→ **Prevents T cell activation**

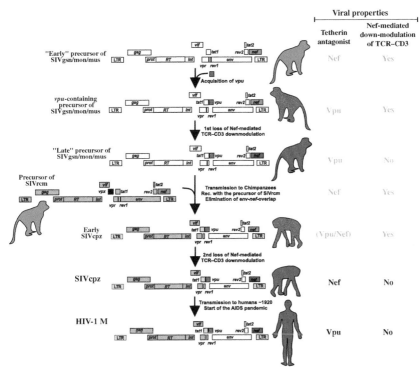

FIGURE 1.5 Schematic presentation of events preceding the evolution of pandemic HIV-1 group M strains. As indicated, *vpu* was most likely achieved by a common precursor of SIVgsn/mus/mon that later recombined with the precursor of SIVrcm in chimpanzees and subsequently transmitted to humans. Hosts infected with viruses that have no *vpu* and modulate CD3 are indicated in green, hosts infected with viruses containing *vpu* and probably able to down-modulate CD3 are indicated in gray, and hosts infected with viruses that have *vpu* and are unable to modulate CD3 are indicated in red. Please note that the properties of ancient viruses (indicated in gray) are hypothetical and based on data derived from present-day viruses. Initially, SIVcpz was equipped with two potential tetherin antagonists (Vpu and Nef), but subsequently only Nef and not Vpu evolved to become an effective tetherin antagonist in chimpanzees (reviewed in [145]). Pandemic HIV-1 group M strains regained Vpu-mediated anti-tetherin activity after zoonotic transmission to humans because the human tetherin orthologue contains a deletion in its cytoplasmic domain that renders it resistant to Nef. *Modified from Kirchhoff (2009) [15].*

Furthermore, the acquisition of a *vpu* gene "complicates" Env expression because both are expressed from the same bicistronic mRNA, and the latter is produced after leaky scanning of the *vpu* initiation codon [142,143]. Thus, Vpu and Env have to be expressed in a highly coordinated manner, and perhaps this may in part explain why HIV-1 virions contain fewer Env trimers than SIVmac virions, which do not have a *vpu* gene [144]. Although virus–host adaptation seems suboptimal for some *vpu*-containing viruses, it was obviously advantageous for the common precursor of SIVgsn/mus/mon to keep this novel accessory gene.

Most likely, Vpu had already evolved its two best established activities (i.e., degradation of the viral CD4 receptor and enhancement of the release of progeny virions by antagonizing tetherin) prior to the diversification of these monkey species, because Vpu proteins from all known SIVs nowadays found in *Cercopithecus* species also perform these two functions [120,139]. Whether these SIV Vpus also protect infected cells from NK and NKT cell-mediated killing through down-modulation of NTB-A and CD1d remains to be examined. It seems that the acquisition of *vpu* by these SIVs also facilitated changes in Nef function, since, in contrast to the great majority of primate lentiviral Nef proteins, those of SIVgsn, SIVmus and SIVmon are unable to down-modulate TCR−CD3 to suppress T cell activation and programmed death [114,168].

Another important step in the evolutionary history of HIV-1 was the recombination of the ancient *Cercopithecus* virus with the precursor of a virus nowadays found in red-capped mangabeys [40,114]. Chimpanzees prey on small monkeys, and this is most likely how one ape became co-infected by both SIVs. Phylogenetic analyses suggest that the 5' half of the SIVcpz genome as well as the *nef* gene originated from the precursor of SIVrcm, and the 3' half of the genome from the ancestor of SIVgsn/mus/mon [40,114] (Figure 1.5). The recombination event eliminated the overlap between the *env* and *nef* open reading frames found in the genomes of other primate lentiviruses. Furthermore, it equipped the precursor of SIVcpz with two potential tetherin antagonists because the ancestor of SIVrcm most likely used Nef (because current SIVrcm strains do), and the precursor of SIVgsn/mus/mon lineage most probably used Vpu (because the descendants do) (reviewed in [145]). Presumably, however, both of them were initially inactive, because tetherin evolved under positive selection pressure and the viral antagonists are usually species-specific. Subsequently, Nef rather than Vpu evolved anti-tetherin activity because the cytoplasmic domain of tetherin that interacts with Nef is somewhat less divergent between chimpanzees and monkeys than the transmembrane domain targeted by Vpu [145]. Nef-mediated tetherin antagonism was maintained or readily reacquired after zoonotic transmission of SIVcpz from chimpanzees to gorillas because the cytoplasmic domains of gorilla and chimpanzee tetherins are highly similar. This situation was different after zoonotic transmission of SIVcpz and SIVgor to humans because human tetherin contains a 5-amino-acid deletion in its cytoplasmic domain that renders it resistant to Nef [119−121]. Pandemic HIV-1 M strains cleared this hurdle perfectly by regaining efficient Vpu-mediated anti-tetherin activity. In contrast, the Vpus from non-pandemic HIV-1 group O and P strains are poor tetherin antagonists, and those of HIV-1 group N strains gained modest anti-tetherin activity but do not degrade CD4 [120] (summarized in Figure 1.6). Thus, only pandemic HIV-1 strains evolved a fully functional Vpu protein during adaptation to humans, which may potentially explain its effective spread in the human population.

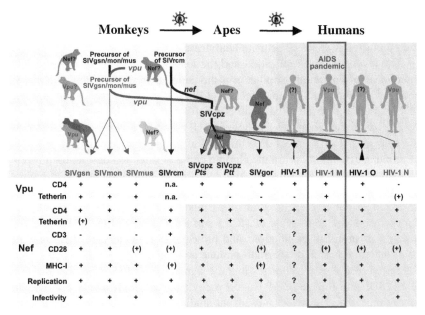

Monkeys ➤ Apes ➤ Humans

		SIVgsn	SIVmon	SIVmus	SIVrcm	SIVcpz Pts	SIVcpz Ptt	SIVgor	HIV-1 P	HIV-1 M	HIV-1 O	HIV-1 N
Vpu	CD4	+	+	+	n.a.	+	+	+	+	+	+	-
	Tetherin	+	+	+	n.a.	-	-	-	-	+	-	(+)
Nef	CD4	+	+	+	+	+	+	+	+	+	+	+
	Tetherin	(+)	-	-	+	+	+	+	-	-	-	-
	CD3	-	-	-	+	-	-	-	?	-	-	-
	CD28	+	+	(+)	(+)	+	+	(+)	?	(+)	(+)	(+)
	MHC-I	+	+	+	(+)	+	+	(+)	?	+	+	+
	Replication	+	+	+	+	+	+	+	?	+	+	+
	Infectivity	+	+	+	+	+	+	+	?	+	+	+

FIGURE 1.6   Overview on Vpu and Nef function in HIV-1 and its closest SIV counterparts. SIVcpz represents a recombinant of the precursors of viruses nowadays found in red-capped mangabeys and *Cercopithecus* monkeys, and was transmitted to humans and gorillas. Vpu was first acquired by a common precursor of SIVgsn/mus/mon, and then transferred from monkeys to apes and to humans by zoonotic primate lentiviral transmissions. The events that led to the emergence of pandemic HIV-1 group M strains are indicated by thick lines. Nef-mediated tetherin antagonism is indicated by blue and Vpu-mediated tetherin antagonism by red lines, respectively. +, active; (+), poorly active; −, inactive; n.a., not applicable because these viruses do not have a *vpu* gene. *Reproduced from Kirchhoff (2010) [55], with permission.*

POSSIBLE RELEVANCE OF VPU AND LACK OF NEF-MEDIATED DOWN-MODULATION OF TCR−CD3 FOR VIRAL PATHOGENESIS

As outlined in the previous paragraph, HIV-1 differs by the presence of a *vpu* gene and fundamental differences in Nef function from SIVs that replicate to high levels in their natural hosts without causing disease. The relative importance of these distinct viral properties for the levels of infection-associated immune activation and the clinical outcome of infection compared to intrinsic host factors remains largely a matter of speculation. It is evident, however, that both viral and host factors play a role in the pathogenesis of AIDS. This is perhaps most obvious from the fact that HIV-1 is more virulent than HIV-2 in the same human host, and that the same viral lineage (SIVsmm/mac/HIV-2) is usually non-pathogenic in its well-adapted natural SM host, moderately pathogenic in the recent human host, and highly virulent in the non-adapted rhesus macaque host (reviewed in [146,147]). As discussed below, accumulating data suggest that a complex interplay of viral and host factors determines the outcome of infection, and that the major protective mechanisms may not be the same in different hosts of primate lentiviruses.

The levels of viral replication and the loss of CD4+ T cells during acute infection are remarkably similar in pathogenic HIV-1 and in non-pathogenic natural SIVsmm and SIVagm infection [148−150]. Thus, these natural hosts of SIV learned to tolerate rather than efficiently control their respective viruses. A key difference between pathogenic HIV-1 and non-pathogenic natural SIVsmm and SIVagm infection is that the latter can avoid damaging high levels of immune activation during the chronic phase of infection despite high levels of virus replication. Importantly, high levels of inflammation are the strongest correlate of disease progression in HIV-1 and HIV-2 infection [151,152]. Various host factors, such as an intact mucosal barrier, effective regulatory T cell responses, low levels of CCR5 surface expression on CD4+ T cells, differences in T cell populations and protection of memory T cells, may all contribute to this lack of aberrant immune activation [13−16]. It has also been suggested that adaptive changes in TLR signaling and IFN-α production may allow SIVsmm-infected SMs to prevent damaging high levels of immune activation [153]. However, subsequent studies demonstrated strong but transient IFN-α responses during acute non-pathogenic SIVagm and SIVsmm infection [154,155]. Thus, SM and AGM plasmacytoid dendritic cells are well capable of producing IFN-α in response to SIV infection, and the major difference between pathogenic HIV-1 and non-pathogenic SIVagm and SIVsmm infection seems to be established during the transition from acute to chronic infection [154−156]. Thus, one key question is: what allows SIV-infected SMs or AGMs to avoid aberrant immune activation during chronic infection despite high levels of viral replication or, *vice versa*, why does HIV-1 cause high levels of chronic inflammation and AIDS?

One possibility is that the acquisition of a *vpu* gene resulted in the evolution of primate lentiviruses with increased virulence [15]. In agreement with this possibility, preliminary evidence suggests that *vpu* encoding SIVs may not co-exist in a well-balanced benign relationship with their natural primate hosts. Most importantly, SIVcpz is associated with an increased mortality rate and causes AIDS in naturally infected chimpanzees [19]. The clinical outcome of natural infections with SIVgsn/mus/mon remains to be clarified, but their low prevalence in the wild (only about 2−4 percent) compared to the 50−90 percent of "regular" SIV infections [23,24] is a clear indicator of suboptimal virus−host adaptation. The exact role of Vpu in viral replication and pathogenesis *in vivo* remains to be determined. Some preliminary data suggest that the two best-established Vpu activities (i.e., CD4 degradation and tetherin antagonism) may not be absolutely required for efficient viral spread and disease progression *in vivo* because HIV-1 groups O and N can cause AIDS [157], although the former seems to lack effective anti-tetherin activity and the latter the Vpu-mediated CD4 degradation function [120,139]. However, additional studies are required to exclude the possibility that HIV-1 O strains evolved a different tetherin antagonist different from Nef or Vpu. Notably, tetherin antagonism may be less important for cell-to-cell spread of virus (a potent means of virus replication *in vivo*) than for the spread of cell-free virions [158]. Some studies suggest that Vpu-defective HIV-1 mutants may even show enhanced cell-to-cell transmission [159,160], whereas others have reported that tetherin also restricts cell-to-cell spread [161]. In *in vitro*-infected peripheral blood mononuclear cell (PBMC) cultures and in *ex vivo*-infected human lymphoid tissues a defective *vpu* gene does not fully impair but significantly reduces HIV-1 replication, particularly in the presence of IFN-α that induces tetherin [162,163]. Further experimentation is necessary, but altogether these data raise the possibility that effective tetherin antagonism may be more important for virus transmission than for viral pathogenesis. Finally, Vpu-mediated degradation of CD4 may be advantageous but not absolutely critical for viral replication *in vivo* because Env and Nef also help the virus to keep CD4 away from the cell surface, and the latter seems to have the major effect (reviewed in [164]).

An interesting question is whether Vpu directly affects the virulence of primate lentiviruses and the levels of infection associated immune activation independently of the viral loads. Indeed, it has been suggested that HIV-1 is particularly effective in inducing IFN-α[165]. To our current knowledge, the main mechanism of type I interferon induction is Env-mediated binding of HIV-1 virions to CD4 on plasmacytoid dendritic cells (pDCs) and subsequent endocytosis of the viral particles to trigger Toll-like receptors (i.e., TLR7/9) [166,167]. Vpu may affect the uptake of virions by pDCs, and thus IFN production, in several ways. On the one hand, Vpu should increase this process by enhancing the functionality of gp120 trimers incorporated into budding virions by CD4 degradation, thus preventing the formation of inactive CD4/gp120 complexes, and by promoting virion release by antagonizing tetherin [164]. On the other hand, the necessity of *vpu*-containing viruses to balance Vpu and Env expression may result in the incorporation of reduced quantities of the viral Env trimers into the virions, and thus reduce virion uptake by pDCs. Thus, both enhancing and suppressive effects of *vpu* on the capability of HIV-1 virions to induce interferons seem plausible, and further studies on a possible role of Vpu in immune activation seem warranted.

The acquisition of Vpu may also have affected the levels of virus-induced immune activation indirectly, because it apparently facilitated changes in Nef function—specifically, the loss of down-modulation of TCR−CD3 [15]. Analysis of a large number of primate lentiviruses revealed a striking concordance between the presence of a *vpu* gene and the inability of Nef to down-modulate CD3 [114]. Although some exceptions do exist [168], this correlation is most likely not just coincidence because phylogenetic data suggest that Nef-mediated down-modulation of TCR−CD3 was actually lost twice during primate lentivirus evolution—first after the acquisition of a *vpu* gene by the common ancestor of SIVgsn/mus/mon, and a second time after recombination of two ancient SIVs in chimpanzees [114] (Figure 1.5). Further experimentation is necessary to obtain more definitive insights into possible links between Vpu and Nef function, but it is tempting to speculate that Vpu, as an effective virion release factor and tetherin antagonist, may have facilitated the evolution of viruses that enhance rather than block T cell activation, as it may allow them to cope with the higher activation of the host immune system and may allow effective production of progeny virions despite the shortened lifespan of the infected cells [15].

Nef-mediated suppression of T cell activation may be beneficial for both sides. It may promote virus spread because inefficient CD4+ helper T cell activation should weaken the antiviral immune response. Furthermore, reduced T cell activation and apoptosis may reduce the damage associated with effective viral replication, and thus help the virally infected host to maintain a functional immune system. In support of a protective role in primate lentiviral infections, it has been shown that inefficient modulation of TCR−CD3 correlates with loss of CD4+ T cells in natural SIVsmm infection [169]. Thus, Nef may help the natural hosts of SIV to prevent the escalation of immune activation. Even in poorly or non-adapted HIV-1 and SIVmac infections Nef most likely accelerates disease progression, mainly because it enhances the viral loads by several orders of magnitude and not because it enhances virulence directly.

In vitro, HIV-1 Nef proteins differ fundamentally from those of SIVagm, SIVsmm and HIV-2 in their effect on the responsiveness of virally infected primary T cells to TCR-mediated stimulation (Figure 1.7). Virally infected T cells expressing the latter three Nef proteins do not respond to TCR−CD3 stimulation. In agreement with its key role in TCR signaling, CD3 down-modulation is required and sufficient for this effect [169]. As a consequence, T cells infected with viruses capable of CD3 down-modulation show lower levels of apoptosis and express low levels of transcription factors such as NF-AT, death receptors and activation markers [114,169]. In contrast, HIV-1-infected T cells respond strongly to stimulation and show marked increases in the transcription of the viral genome and various cellular genes, as well as in activation-induced cell death [114,169]. Notably, these effects have been confirmed in primary cells. Nef proteins that down-modulate TCR−CD3 disrupt the formation of the immunological synapse between infected T cells and antigen-presenting macrophages or dendritic cells. In contrast, HIV-1 Nefs fail to suppress synapse formation and TCR signaling [170]. Thus, the majority of primate lentiviruses may disrupt the interaction between virally infected T cells and antigen-presenting cells, whereas HIV-1 just deregulates it.

It is conceivable that viruses that render infected T cells hyper-responsive to stimulation may cause higher levels of immune activation than those that block T cell activation. It is largely unclear, however, how the hyper-responsiveness of infected T cells to stimulation relates to the overall levels of infection-associated inflammation. Obviously, the accelerated death of HIV-1-infected

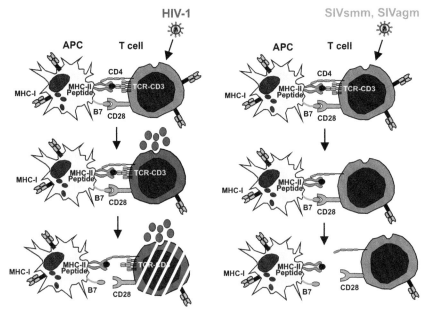

FIGURE 1.7 Model for the manipulation of T cell/APC interaction by HIV-1 (left) and SIVsmm or SIVagm (right). HIV-1 Nef proteins down-modulate CD4 and (less effectively) MHC-I from the cell surface, but do not downregulate TCR−CD3 and have only weak effects on CD28. Consequently, the responsiveness of HIV-1-infected T cells to stimulation by APCs is deregulated, and they show high levels of activation, cytokine secretion and apoptotic death. In comparison, SIVsmm and SIVagm Nefs efficiently down-modulate TCR−CD3 and (usually) CD28 from the cell surface and disrupt the interaction of virally infected T cells with APCs. As a consequence these T cells do not respond to TCR−CD3 mediated stimulation and show low levels of activation and apoptosis at least in cocultures of APCs and virally infected primary T cells *in vivo* [114, 170].

cells itself may drive immune activation and exhaustion. The finding that the half-life of the infected cells is similar in pathogenic and non-pathogenic infection seems to argue against this possibility [150,171]. However, these studies only determined the overall decline in virally infected cells, and enhanced proliferation of HIV-1-infected cells may potentially compensate for the enhanced levels of apoptosis. A different lifespan of infected T cells and thus time frame of virus production would also help to explain why the viral loads are similar in pathogenic and non-pathogenic infection, although T cells that are more strongly activated should produce greater amounts of virus. In addition, the different phenotypes of T cells infected with HIV-1 or SIVsmm and SIVagm may also affect the function and survival of bystander T cells. Helper CD4+ T cells that are a main target cell of SIV and HIV infection orchestrate the immune response, and it is their main task to manipulate other cells. Thus, hyperactivated virally infected helper CD4+ T cells may contribute to high levels of immune activation by sequestering cytokines that induce the migration, inflammatory response and death of uninfected bystander cells. While Nef may usually function to uncouple T cell activation from interaction with antigen-presenting cells, it may also help to prevent the escalation of immune activation in some natural SIV infections. Obviously, however, efficient downregulation of TCR−CD3 is unable to prevent disease progression in the non-adapted macaque host that is highly susceptible to disease, because SIVmac rapidly causes simian AIDS in this experimental host although its Nef protein down-modulates TCR−CD3 with high efficiency. Similarly, it has been reported that TCR−CD3 down-modulation by Nef does not protect against progression in HIV-2 infection [172]. Notably, however, *nef* alleles that render T cells hyper-responsive to stimulation increase the virulence of SIVmac even further and are associated with acute pathogenicity [173]. Furthermore, even in HIV-2 infected individuals with undetectable viral loads the efficiency of Nef-mediated down-modulation of CD3 correlated with the levels of immune activation [172]. Thus, this Nef function can obviously influence the activation state of the immune system of infected individuals, which is a major determinant of progression to AIDS in HIV-2-infected individuals. In fact, we found that the efficiency of CD3 modulation by Nef correlates with the CD4+ T cell counts in viremic HIV-2-infected individuals (Khalid and Kirchhoff, unpublished observations). In further support of a role of Nef-mediated CD3 down-modulation in well-balanced virus−host relationships, infection of macaques with SIVmac constructs expressing HIV-1 *nef* alleles results in an "all or nothing" phenotype—i.e., elimination of the virus or high viral loads and disease [174,175]. Altogether, these results emphasize that Nef is only one of many factors that affect the clinical outcome of primate lentiviral infection, and that it acts as a modulator and not as the sole determinant of infection-associated immune activation. Nonetheless, the experimental data are in agreement with the possibility that (at similar levels of replication) primate lentiviruses that suppress T cell activation are less pathogenic than those that have lost the CD3 down-modulation function [176].

WHY DID LENTIVIRUSES THAT DO NOT SUPPRESS T CELL ACTIVATION EMERGE AT ALL?

Some SIVs that lack *vpu* and down-modulate CD3 seem to have achieved an ideally balanced relationship with their primate hosts, because they maintain high viral loads and spread efficiently without causing disease. The fact that most SIVs down-modulate TCR−CD3 suggests that these viruses are evolutionary older than the *vpu* containing viruses lacking this function. If the former virus−host relationships are "perfect", then why did *vpu* containing viruses emerge in the first place? At least for the common precursor of SIVgsn/mus/mon and for SIVcpz it was obviously advantageous to keep *vpu* and to lose the ability of Nef to suppress T cell activation. One straightforward explanation is that these lentiviruses had not yet established a well-balanced virus–host relationship when *vpu* was acquired. Furthermore, a different host environment may change the selective pressure on the virus and demand different viral properties for effective viral persistence. For effective viral replication, primate lentiviruses must evoke levels of T cell activation sufficient for effective viral transcription but also low enough to avoid apoptosis prior to completion of the viral replication cycle. Obviously, they must also avoid an escalation of immune activation to levels killing the host before virus transmission. It is evident that different primate species respond differently to SIV infection. For example, after infection with the same virus, rhesus macaques develop and maintain high levels of immune activation and progress to AIDS, whereas SMs show only a transient increase in inflammation and avoid disease progression [177,178]. The reasons for this are poorly understood, but may involve differences in T cell subsets and in the innate immune response [13–16]. Possibly, Nef evolved to compensate such species-dependent differences in the responsiveness of virally infected T cells to stimulation. As mentioned above, some Nef functions, such as down-modulation of CD4 and MHC-I, as well as the enhancement of viral infectivity and replication, are almost generally conserved and thus advantageous for the virus. In contrast, primate lentiviruses show major differences in functions that may affect T cell activation. Besides CD3 down-modulation, many primate lentiviral Nefs also modulate the surface expression of CD28 [179,180] and CXCR4 [181] to alter the functionality and migration of T cells. Notably, many HIV-2 and SIVmac Nef alleles down-modulate CD28 and CXCR4 substantially more efficiently than those of HIV-1 [114,181]. Thus, lack of CD3 down-modulation is not compensated by increased activity in other functions that affect the responsiveness to stimulation. On the contrary, *nef* alleles that are unable to modulate TCR–CD3 are usually also less effective in down-modulating CD28 [114]. If the above hypothesis is true, a host containing highly reactive T cells should select for a virus that is more active in suppressing T cell activation. The observation that the SIVmac239 Nef allele evolved to become more effective in down-modulating TCR–CD3 and CD28 than primary SIVsmm Nefs during the passage of SIVmac239 in rhesus macaques that show high levels of immune activation and are particularly sensitive to SIV-induced disease is in agreement with this possibility. The possible evolution of a more virulent subset of primate lentiviruses seems counterintuitive, because a virus that kills its host basically also commits "suicide" since it cannot be further transmitted. However, this disadvantage may be modest if the progression to fatal disease is slow and the pathogen can still be transmitted for years. Furthermore, high viral loads that increase the efficiency of virus transmission may compensate for a reduced lifespan of the infected host. HIV-1 gives a sobering example of this, because it has caused a global pandemic and is still spreading, whereas HIV-2 infections are less common and seem to be declining, although the latter virus is less pathogenic in humans.

VIRAL CORECEPTOR TROPISM AND PATHOGENESIS

To our current knowledge, all primate lentiviruses use CD4 as the primary receptor and a seven-transmembrane G-protein-coupled receptor as a coreceptor to enter its target cells. CD4 is mainly expressed by T helper cells and, at lower levels, by macrophages and dendritic cells. Thus, these viruses can infect, manipulate and eliminate exactly those cell types that play key roles in the immune system. The main coreceptor for HIV-1 is CCR5, although virus variants that show a coreceptor switch or expansion to CXCR4 are detected in about 50 percent of all AIDS cases [182,183]. The physiological importance of CCR5 is evident from the fact that individuals harboring homozygous deletions of 32 bp (CCR5-Δ32) that are found in about 1 percent of the Caucasian population show a reduced risk for HIV-1 infection by sexual intercourse [184,185]. Strikingly, immune reconstitution of an AIDS patient, who had also developed myeloid leukemia, with cells from a matching Δ32/Δ32 donor resulted in undetectable viral loads in the absence of antiretroviral treatment for several years after bone marrow transplantation [186]. Furthermore, an inhibitor of CCR5 (Maraviroc) has been approved for the treatment of HIV-infected individuals in the clinic [187].

CCR5 also seems to be the major coreceptor of most other primate lenti-viruses, although some of them can also use a wide variety of alternative coreceptors, such as CCR1, CCR2b, CCR3, CXCR6, CCR8, GPR1, GPR15/Bob, STRL-33/Bonzo and ChemR23, for virus entry—at least in cell culture [188,189]. The role of the alternative coreceptors for viral replication in "regular" HIV and SIV infections *in vivo* is largely unclear [190]. It is note-worthy, however, that SIVs can replicate efficiently in some natural hosts without using CCR5. For example, it has long been known that SIVrcm may use CCR2b as the major entry cofactor [191]. More recently, it has been shown that a significant number of SMs (8 percent) are homozygous for a 2 bp deletion (Δ2) in CCR5, resulting in a truncated molecule that is not expressed on the cell surface [192]. The average viral loads in these animals were only slightly lower compared to those derived from SMs with the wild-type CCR5 alleles, and the SIVsmm strains used CXCR6, GPR15 and GPR1 as alternative coreceptors. Effective and promiscuous alternative coreceptor usage has also been observed for HIV-2 and SIVagm [193,194]. Furthermore, the molecular SIVmac239 clone, which is commonly used for studies in the SIV/macaque model, effi-ciently utilizes GPR15/Bob and STRL-33/Bonzo in addition to CCR5 [195]. Altogether, usage of chemokine receptors other than CCR5 and CXCR4 as entry cofactors seems more common among primate lentiviruses than antici-pated, and this warrants further investigation.

It is well known that the emergence of CXCR4-tropic HIV-1 variants is associated with a rapid decline in CD4+ T cell counts and rapid progression to AIDS (reviewed in [196]). Thus, while the coreceptor switch/expansion is not obligatory for disease progression, it is associated with a very poor prognosis in the absence of therapy. Initially, it was thought that CXCR4-tropic HIV-1 strains are more cytopathic than those using CCR5. Subsequently, however, it has been shown that CCR5- and CXCR4-tropic HIV-1 are equally cytopathic for their T cell targets in human lymphoid tissues [197]. Since a much larger fraction of T cells (~80 percent) expresses CXCR4 than CCR5 (~20 percent), depletion of the latter does not substantially change the total CD4+ T cell counts [197]. The emergence of CXCR4-tropic viruses in SIV infections seems rare, but is occasionally observed [198,199]. Quite strikingly, the emergence of SIVsmm capable of utilizing CXCR4 and other coreceptors was associated with an almost complete loss of CD4+ T cells in two SMs but not with the development of any opportunistic infections or other signs of disease during several years of follow-up [148,198]. Recent data suggest that double-negative T cells may functionally compensate for the loss of CD4+ helper T cells in this species [199]. It will be of great interest to clarify how common and effective "CD4-independent" T helper-like functions are.

Another interesting question is why CXCR4-tropic SIVs do not emerge more frequently, although monkey CXCR4 molecules can clearly function as effective coreceptors of SIV and the coreceptor switch/expansion usually requires only a limited number of changes in the V3 loop region of the viral Env protein. One plausible explanation is that CXCR4-tropic viruses are easier to neutralize, and thus only emerge after the development of immunodeficiency. However, after experimental infection with CXCR4-tropic SIV strains the coreceptor tropism was often maintained and associated with effective viral replication [200,201]. Notably, the drastic loss of CD4+ T cells in the two SMs infected with SIVsmm strains showing broad coreceptor usage was associated with a strong decline in viral RNA levels, most likely because of limited target-cell availability [148,198]. Thus, while broad coreceptor usage may provide a short-term advantage for these viruses in the individual hosts they should not spread efficiently in the population because they do not maintain high viral loads.

LATEST ADVANCES

Two elegant recent studies have identified SAMHD1 as the long-sought HIV-1 restriction factor that is expressed in myeloid cell types and counteracted by the Vpx protein of the SIVsmm/HIV-2 lineage [202,203]. SAMHD1 was first identified as an IFN-γ inducible factor from human DCs [204], and mutations in *SAMHD1* are associated with the Aicardi-Goutières syndrome, an autosomal recessive encephalopathy associated with perturbances of the type I IFN metabolism [205]. The precise mechanisms of SAMHD1-mediated restriction of HIV-1 in myeloid-lineage cells and of its antagonism by Vpx need further study. The recent studies show that SAMHD1 blocks HIV-1 infection at an early step of the viral life cycle and results in increased levels of viral RNA [202,203]. Mutations in the HD domain disrupt its antiviral activity, suggesting that phosphodiesterase activity is critical for restriction [203]. The results of

Hrecka and colleagues suggest that Vpx targets SAMHD1 for proteasomal degradation through interactions with the CUL4A/DCAF1 E3 ubiquitin ligase complex [202]. Vpx originated from Vpr [56,57], and why the HIV-1 Vpr has apparently not evolved anti-SAMHD1 activity is an interesting question. One possibility is that HIV-1 is sensed more effectively by infected DCs than other primate lentiviruses because its capsid interacts with cyclophilin A [206], and that the lack of a SAMHD1 antagonist helps HIV-1 to avoid DC-dependent antiviral immune responses. This needs further study, but raises the interesting possibility that reducing SAMHD1 function may help to increase innate and adaptive immune responses to HIV-1.

SUMMARY AND PERSPECTIVES

In summary, lentiviruses have most likely been infecting NHPs for millions of years. Today, they are widely distributed in African NHPs and have obviously sometimes achieved an ideally balanced relationship with their primate hosts (schematically indicated in Figure 1.8). Accumulating evidence also suggests, however, that SIV and HIV strains are highly divergent not only in their genomic sequences (which sometimes only show 30 percent homology) but also in their biological properties, and it has become clear that not all natural SIV infections are non-pathogenic. In analogy to visits by unwelcome guests, the question of how well primate lentiviruses can be tolerated depends on a variety of factors; in simple terms: How well do they behave? How many are there? How big are the resources to accommodate them? Is it possible to control them or even to kick them out? It is conceivable that it may be easier for the infected host to tolerate viruses that suppress the responsiveness of virally infected T cells to stimulation compared to those that render them hyper-responsive. In the former case, the virally infected cells are basically taken out of the system, they hardly interact with antigen-presenting cells, and they may die and need to be replaced only at a relatively slow rate. In the latter case, the virally infected cells express high levels of death receptors and cytokines, and may thus affect the survival and function of bystander cells. Furthermore, they undergo activation-induced cell death. At first sight, it may seem counterintuitive that a stronger effect on T cell function (by combined Nef-mediated down-modulation of CD3, CD4, CD28 and CXCR4) may help the natural hosts of SIV to maintain a functional immune system. However, it is plausible that the functionality of the minor percentage of virally infected cells will hardly affect the overall immune competence of the host. In contrast, the rate at which these cells die and need to be replaced may significantly accelerate exhaustion of the immune system. However, most of these results come from cell culture models, and further *in vivo* studies are obligatory to further elucidate the importance of these viral factors compared to intrinsic host properties. We have generated SIVagm constructs that express a functional Vpu and a Nef protein unable to down-modulate TCR−CD3. Such constructs should help to clarify

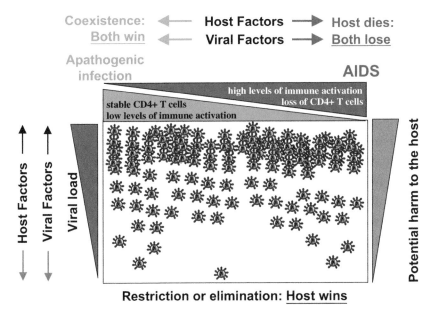

FIGURE 1.8 Virus–host interactions and the virological and clincal outcome of primate lentiviral infections. Both host factors (such as the CTL response and genetic factors) as well as viral properties (e.g., the capability to antagonize host restriction factors and to use virus dependency factors) determine the viral load. Elimination of the invading pathogen after cross-species transmission will usually go unnoticed because no trace is left. If the virus manages to become established and to replicate efficiently in a new species, the clinical outcome of infection once again depends on a variety of host factors (e.g., responsiveness to infection, T cell populations, TLR signaling) and viral properties (e.g., coreceptor tropism and accessory gene function). AIDS and death in poorly or non-adapted hosts, like HIV-1-infected humans or SIVmac-infected macaques, is disadvantageous for both sides because the death of the host implies the end of virus replication and spread. Thus, in the long term, well-balanced virus–host relationships may become established where the virus replicates to high levels and spreads efficiently without harming the host, as in SIVagm-infected AGMs and in SIVsmm-infected SMs. The identification of host and viral factors that allow benign virus–host relationships has become a major focus of AIDS research.

the relevance of viral properties that are characteristic for HIV-1 for immune activation and viral pathogenesis *in vivo*. While important progress has been made, many key questions remain: Why have apparently only 3 of 40 SIV-infected NHPs transmitted their virus to humans? Why is only one of at least a dozen NHP-human transmissions responsible for the AIDS pandemic? What is the risk of further zoonotic transmissions of primate lentiviruses to humans? What is the contribution of different viral and host properties to the clinical outcome of infection? Will the increasing knowledge about host restriction and virus dependency factors lead to novel and effective therapeutic and preventive strategies? In any case, our understanding of the natural history, biological properties and evolution of primate lentiviruses is far from complete, and further studies are highly warranted.

ACKNOWLEDGMENTS

We thank Kristina Wohllaib, Dré van der Merwe, Christine Goffinet, Anke Specht and Daniel Sauter for critical reading of the manuscript. We apologize to the authors of many interesting studies that could not be cited due to space limitations. The authors are supported by grants from the Deutsche Forschungsgemeinschaft and the Landesstiftung Baden-Würtemberg.

REFERENCES

[1] Hahn BH, Shaw GM, De Cock KM, Sharp PM. AIDS as a zoonosis: Scientific and public health implications. Science 2000;287:607–14.

[2] Van Heuverswyn F, Peeters M. The origins of HIV and implications for the global epidemic. Curr Infect Dis Rep 2007;9:338–46.

[3] Sharp PM, Hahn BH. The evolution of HIV-1 and the origin of AIDS. Phil Trans R Soc B 2010;365:2487–94.

[4] Pandrea I, Apetrei C. Where the wild things are: Pathogenesis of SIV infection in African nonhuman primate hosts. Curr HIV/AIDS Rep 2010;1:28–36.

[5] Paiardini M, Pandrea I, Apetrei C, Silvestri G. Lessons learned from the natural hosts of HIV-related viruses. Annu Rev Med 2009;60:485–95.

[6] Keele BF, Van Heuverswyn F, Li Y, Bailes E, Takehisa J, Santiago ML, et al. Chimpanzee reservoirs of pandemic and nonpandemic HIV-1. Science 2006;313:523–6.

[7] Korber B, Muldoon M, Theiler J, Gao F, Gupta R, Lapedes A, et al. Timing the ancestor of the HIV-1 pandemic strains. Science 2000;288:1789–96.

[8] Gao F, Yue L, White AT, Pappas PG, Barchue J, Hanson AP, et al. Human infection by genetically diverse SIVsm-related HIV-2 in West Africa. Nature 1992;358:495–9.

[9] Hirsch VM, Olmsted RA, Murphey-Corb M, Purcell RH, Johnson PR. An African primate lentivirus (SIVsm) closely related to HIV-2. Nature 1989;339:389–92.

[10] Worobey M, Telfer P, Souquière S, Hunter M, Coleman CA, Metzger MJ, et al. Island biogeography reveals the deep history of SIV. Science 2010;329:1487.

[11] Gifford RJ, Katzourakis A, Tristem M, Pybus OG, Winters M, Shafer RW. A transitional endogenous lentivirus from the genome of a basal primate and implications for lentivirus evolution. Proc Natl Acad Sci USA 2008;23:20362–7.

[12] Gilbert C, Maxfield DG, Goodman SM, Feschotte C. Parallel germline infiltration of a lentivirus in two Malagasy lemurs. PLoS Genet 2009;5:e1000425.

[13] Silvestri G, Paiardini M, Pandrea I, Lederman MM, Sodora DL. Understanding the benign nature of SIV infection in natural hosts. J Clin Invest 2007;117:3148–54.

[14] Sodora DL, Allan JS, Apetrei C, Brenchley JM, Douek DC, Else JG, et al. Toward an AIDS vaccine: lessons from natural simian immunodeficiency virus infections of African nonhuman primate hosts. Nat Med 2009;15:861–5.

[15] Kirchhoff F. Is the high virulence of HIV-1 an unfortunate coincidence of primate lentiviral evolution? Nat Rev Microbiol 2009;7:467–76.

[16] Brenchley JM, Silvestri G, Douek DC. Nonprogressive and progressive primate immuno-deficiency lentivirus infections. Immunity 2010;32:737–42.

[17] Santiago ML, Rodenburg CM, Kamenya S, Bibollet-Ruche F, Gao F, Bailes E, et al. SIVcpz in wild chimpanzees. Science 2002;295:465.

[18] Santiago ML, Lukasik M, Kamenya S, Li Y, Bibollet-Ruche F, Bailes E, et al. Foci of endemic simian immunodeficiency virus infection in wild-living eastern chimpanzees (*Pan troglodytes schweinfurthii*). J Virol 2003;77:7545–62.

[19] Keele BF, Jones JH, Terio KA, Estes JD, Rudicell RS, Wilson ML, et al. Increased mortality and AIDS-like immunopathology in wild chimpanzees infected with SIVcpz. Nature 2009;460:515−9.

[20] Van Heuverswyn F, Li Y, Neel C, Bailes E, Keele BF, Liu W, et al. SIV infection in wild gorillas. Nature 2006;444:164.

[21] Takehisa J, Kraus MH, Decker JM, Li Y, Keele BF, Bibollet-Ruche F, et al. Generation of infectious molecular clones of simian immunodeficiency virus from fecal consensus sequences of wild chimpanzees. J Virol 2007;81:7463−75.

[22] VandeWoude S, Apetrei C. Going wild: lessons from T-lymphotropic naturally occurring lentiviruses. Clin Microbiol Rev 2006;19:728−62.

[23] Aghokeng AF, Liu W, Bibollet-Ruche F, Loul S, Mpoudi-Ngole E, Laurent C, et al. Widely varying SIV prevalence rates in naturally infected primate species from Cameroon. Virology 2006;345:174−89.

[24] Aghokeng AF, Ayouba A, Mpoudi-Ngole E, Loul S, Liegeois F, Delaporte E, et al. Extensive survey on the prevalence and genetic diversity of SIVs in primate bushmeat provides insights into risks for potential new cross-species transmissions. Infect Genet Evol 2010;10:386−96.

[25] Fultz PN, Gordon TP, Anderson DC, McClure HM. Prevalence of natural infection with simian immunodeficiency virus and simian T-cell leukemia virus type I in a breeding colony of sooty mangabey monkeys. AIDS 1990;4:619−25.

[26] Pandrea I, Onanga R, Souquiere S, Mouinga-Ondéme A, Bourry O, Makuwa M, et al. Paucity of CD4+CCR5+ T-cells may prevent breastfeeding transmission of SIV in natural non-human primate hosts. J Virol 2008;82:5501−9.

[27] Chahroudi A, Meeker T, Lawson B, Ratcliffe S, Else J, Silvestri G. Mother-to-infant transmission of SIV is rare in sooty mangabeys and is associated with low viremia. J Virol [Epub ahead of print] 2011.

[28] Salemi M, De Oliveira T, Courgnaud V, Moulton V, Holland B, Cassol S, et al. Mosaic genomes of the six major primate lentivirus lineages revealed by phylogenetic analyses. J Virol 2003;77:7202−13.

[29] Allan JS, Short M, Taylor ME, Su S, Hirsch VM, Johnson PR, et al. Species-specific diversity among simian immunodeficiency viruses from African green monkeys. J Virol 1991;65:2816−28.

[30] Muller MC, Saksena NK, Nerrienet E, Chappey C, Herve VM, Durand JP, et al. Simian immunodeficiency viruses from central and western Africa: Evidence for a new species-specific lentivirus in tantalus monkeys. J Virol 1993;67:1227−35.

[31] Jin MJ, Hui H, Robertson DL, Müller MC, Barré-Sinoussi F, Hirsch VM, et al. Mosaic genome structure of simian immunodeficiency virus from west African green monkeys. EMBO J 1994;13:2935−47.

[32] Daniel MD, Letvin NL, King NW, Kannagi M, Sehgal PK, Hunt RD, et al. Isolation of T-cell tropic HTLV-III-like retrovirus from macaques. Science 1985;228:1201−4.

[33] Bibollet-Ruche F, Galat-Luong A, Cuny G, Sarni-Manchado P, Galat G, Durand JP, et al. Simian immunodeficiency virus infection in a patas monkey (*Erythrocebus patas*): Evidence for cross-species transmission from African green monkeys (*Cercopithecus aethiops sabaeus*) in the wild. J Gen Virol 1996;77:773−81.

[34] Jin MJ, Rogers J, Phillips-Conroy JE, Allan JS, Desrosiers RC, Shaw GM, et al. Infection of a yellow baboon with simian immunodeficiency virus from African green monkeys: evidence for cross-species transmission in the wild. J Virol 1994;68: 8454−60.

[35] Tomonaga K, Katahira J, Fukasawa M, Hassan MA, Kawamura M, Akari H, et al. Isolation and characterization of simian immunodeficiency virus from African white-crowned mangabey monkeys (*Cercocebus torquatus lunulatus*). Arch Virol 1993;129:77−92.

[36] Chen J, Powell D, Hu WS. High frequency of genetic recombination is a common feature of primate lentivirus replication. J Virol 2006;80:9651−8.

[37] Mostowy R, Kouyos RD, Fouchet D, Bonhoeffer S. The role of recombination for the coevolutionary dynamics of HIV and the immune response. PLoS One 2011;6:e16052.

[38] Wooley DP, Smith RA, Czajak S, Desrosiers RC. Direct demonstration of retroviral recombination in a rhesus monkey. J Virol 1997;71:9650−3.

[39] Souquiere S, Bibollet-Ruche F, Robertson DL, Makuwa M, Apetrei C, Onanga R, et al. Wild *Mandrillus sphinx* are carriers of two types of lentivirus. J Virol 2001;75:7086−96.

[40] Bailes E, Gao F, Bibollet-Ruche F, Courgnaud V, Peeters M, Marx PA, et al. Hybrid origin of SIV in chimpanzees. Science 2003;300:1713.

[41] Dazza MC, Ekwalanga M, Nende M, Shamamba KB, Bitshi P, Paraskevis D, et al. Characterization of a novel vpu-harboring simian immunodeficiency virus from a Dent's Mona monkey (*Cercopithecus mona denti*). J Virol 2005;79:8560−71.

[42] Wertheim JO, Worobey MA. Challenge to the ancient origin of SIVagm based on African green monkey mitochondrial genomes. PLoS Pathog 2007;3:e95.

[43] Sharp PM, Bailes E, Gao F, Beer BE, Hirsch VM, Hahn BH. Origins and evolution of AIDS viruses: estimating the time-scale. Biochem Soc Trans 2000;28:275−82.

[44] Bjork A, Liu W, Wertheim JO, Hahn BH, Worobey M. Evolutionary history of chimpanzees inferred from complete mitochondrial genomes. Mol Biol Evol 2011;28:615−23.

[45] Chen Z, Telfer P, Gettie A, Reed P, Zhang L, Ho DD, et al. Genetic characterization of new west African simian immunodeficiency virus SIVsm: geographic clustering of household-derived SIV strains with human immunodeficiency virus type 2 subtypes and genetically diverse viruses from a single feral sooty mangabey troop. J Virol 1996;70:3617−27.

[46] Santiago ML, Range F, Keele BF, Li Y, Bailes E, Bibollet-Ruche F, et al. Simian immunodeficiency virus infection in free-ranging sooty mangabeys (*Cercocebus atys atys*) from the Tai Forest, Cote d'Ivoire: Implications for the origin of epidemic human immunodeficiency virus type 2. J Virol 2005;79:12515−27.

[47] Gao F, Yue L, Robertson DL, Hill SC, Hui H, Biggar RJ, et al. Genetic diversity of human immunodeficiency virus type 2: Evidence for distinct sequence subtype with differences in virus biology. J Virol 1994;68:7433−47.

[48] Damond F, Worobey M, Campa P, Farfara I, Colin G, Matherson S, et al. Identification of a highly divergent HIV type 2 and proposal for a change in HIV type 2 classification. AIDS Res Hum Retroviruses 2004;20:666−72.

[49] Huet T, Cheynier R, Meyerhans A, Roelants G, Wain-Hobson S. Genetic organization of a chimpanzee lentivirus related to HIV-1. Nature 1990;345:356−8.

[50] Peeters M, Honore C, Huet T, Bedjabaga L, Ossari S, Bussi P, et al. Isolation and partial characterization of an HIV-related virus occurring naturally in chimpanzees in Gabon. AIDS 1989;3:625−30.

[51] Prince AM, Brotman B, Lee D-H, Andrus L, Valinsky J, Marx PA. Lack of evidence for HIV type 1-related SIVcpz infection in captive and wild chimpanzees (*Pan troglodytes verus*) in West Africa. AIDS Res Hum Retroviruses 2002;18:657−60.

[52] Takehisa J, Kraus MH, Ayouba A, Bailes E, Van Heuverswyn F, Decker JM, et al. Origin and biology of simian immunodeficiency virus infecting wild western gorillas. J Virol 2009;83:1635−48.

[53] Plantier JC, Leoz M, Dickerson JE, De Oliveira F, Cordonnier F, Lemée V, et al. A new human immunodeficiency virus derived from gorillas. Nat Med 2009;15:871−2.

[54] Watts JM, Dang KK, Gorelick RJ, Leonard CW, Bess JW, Swanstrom R, et al. Architecture and secondary structure of an entire HIV-1 RNA genome. Nature 2009;460:711−6.

[55] Kirchhoff F. Immune evasion and counteraction of restriction factors by HIV-1 and other primate lentiviruses. Cell Host Microbe 2010;8:55−67.

[56] Sharp PM, Bailes E, Stevenson M, Emerman M, Hahn BH. Gene acquisition in HIV and SIV. Nature 1996;383:586−7.

[57] Tristem M, Marshall C, Karpas A, Petrik J, Hill F. Origin of vpx in lentiviruses. Nature 1990;347:341−2.

[58] Courgnaud V, Abela B, Pourrut X, Mpoudi-Ngole E, Loul S, Delaporte E, et al. Identification of a new simian immunodeficiency virus lineage with a *vpu* gene present among different *Cercopithecus* monkeys (*C. mona, C. cephus,* and *C. nictitans*) from Cameroon. J Virol 2003;77:12523−34.

[59] Bushman FD, Malani N, Fernandes J, D'Orso I, Cagney G, Diamond TL, et al. Host cell factors in HIV replication: Meta-analysis of genome-wide studies. PLoS Pathog 2009;5:e1000437.

[60] Lever AM, Jeang KT. Insights into cellular factors that regulate HIV-1 replication in human cells. Biochemistry 2011;50:920−31.

[61] McNatt MW, Zang T, Hatziioannou T, Bartlett M, Fofana IB, Johnson WE, et al. Species-specific activity of HIV-1 Vpu and positive selection of tetherin transmembrane domain variants. PLoS Pathog 2009;5:e1000300.

[62] Sawyer SL, Emerman M, Malik HS. Ancient adaptive evolution of the primate antiviral DNA-editing enzyme APOBEC3G. PLoS Biol 2004;2:E275.

[63] Sawyer SL, Emerman M, Malik HS. Discordant evolution of the adjacent antiretroviral genes TRIM22 and TRIM5 in mammals. PLoS Pathog 2007;3:e197.

[64] Bozek K, Lengauer T. Positive selection of HIV host factors and the evolution of lentivirus genes. BMC Evol Biol 2010;10:186.

[65] Wain LV, Bailes E, Bibollet-Ruche F, Decker JM, Keele BF, Van Heuverswyn F, et al. Adaptation of HIV-1 to its human host. Mol Biol Evol 2007;24:1853−60.

[66] Bieniasz PD. Intrinsic immunity: A front-line defense against viral attack. Nat Immunol 2004;5:1109−15.

[67] Chiu YL, Greene WC. APOBEC3G: An intracellular centurion. Philos. Trans R Soc B 2009;364:689−703.

[68] Malim MH, Emerman M. HIV-1 accessory proteins-ensuring viral survival in a hostile environment. Cell Host Microbe 2008;3:388−98.

[69] Neil S, Bieniasz P. Human immunodeficiency virus, restriction factors, and interferon. J Interferon Cytokine Res 2009;29:569−80.

[70] Strebel K, Luban J, Jeang KT. Human cellular restriction factors that target HIV-1 replication. BMC Med 2009;7:48.

[71] Huthoff H, Towers GJ. Restriction of retroviral replication by APOBEC3G/F and TRIM5alpha. Trends Microbiol 2008;16:612−9.

[72] Williams KC, Burdo TH. HIV and SIV infection: The role of cellular restriction and immune responses in viral replication and pathogenesis. Acta Pathol Microbiol Immunol 2009;117:400−12.

[73] Stremlau M, Owens CM, Perron MJ, Kiessling M, Autissier P, Sodroski J. The cytoplasmic body component TRIM5alpha restricts HIV-1 infection in Old World monkeys. Nature 2004;427:848−53.

[74] Kratovac Z, Virgen CA, Bibollet-Ruche F, Hahn BH, Bieniasz PD, Hatziioannou T. Primate lentivirus capsid sensitivity to TRIM5 proteins. J Virol 2008;82:6772−7.

[75] Yap MW, Nisole S, Stoye JP. A single amino acid change in the SPRY domain of human Trim5alpha leads to HIV-1 restriction. Curr Biol 2005;15:73−8.

[76] Sheehy AM, Gaddis NC, Choi JD, Malim MH. Isolation of a human gene that inhibits HIV-1 infection and is suppressed by the viral Vif protein. Nature 2002;418:646−50.

[77] Mariani R, Chen D, Schröfelbauer B, Navarro F, König R, Bollman B, et al. Species-specific exclusion of APOBEC3G from HIV-1 virions by Vif. Cell 2003;114:21−31.

[78] Stopak K, de Noronha C, Yonemoto W, Greene WC. HIV-1 Vif blocks the antiviral activity of APOBEC3G by impairing both its translation and intracellular stability. Mol Cell 2003;12:591−601.

[79] Bishop KN, Verma M, Kim EY, Wolinsky SM, Malim MH. APOBEC3G inhibits elongation of HIV-1 reverse transcripts. PLoS Pathog 2008:e1000231.

[80] Wissing S, Galloway NL, Greene WC. HIV-1 Vif versus the APOBEC3 cytidine deaminases: an intracellular duel between pathogen and host restriction factors. Mol Aspects Med 2010;31:383−97.

[81] Holmes RK, Koning FA, Bishop KN, Malim MH. APOBEC3F can inhibit the accumulation of HIV-1 reverse transcription products in the absence of hypermutation. Comparisons with APOBEC3G. J Biol Chem 2007;282:2587−95.

[82] Neil SJ, Zang T, Bieniasz PD. Tetherin inhibits retrovirus release and is antagonized by HIV-1 Vpu. Nature 2008;451:425−30.

[83] Van Damme N, Goff D, Katsura C, Jorgenson RL, Mitchell R, Johnson MC, et al. The interferon-induced protein BST-2 restricts HIV-1 release and is downregulated from the cell surface by the viral Vpu protein. Cell Host Microbe 2008;3:245−52.

[84] Kupzig S, Korolchuk V, Rollason R, Sugden A, Wilde A, Banting G. Bst-2/HM1.24 is a raft-associated apical membrane protein with an unusual topology. Traffic 2003;4: 694−709.

[85] Perez-Caballero D, Zang T, Ebrahimi A, McNatt MW, Gregory DA, Johnson MC, et al. Tetherin inhibits HIV-1 release by directly tethering virions to cells. Cell 2009;139: 499−511.

[86] Schoggins JW, Wilson SJ, Panis M, Murphy MY, Jones CT, Bieniasz P, et al. A diverse range of gene products are effectors of the type I interferon antiviral response. Nature [Epub ahead of print] 2011.

[87] Goujon C, Rivière L, Jarrosson-Wuilleme L, Bernaud J, Rigal D, Darlix JL, et al. SIVSM/HIV-2 Vpx proteins promote retroviral escape from a proteasome-dependent restriction pathway present in human dendritic cells. Retrovirology 2007;4:2.

[88] Sharova N, Wu Y, Zhu X, Stranska R, Kaushik R, Sharkey M, et al. Primate lentiviral Vpx commandeers DDB1 to counteract a macrophage restriction. PLoS Pathog 2008;4: e1000057.

[89] Kaushik R, Zhu X, Stranska R, Wu Y, Stevenson M. A cellular restriction dictates the permissivity of nondividing monocytes/macrophages to lentivirus and gammaretrovirus infection. Cell Host Microbe 2009;6:68−80.

[90] Rotger M, Dang KK, Fellay J, Heinzen EL, Feng S, Descombes P, et al. Swiss HIV Cohort Study; Center for HIV/AIDS Vaccine Immunology. Genome-wide mRNA expression correlates of viral control in CD4+ T-cells from HIV-1-infected individuals. PLoS Pathog 2010;26:e1000781.

[91] Malim MH. APOBEC proteins and intrinsic resistance to HIV-1 infection. Philos Trans R Soc Lond B Biol Sci 2009;12:675−87.

[92] Gaddis NC, Sheehy AM, Ahmad KM, Swanson CM, Bishop KN, Beer BE, et al. Further investigation of simian immunodeficiency virus Vif function in human cells. J Virol 2004;78:12041−6.

[93] Planelles V, Benichou S. Vpr and its interactions with cellular proteins. Curr Top Microbiol Immunol 2009;339:177−200.

[94] Le Rouzic E, Belaïdouni N, Estrabaud E, Morel M, Rain JC, Transy C, et al. HIV-1 Vpr arrests the cell cycle by recruiting DCAF1/VprBP, a receptor of the Cul4−DDB1 ubiquitin ligase. Cell Cycle 2007;6:182−8.

[95] Connor RI, Chen BK, Choe S, Landau NR. Vpr is required for efficient replication of human immunodeficiency virus type-1 in mononuclear phagocytes. Virology 1995;206:935−44.

[96] Balliet JW, Kolson DL, Eiger G, Kim FM, McGann KA, Srinivasan A, et al. Distinct effects in primary macrophages and lymphocytes of the human immunodeficiency virus type 1 accessory genes *vpr*, *vpu*, and *nef*: mutational analysis of a primary HIV-1 isolate. Virology 1994;200:623−31.

[97] Ariën KK, Verhasselt B. HIV Nef: Role in pathogenesis and viral fitness. Curr HIV Res 2008;6:200−8.

[98] Kirchhoff F, Schindler M, Specht A, Arhel N, Münch J. Role of Nef in primate lentiviral immunopathogenesis. Cell Mol Life Sci 2008;65:2621−36.

[99] Deacon NJ, Tsykin A, Solomon A, Smith K, Ludford-Menting M, Hooker DJ, et al. Genomic structure of an attenuated quasi species of HIV-1 from a blood transfusion donor and recipients. Science 1995;270:988−91.

[100] Kestler HW, Ringler DJ, Mori K, Panicali DL, Sehgal PK, Daniel MD, et al. Importance of the *nef* gene for maintenance of high virus loads and for development of AIDS. Cell 1991;65:651−62.

[101] Kirchhoff F, Greenough TC, Brettler DB, Sullivan JL, Desrosiers RC. Absence of intact nef sequences in a long-term, nonprogressing survivor of HIV-1 infection. N Engl J Med 1995;332:228−32.

[102] Arhel NJ, Kirchhoff F. Implications of Nef: host cell interactions in viral persistence and progression to AIDS. Curr Top Microbiol Immunol 2009;33:147−75.

[103] Roeth JF, Collins KL. Human immunodeficiency virus type 1 Nef: Adapting to intracellular trafficking pathways. Microbiol Mol Biol Rev 2006;70:548−63.

[104] Renkema GH, Saksela K. Interactions of HIV-1 NEF with cellular signal transducing proteins. Front Biosci 2000;5:268−83.

[105] Stumptner-Cuvelette P, Morchoisne S, Dugast M, Le Gall S, Raposo G, Schwartz O, et al. HIV-1 Nef impairs MHC class II antigen presentation and surface expression. Proc Natl Acad Sci USA 2001;98:12144−9.

[106] Schindler M, Würfl S, Benaroch P, Greenough TC, Daniels R, Easterbrook P, et al. Down-modulation of mature major histocompatibility complex class II and up-regulation of invariant chain cell surface expression are well-conserved functions of human and simian immunodeficiency virus nef alleles. J Virol 2003;77:10548−56.

[107] Djordjevic JT, Schibeci SD, Stewart GJ, Williamson P. HIV type 1 Nef increases the association of T cell receptor (TCR)-signaling molecules with T cell rafts and promotes activation-induced raft fusion. AIDS Res Hum Retrovir 2004;20:547−55.

[108] Fenard D, Yonemoto W, de Noronha C, Cavrois M, Williams SA, Greene WC. Nef is physically recruited into the immunological synapse and potentiates T cell activation early after TCR engagement. J Immunol 2005;175:6050−7.

[109] Fortin JF, Barat C, Beausejour Y, Barbeau B, Tremblay MJ. Hyper-responsiveness to stimulation of HIV-infected CD4+ T cells requires Nef and Tat virus gene products and

results from higher NFAT, NF-kappaB, and AP-1 induction. J Biol Chem 2004;279:39520−31.

[110] Manninen A, Renkema GH, Saksela K. Synergistic activation of NFAT by HIV-1 Nef and the Ras/MAPK pathway. J Biol Chem 2000;275:16513−7.

[111] Schrager JA, Marsh JW, HIV-1 Nef increases T cell activation in a stimulus-dependent manner. Proc Natl Acad Sci USA 1999;96:8167−72.

[112] Simmons A, Aluvihare V, McMichael A. Nef triggers a transcriptional program in T cells imitating single-signal T cell activation and inducing HIV virulence mediators. Immunity 2001;14:763−77.

[113] Wang JK, Kiyokawa E, Verdin E, Trono D. Nef protein of HIV-1 associates with rafts and primes T cells for activation. Proc Natl Acad Sci USA 2000;97:394−9.

[114] Schindler M, Münch J, Kutsch O, Li H, Santiago ML, Bibollet-Ruche F, et al. Nef-mediated suppression of T cell activation was lost in a lentiviral lineage that gave rise to HIV-1. Cell 2006;125:1055−67.

[115] Lenassi M, Cagney G, Liao M, Vaupotic T, Bartholomeeusen K, Cheng Y, et al. HIV Nef is secreted in exosomes and triggers apoptosis in bystander CD4+ T cells. Traffic 2010;11:110−22.

[116] Qiao X, He B, Chiu A, Knowles DM, Chadburn A, Cerutti A. Human immunodeficiency virus 1 Nef suppresses CD40-dependent immunoglobulin class switching in bystander B cells. Nat Immunol 2006;7:302−10.

[117] James CO, Huang MB, Khan M, Garcia-Barrio M, Powell MD, Bond VC. Extracellular Nef protein targets CD4(+) T cells for apoptosis by interacting with CXCR4 surface receptors. J Virol 2004;78:3099−109.

[118] Pizzato M, Helander A, Popova E, Calistri A, Zamborlini A, Palù G, et al. Dynamin 2 is required for the enhancement of HIV-1 infectivity by Nef. Proc Natl Acad Sci USA 2007;104:6812−7.

[119] Jia B, Serra-Moreno R, Neidermyer W, Rahmberg A, Mackey J, Fofana IB, et al. Species-specific activity of SIV Nef and HIV-1 Vpu in overcoming restriction by tetherin/BST2. PLOS Pathog 2009;5:1000429.

[120] Sauter D, Schindler M, Specht A, Landford WN, Münch J, Kim KA, et al. Tetherin-driven evolution of Vpu and Nef function and the emergence of pandemic and non-pandemic HIV-1 strains. Cell Host Microbe 2009;6:409−21.

[121] Zhang F, Wilson SJ, Landford WC, Virgen B, Gregory D, Johnson MC, et al. Nef proteins from Simian Immunodeficiency Viruses are tetherin antagonists. Cell Host Microbe 2009;6:54−67.

[122] Goujon C, Rivière L, Jarrosson-Wuilleme L, Bernaud J, Rigal D, Darlix JL, et al. SIVSM/HIV-2 Vpx proteins promote retroviral escape from a proteasome-dependent restriction pathway present in human dendritic cells. Retrovirology 2007;4:2.

[123] Fletcher TM, Brichacek B, Sharova N, Newman MA, Stivahtis G, Sharp PM, et al. Nuclear import and cell cycle arrest functions of the HIV-1 Vpr protein are encoded by two separate genes in HIV-2/SIV(SM) 3rd ed. EMBO J 1996;15:6155−65.

[124] Srivastava S, Swanson SK, Manel N, Florens L, Washburn MP, Skowronski J. Lentiviral Vpx accessory factor targets VprBP/DCAF1 substrate adaptor for Cullin 4 E3 ubiquitin ligase to enable macrophage infection. PLoS Pathog 2008;4:e1000059.

[125] Ayinde D, Maudet C, Transy C, Margottin-Goguet F. Limelight on two HIV/SIV accessory proteins in macrophage infection: Is Vpx overshadowing Vpr? Retrovirology 2010;7:35.

[126] Gibbs JS, Lackner AA, Lang SM, Simon MA, Sehgal PK, Daniel MD, et al. Progression to AIDS in the absence of a gene for vpr or vpx. J Virol 1995;69:2378−83.

[127] Ruiz A, Guatelli JC, Stephens EB. The vpu protein: new concepts in virus release and CD4 down-modulation. Curr HIV Res 2010;8:240−52.

[128] Dubé M, Bego MG, Paquay C, Cohen ÉA. Modulation of HIV-1−host interaction: role of the Vpu accessory protein. Retrovirology 2010;7:114.

[129] Andrew A, Strebel K. HIV-1 Vpu targets cell surface markers CD4 and BST-2 through distinct mechanisms. Mol Aspects Med 2010;5:407−17.

[130] Guatelli JC. Interactions of viral protein U (Vpu) with cellular factors. Curr Top Microbiol Immunol 2009;339:27−45.

[131] Bour S, Schubert U, Strebel K. The human immunodeficiency virus type 1 Vpu protein specifically binds to the cytoplasmic domain of CD4: Implications for the mechanism of degradation. J Virol 1995;69:1510−20.

[132] Willey RL, Maldarelli F, Martin MA, Strebel K. Human immunodeficiency virus type 1 Vpu protein induces rapid degradation of CD4. J Virol 1992;66:7193−200.

[133] Mitchell RS, Katsura C, Skasko MA, Fitzpatrick K, Lau D, Ruiz A, et al. Vpu antagonizes BST-2-mediated restriction of HIV-1 release via beta-TrCP and endo-lysosomal trafficking. PLoS Pathog 2009;5:1000450.

[134] Douglas JL, Viswanathan K, McCarroll MN, Gustin JK, Früh K, Moses AV. Vpu directs the degradation of the human immunodeficiency virus restriction factor BST-2/Tetherin via a {beta}TrCP-dependent mechanism. J Virol 2009;83:7931−47.

[135] Goffinet C, Allespach I, Homann S, Tervo HM, Habermann A, Rupp D, et al. HIV-1 antagonism of CD317 is species specific and involves Vpu-mediated proteasomal degradation of the restriction factor. Cell Host Microbe 2009;5:285−97.

[136] Gupta RK, Hué S, Schaller T, Verschoor E, Pillay D, Towers GJ. Mutation of a single residue renders human tetherin resistant to HIV-1 Vpu-mediated depletion. PLoS Pathog 2009;5:1000443.

[137] Mangeat B, Gers-Huber G, Lehmann M, Zufferey M, Luban J, Piguet V. HIV-1 Vpu neutralizes the antiviral factor Tetherin/BST-2 by binding it and directing its beta-TrCP2-dependent degradation. PLoS Pathog 2009;5:e1000574.

[138] Dubé M, Roy BB, Guiot-Guillain P, Binette J, Mercier J, Chiasson A, et al. Antagonism of tetherin restriction of HIV-1 release by Vpu involves binding and sequestration of the restriction factor in a perinuclear compartment. PLoS Pathog 2010;6: e1000856.

[139] Yang SJ, Lopez LA, Hauser H, Exline CM, Haworth KG, Cannon PM. Anti-tetherin activities in Vpu-expressing primate lentiviruses. Retrovirology 2010;7:13.

[140] Moll M, Andersson SK, Smed-Sörensen A, Sandberg JK. Inhibition of lipid antigen presentation in dendritic cells by HIV-1 Vpu interference with CD1d recycling from endosomal compartments. Blood 2010;116:1876−84.

[141] Shah AH, Sowrirajan B, Davis ZB, Ward JP, Campbell EM, Planelles V, et al. Degranulation of natural killer cells following interaction with HIV-1-infected cells is hindered by downmodulation of NTB-A by Vpu. Cell Host Microbe 2010;8:397−409.

[142] Anderson JL, Johnson AT, Howard JL, Purcell DF. Both linear and discontinuous ribosome scanning are used for translation initiation from bicistronic human immunodeficiency virus type 1 env mRNAs. J Virol 2007;81:4664−76.

[143] Schwartz S, Felber BK, Fenyö EM, Pavlakis GN. Env and Vpu proteins of human immunodeficiency virus type 1 are produced from multiple bicistronic mRNAs. J Virol 1990;64:5448−56.

[144] Chertova E, Bess JW, Crise BJ, Sowder RC, Schaden TM, Hilburn JM, et al. Envelope glycoprotein incorporation, not shedding of surface envelope glycoprotein (gp120/SU),

is the primary determinant of SU content of purified human immunodeficiency virus type 1 and simian immunodeficiency virus. J Virol 2002;76:5315−25.

[145] Sauter D, Specht A, Kirchhoff F. Tetherin: Holding on and letting go. Cell 2010;141:392−8.

[146] Silvestri G. Naturally SIV-infected sooty mangabeys: Are we closer to understanding why they do not develop AIDS? J Med Primatol 2005;34:243−52.

[147] Rowland-Jones S. Protective immunity against HIV infection: Lessons from HIV-2 infection. Future Microbiol 2006;1:427−33.

[148] Gordon S, Klatt NR, Bosinger SE, Brenchley JM, Milush JM, Engram JC, et al. Severe depletion of mucosal CD4+ T cells in AIDS-free SIV-infected sooty mangabeys. J Immunol 2007;179:3026−34.

[149] Pandrea I, Gautam R, Ribeiro RM, Brenchley JM, Butler IF, Pattison M, et al. Acute loss of intestinal CD4+ T cells is not predictive of simian immunodeficiency virus virulence. J Immunol 2007;179:3035−46.

[150] Pandrea I, Ribeiro RM, Gautam R, Gaufin T, Pattison M, Barnes M, et al. Simian immunodeficiency virus SIVagm dynamics in African green monkeys. J Virol 2008;82: 3713−24.

[151] Giorgi JV, Hultin LE, McKeating JA, Johnson TD, Owens B, Jacobson LP, et al. Shorter survival in advanced human immunodeficiency virus type 1 infection is more closely associated with T lymphocyte activation than with plasma virus burden or virus chemokine coreceptor usage. J Infect Dis 1999;179:859−70.

[152] Sousa AE, Carneiro J, Meier-Schellersheim M, Grossman Z, Victorino RM. CD4 T cell depletion is linked directly to immune activation in the pathogenesis of HIV-1 and HIV-2 but only indirectly to the viral load. J Immunol 2002;169:3400−6.

[153] Mandl JN, Barry AP, Vanderford TH, Kozyr N, Chavan R, Klucking S, et al. Divergent TLR7 and TLR9 signaling and type I interferon production distinguish pathogenic and nonpathogenic AIDS virus infections. Nat Med 2008;14:1077−87.

[154] Bosinger SE, Li Q, Gordon SN, Klatt NR, Duan L, Xu L, et al. Global genomic analysis reveals rapid control of a robust innate response in SIV-infected sooty mangabeys. J Clin Invest 2009;119:3556−72.

[155] Jacquelin B, Mayau V, Targat B, Liovat AS, Kunkel D, Petitjean G, et al. Nonpathogenic SIV infection of African green monkeys induces a strong but rapidly controlled type I IFN response. J Clin Invest 2009;119:3544−55.

[156] Estes JD, Gordon SN, Zeng M, Chahroudi AM, Dunham RM, Staprans SI, et al. Early resolution of acute immune activation and induction of PD-1 in SIV-infected sooty mangabeys distinguishes nonpathogenic from pathogenic infection in rhesus macaques. J Immunol 2008;180:6798−807.

[157] Mauclère P, Loussert-Ajaka I, Damond F, Fagot P, Souquières S, Monny Lobe M, et al. Serological and virological characterization of HIV-1 group O infection in Cameroon. AIDS 1997;15:445−53.

[158] Vendrame D, Sourisseau M, Perrin V, Schwartz O, Mammano F. Partial inhibition of human immunodeficiency virus replication by type I interferons: Impact of cell-to-cell viral transfer. J Virol 2009;83:10527−37.

[159] Gummuluru S, Kinsey CM, Emerman M. An *in vitro* rapid-turnover assay for human immunodeficiency virus type 1 replication selects for cell-to-cell spread of virus. J Virol 2000;74:10882−91.

[160] Jolly C, Booth NJ, Neil SJ. Cell−cell spread of human immunodeficiency virus type 1 overcomes tetherin/BST-2-mediated restriction in T cells. J Virol 2010;84: 12185−99.

[161] Casartelli N, Sourisseau M, Feldmann J, Guivel-Benhassine F, Mallet A, Marcelin AG, et al. Tetherin restricts productive HIV-1 cell-to-cell transmission. PLoS Pathog 2010;6:e1000955.

[162] Rücker E, Grivel JC, Münch J, Kirchhoff F, Margolis L. Vpr and Vpu are important for efficient human immunodeficiency virus type 1 replication and CD4+ T-cell depletion in human lymphoid tissue *ex vivo*. J Virol 2004;78:12689−93.

[163] Schindler M, Rajan D, Banning C, Wimmer P, Koppensteiner H, Iwanski A, et al. Vpu serine 52 dependent counteraction of tetherin is required for HIV-1 replication in macrophages, but not in *ex vivo* human lymphoid tissue. Retrovirology 2010;7:1.

[164] Lama J. The physiological relevance of CD4 receptor down-modulation during HIV infection. Curr HIV Res 2003;1:167−84.

[165] Boasso A, Shearer GM. Chronic innate immune activation as a cause of HIV-1 immunopathogenesis. Clin Immunol 2008;126:235−42.

[166] Beignon AS, McKenna K, Skoberne M, Manches O, DaSilva I, Kavanagh DG, et al. Endocytosis of HIV-1 activates plasmacytoid dendritic cells via Toll-like receptor−viral RNA interactions. J Clin Invest 2005;115:3265−75.

[167] Haupt S, Donhauser N, Chaipan C, Schuster P, Puffer B, Daniels RS, et al. CD4 binding affinity determines human immunodeficiency virus type 1-induced alpha interferon production in plasmacytoid dendritic cells. J Virol 2008;82:8900−5.

[168] Schmökel J, Sauter D, Schindler M, Leendertz FH, Bailes E, Dazza MC, et al. The presence of a *vpu* gene and the lack of Nef-mediated downmodulation of T cell receptor-CD3 are not always linked in primate lentiviruses. J Virol 2011;85:742−52.

[169] Schindler M, Schmökel J, Specht A, Li H, Münch J, Khalid M, et al. Inefficient Nef-mediated downmodulation of CD3 and MHC-I correlates with loss of CD4+ T cells in natural SIV infection. PLOS Pathogens 2008;4:e1000107.

[170] Arhel N, Lehmann M, Clauss K, Nienhaus GU, Piguet V, Kirchhoff F. The inability to disrupt the immunological synapse between infected human T cells and APCs distinguishes HIV-1 from most other primate lentiviruses. J Clin Invest 2009;119:2965−75.

[171] Gordon S, Dunham RM, Engram JC, Estes J, Wang Z, Klatt NR, et al. Short-lived infected cells support virus replication in sooty mangabeys naturally infected with simian immunodeficiency virus: Implications for AIDS pathogenesis. J Virol 2008;82:3725−35.

[172] Feldmann J, Leligdowicz A, Jaye A, Dong T, Whittle H, Rowland-Jones SL. Downregulation of the T-cell receptor by human immunodeficiency virus type 2 Nef does not protect against disease progression. J Virol 2009;83:12968−72.

[173] Du Z, Lang SM, Sasseville VG, Lackner A, Ilyinskii PO, Daniel MDJJ, et al. Identification of a nef allele that causes lymphocyte activation and acute disease in macaque monkeys. Cell 1995;82:665−74.

[174] Alexander L, Du Z, Howe AY, Czajak S, Desrosiers RC. Induction of AIDS in rhesus monkeys by a recombinant simian immunodeficiency virus expressing nef of human immunodeficiency virus type 1. J Virol 1999;73:5814−25.

[175] Kirchhoff F, Münch J, Carl S, Stolte N, Mätz-Rensing K, Fuchs D, et al. The HIV-1 *nef* gene can to a large extent replace SIV *nef in vivo*. J Virol 1999;73:8371−83.

[176] Mandell CP, Reyes RA, Cho K, Sawai ET, Fang AL, Schmidt KA, et al. SIV/HIV Nef recombinant virus (SHIVnef) produces simian AIDS in rhesus macaques. Virology 1999;265:235−51.

[177] Kaur A, Grant RM, Means RE, McClue H, Feinberg M, Johnson RP. Diverse host responses and outcomes following SIVmac239 infection in sooty mangabeys and rhesus macaques. J Virol 1998;72:9597−611.

[178] Silvestri G, Fedanov A, Germon S, Kozyr N, Kaiser WJ, Garber DA, et al. Divergent host responses during primary simian immunodeficiency virus SIVsm infection of natural sooty mangabey and nonnatural rhesus macaque hosts. J Virol 2005;79:4043−54.

[179] Bell I, Schaefer TM, Trible RP, Amedee A, Reinhart TA. Down-modulation of the costimulatory molecule, CD28, is a conserved activity of multiple SIV Nefs and is dependent on histidine 196 of Nef. Virology 2001;283:148−58.

[180] Swigut T, Shohdy N, Skowronski J. Mechanism for downregulation of CD28 by Nef. EMBO J 2001;20:1593−604.

[181] Hrecka K, Swigut T, Schindler M, Kirchhoff F, Skowronski J. Nef proteins from diverse groups of primate lentiviruses downmodulate CXCR4 to inhibit migration to SDF-1 chemokine. J Virol 2005;79:10650−9.

[182] Scarlatti G, Tresoldi E, Bjorndal A, Fredriksson R, Colognesi C, Allikmets R, et al. In vivo evolution of HIV-1 co-receptor usage and sensitivity to chemokine-mediated suppression. Nat Med 1997;3:1259−65.

[183] Dean M, Carrington M, Winkler C, Huttley GA, Smith MW, Allikmets R, et al. Genetic restriction of HIV-1 infection and progression to AIDS by a deletion allele of the CCR5 structural gene. Science 1996;273:1856−62.

[184] Liu R, Paxton WA, Choe S, Ceradini D, Martin SR, Horuk R, et al. Homozygous defect in HIV-1 coreceptor accounts for resistance of some multiply-exposed individuals to HIV-1 infection. Cell 1996;86:367−77.

[185] Samson M, Libert F, Doranz BJ, Rucker J, Liesnard C, Farber CM, et al. Resistance to HIV-1 infection in caucasian individuals bearing mutant alleles of the CCR-5 chemokine receptor gene. Nature 1996;382:722−5.

[186] Hütter G, Nowak D, Mossner M, Ganepola S, Müssig A, Allers K, et al. Long-term control of HIV by CCR5 delta32/delta32 stem-cell transplantation. N Engl J Med 2009;360:692−8.

[187] Emmelkamp JM, Rockstroh JK. Maraviroc, risks and benefits: A review of the clinical literature. Expert Opin Drug Saf 2008;7:559−69.

[188] Rucker J, Edinger AL, Sharron M, Samson M, Lee B, Berson JF, et al. Utilization of chemokine receptors, orphan receptors, and herpesvirus-encoded receptors by diverse human and simian immunodeficiency viruses. J Virol 1997;71:8999−9007.

[189] Deng HK, Unutmaz D, KewalRamani VN, Littman DR. Expression cloning of new receptors used by simian and human immunodeficiency viruses. Nature 1997;388:296−300.

[190] Pohlmann S, Stolte N, Münch J, Ten Haaft P, Heeney JL, Stahl-Hennig C, et al. Co-receptor usage of BOB/GPR15 in addition to CCR5 has no significant effect on replication of simian immunodeficiency virus in vivo. J Infect Dis 1999;180:1494−502.

[191] Chen Z, Kwon D, Jin Z, Monard S, Telfer P, Jones MS, et al. Natural infection of a homozygous delta24 CCR5 red-capped mangabey with an R2b-tropic simian immunodeficiency virus. J Exp Med 1998;188:2057−65.

[192] Riddick NE, Hermann EA, Loftin LM, Elliott ST, Wey WC, Cervasi B, et al. A novel CCR5 mutation common in sooty mangabeys reveals SIVsmm infection of CCR5-null natural hosts and efficient alternative coreceptor use in vivo. PLoS Patho 2010;6. pii: e1001064.

[193] Mörner A, Björndal A, Albert J, Kewalramani VN, Littman DR, Inoue R, et al. Primary human immunodeficiency virus type 2 (HIV-2) isolates, like HIV-1 isolates, frequently use CCR5 but show promiscuity in coreceptor usage. J Virol 1999;73:2343−9.

[194] Gnanadurai CW, Pandrea I, Parrish NF, Kraus MH, Learn GH, Salazar MG, et al. Genetic identity and biological phenotype of a transmitted/founder virus representative of

nonpathogenic simian immunodeficiency virus infection in African green monkeys. J Virol 2010;84:12245−54.

[195] Kirchhoff F, Pöhlmann S, Hamacher M, Means RE, Kraus T, Überla K, et al. Simian immunodeficiency virus variants with differential T-cell and macrophage tropism use CCR5 and an unidentified cofactor expressed in CEMx174 cells for efficient entry. J Virol 1997;71:6509−16.

[196] Cheng-Mayer C, Tasca S, Ho SH. Coreceptor switch in infection of nonhuman primates. Curr HIV Res 2009;7:30−8.

[197] Grivel JC, Margolis LB. CCR5- and CXCR4-tropic HIV-1 are equally cytopathic for their T-cell targets in human lymphoid tissue. Nat Med 1999;5:344−6.

[198] Milush JM, Reeves JD, Gordon SN, Zhou D, Muthukumar A, Kosub DA, et al. Virally induced CD4+ T cell depletion is not sufficient to induce AIDS in a natural host. J Immunol 2007;179:3047−56.

[199] Milush JM, Mir KD, Sundaravaradan V, Gordon SN, Engram J, Cano CA, et al. Lack of clinical AIDS in SIV-infected sooty mangabeys with significant CD4+ T cell loss is associated with double-negative T cells. J Clin Invest 2011;121:1102−10.

[200] Nishimura Y, Brown CR, Mattapallil JJ, Igarashi T, Buckler-White A, Lafont BA, et al. Resting naive CD4+ T cells are massively infected and eliminated by X4-tropic simian-human immunodeficiency viruses in macaques. Proc Natl Acad Sci USA 2005;102:8000−5.

[201] Harouse JM, Gettie A, Tan RC, Blanchard J, Cheng-Mayer C. Distinct pathogenic sequela in rhesus macaques infected with CCR5 or CXCR4 utilizing SHIVs. Science 1999;284:816−9.

[202] Hrecka K, Hao C, Gierszewska M, Swanson SK, Kesik-Brodacka M, Srivastava S, et al. Vpx relieves inhibition of HIV-1 infection of macrophages mediated by the SAMHD1 protein. Nature 2011;474:658−61.

[203] Laguette N, Sobhian B, Casartelli N, Ringeard M, Chable-Bessia C, Ségéral E, et al. SAMHD1 is the dendritic- and myeloid-cell-specific HIV-1 restriction factor counteracted by Vpx. Nature 2011;474:654−7.

[204] Li N, Zhang W, Cao X. Identification of a human homologue of mouse IFN-gamma induced protein from human dendritic cells. Immunol Lett 2000;74:221−4.

[205] Rice GI, Bond J, Asipu A, Brunette RL, Manfield IW, Carr IM, et al. Mutations involved in Aicardi-Goutières syndrome implicate SAMHD1 as regulator of the innate immune response. Nat Genet 2009;41:829−32.

[206] Manel N, Hogstad B, Wang Y, Levy DE, Unutmaz D, Littman DR. A cryptic sensor for HIV-1 activates antiviral innate immunity in dendritic cells. Nature 2010;467:214−7.

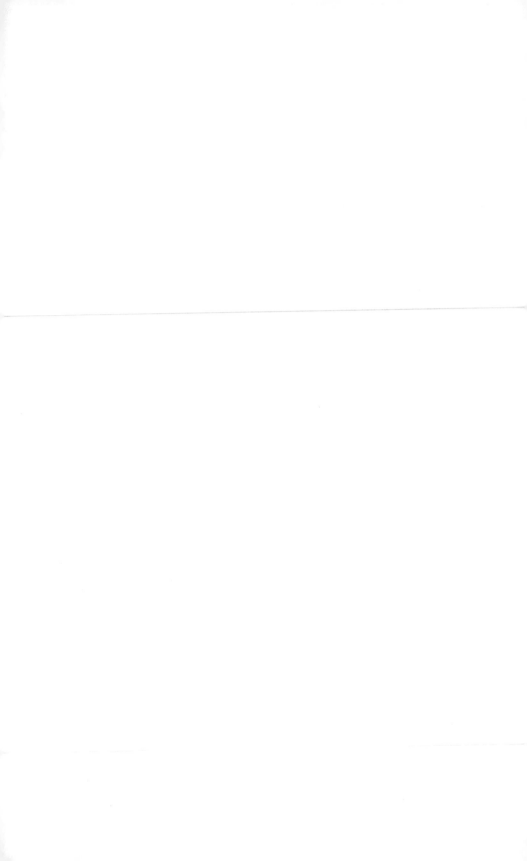

Chapter 2

Natural SIV Infection: Immunological Aspects

Béatrice Jacquelin [1], Roland C. Zahn [2], Françoise Barré-Sinoussi [1], Jörn E. Schmitz [2], Amitinder Kaur [3] and Michaela C. Müller-Trutwin [1]

[1] *Institut Pasteur, Unité Régulation des Infections Rétrovirales, Paris, France,* [2] *Division of Viral Pathogenesis, Beth Israel Deaconess Medical Center, Harvard Medical School, Boston, Massachusetts, USA,* [3] *Division of Immunology, New England Primate Research Center, Southborough, Massachusetts, USA*

Chapter Outline

SIV NATURAL HOSTS

African non-human primates (NHPs) represent the only reservoir of simian immunodeficiency viruses (SIV) in the wild. These lentiviruses are the ancestors of the human immunodeficiency viruses (HIV-1 and HIV-2) [1–3]. Currently, serological evidence of SIV infection has been shown for more than

40 of the 69 different primate species found in Africa, and SIV infection has been confirmed by sequence analysis in the majority of them [4–6]. The first species identified as natural carriers of SIVs were sooty mangabeys (SMs), African green monkeys (AGMs), mandrills and chimpanzees. In most cases, the SIV-infected primate species represents the natural reservoir for a particular SIV virus strain, and the strains are designated as such (e.g., SIV of AGMs, or SIVagm; SIV of SMs, or SIVsmm).

For three of the African NHPs, SMs, AGMs and mandrills, it has been demonstrated that the SIV infection is non-pathogenic. In chimpanzees, it has been shown in field studies that SIV infection can reduce life expectancy [7]. For a few other species, such as l'Hoest monkeys, SIV infection seems to be harmless, but too few animals have been followed to make a definitive scientific statement as to the pathogenicity of the SIV infection in the other species. Only rare cases of AIDS have been described in African monkeys, all of which occurred in captive animals [8–10]. In this chapter we will mainly focus on SIV infection in AGMs and SMs, which have been studied the most with respect to correlates of protection against AIDS.

SEROPREVALENCE OF SIV IN NATURAL HOSTS AND MODES OF TRANSMISSION

Natural transmission of SIV in African NHPs is predominantly horizontal, and thought to occur through sexual contacts or bite wounds. Vertical transmission is extremely rare [11]. SIV seropositivity is indeed virtually absent in very young animals [12–15]. In humans, HIV is spread from mother to child during pregnancy, at delivery or through breastfeeding [16]. Macaque models have been developed to examine the different routes of transmission. They can be infected by the mucosal routes, including the oral route, but very high doses or multiple exposures of SIV are required. Today it is well-accepted that mucosal tissues play a major role in pathogenesis of the infection, but this observation is true regardless of the route of transmission [16]. Until today, natural hosts have mostly been experimentally infected by the intravenous route. Experimental infection of natural hosts has recapitulated the virological and immunological characteristics of the chronic phase of naturally acquired SIV infection. The route of transmission does not seem to influence disease progression in non-natural hosts either. However, the intravenous route may lead to a more rapid transport of the virus to lymph nodes (LNs), and thus the very early events might show a more rapid kinetic.

The average SIV seroprevalence of AGMs, SMs and mandrills in the wild has been reported to be 40–50 percent. The natural habitat of SMs (*Cercocebus atys*) coincides with the geographical region where HIV-2 is prevalent in West Africa (Figure 2.1). Mandrills (*Mandrillus sphinx*) are endemic in Gabon, central Africa (Figure 2.1), and are as of today the only NHP species known to be the reservoir of two types of SIV: SIVmnd-1 and SIVmnd-2 [17]. AGMs are

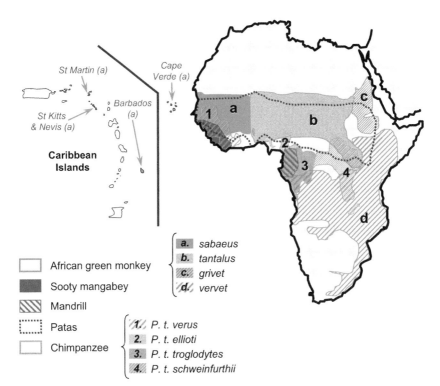

FIGURE 2.1 **Geographic distribution of African NHP species and subspecies infected with SIV.**
Modified from Beer et al. (1999) [179], Lernould (1988) [180] and Sharp and Hahn (2010) [181].

the most geographically dispersed NHPs throughout sub-Saharan Africa, and
are divided into four species, namely vervet (*Chlorocebus pygerythrus*), grivet
(*Chlorocebus aethiops*), sabaeus (*Chlorocebus sabaeus*) and tantalus (*Chlorocebus tantalus*), each of them harboring its own SIVagm subtype [18] (see
Figure 2.1 for their geographic distribution). Three hundred years ago, AGMs
that belonged to the sabaeus subspecies were transferred during slave trade
from West Africa to the Caribbean islands. In contrast to their African relatives,
in which SIV prevalence is up to 80 percent in the adult population, Caribbean
AGMs are negative for SIV [19]. Since there is apparently no vertical transmission of SIVagm in naturally infected AGMs or SMs [11,20], a possible
explanation could be that the founder AGMs were all infants.

Of the four chimpanzee subspecies in Africa, only *Pan troglodytes troglodytes* and *Pan troglodytes schweinfurthii* in Central/West Africa (Figure 2.1) have
been shown to harbor SIVcpz [2], with a prevalence ranging from 4 to 48 percent.
The two West African chimpanzee subspecies, *Pan troglodytes ellioti* and *Pan
troglodytes verus* (Figure 2.1), are free from SIVcpz infection in the wild [2,21].
The reasons for this difference in the distribution of SIVcpz between chimpanzee

subspecies remain unclear, but might be explained by a lack of migration, extinction of infected communities, resistance to SIVcpz infection in *Pan troglodytes ellioti* and *Pan troglodytes verus*, or a combination of these factors [22,23]. In line with this, a glycosylation site polymorphism in the chimpanzee CD4 receptor has recently been identified and seems to be more frequent in West African chimpanzees. This mutation might protect these chimpanzees from naturally acquiring SIVcpz [24]. However, West African chimpanzees have been shown to be susceptible to infection by SIVcpz in captivity [25].

OUTCOME OF SIV INFECTION IN HETEROLOGOUS SPECIES

As explained above, natural hosts such as AGMs, SMs and mandrills are resistant to AIDS pathogenesis following SIV infection. This is also true for AGMs from Caribbean islands [19]. Sometimes, African NHPs experience incidental infections after exposure to SIV in the wild by a NHP who is a member of a different primate species [26–28]—for instance, SIVagm infection of patas monkeys (*Erythrocebus patas*) has been observed [26,29]. Patas monkeys have never been reported as carrying species-specific SIV. Nevertheless, experimental exposure to SIVagm results in an infection pattern similar to that of AGMs [29,30]. Similarly, baboons have not been reported as carriers of a species-specific SIV, but sporadic non-pathogenic SIVagm infections of yellow baboons and chacma baboons have been reported [27,28]. Baboons are also susceptible to HIV-2 infection and, in this case, succumb to AIDS [31].

Epidemiological studies have shown that Asian and New World NHPs are not infected with SIV in their natural habitat. Cross-species transmission of SIV from African to Asian primates can lead to a pathogenic infection. For instance, SIVmac that is derived from SIVsmm induces AIDS in rhesus macaques (RMs) (*Macaca mulatta*), cynomolgus macaques (*Macaca fascicularis*) and pigtailed macaques (*Macaca nemestrina*). They are therefore NHP species widely used in research as pathogenic models of SIV infection. Additionally, macaques show distinct susceptibility to SIV infection and AIDS depending on the species and geographic origin [32]. For instance, SIVagm infection of RMs does not result in AIDS, whereas pigtailed macaques infected with SIVagm, SIV l'hoest or SIVsun can succumb to AIDS [33,34]. Of note, only infection with particular strains of SIVagm, such as SIVagm.ver90, SIVagm.sab92018, but not SIVagm.ver155, is pathogenic in pigtailed macaques [35,36]. This illustrates that the outcome of SIV infection is determined by an interplay of both host and virus determinants. Some of the 11 described SIV strains from SMs show a better fitness in terms of transmission to and replication in the new hosts after cross-species transmission [37,38]. Higher fitness in the new species can be obtained by serial passage of the virus in the new host. This drastically shortens the time of chronic infection until onset of disease progression. SIVsmm viruses adapted to these Asian hosts are called SIVmac [39,40]. It is known that different SIVsmm strains can show intrinsic differences in pathogenicity [37,41].

NATURAL HISTORY OF SIV INFECTION IN NATURAL HOSTS

The term "natural host" used hereafter will refer to the most studied species—i.e., AGM, SM and mandrill—in which infection with their species-specific SIV is non-pathogenic. The natural history of SIV infection in natural hosts is divided into three stages: the acquisition of SIV infection, the primary phase, and the chronic asymptomatic phase. In HIV-infected humans, these three phases are also observed. The duration of the chronic asymptomatic phase varies according to individuals (median duration: 7−10 years in untreated humans and 6 months to 3 years in macaques). The chronic phase in HIV-infected humans and SIVmac-infected macaques is followed by the final stage that corresponds to the clinical phase of AIDS which typically leads to premature death of the infected individual if not treated.

The primary infection in experimentally infected natural hosts corresponds to the time before seroconversion occurs. A similar timeframe is observed in SIVmac-infected macaques. Anti-SIV antibodies are detectable by 2 weeks in SIVmac-infected RMs, and seroconversion is completed by 1 month post-infection [42−44]. This phase can only be studied after an experimental infection. The analysis of the early dynamics of the virus in peripheral blood typically shows massive viral replication, with a peak of viremia occurring 1−2 weeks post-infection. Plasma RNA copy numbers reach between 10^4 and 10^9/ml at the peak. The peak of viremia coincides with a CD4+ T cell depletion in blood [42,45,46] (Figure 2.2). After the peak, there is a sharp decline of RNA viral copy numbers, by 1−3 log, to variable set-point levels [42]. In natural hosts the viremia levels during the chronic phase remain stable, and are similar in AGMs, SMs, mandrills and chimpanzees [43,47−50]. Concomitantly to the CD4+ T cell depletion, there is an increase in the percentage of activated T cells. However, after the third week of infection the activation levels decrease again to baseline and remain normal [51] (Figure 2.2). By the end of primary infection, blood CD4+ T cell levels also return towards baseline levels.

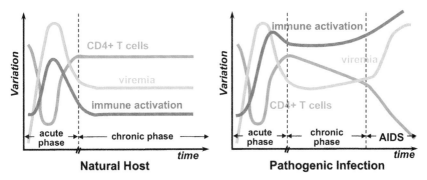

FIGURE 2.2 **Variation of viremia**, CD4+ T cells and immune activation in blood during the course of non-pathogenic SIV infections of natural hosts and pathogenic HIV/SIV infections.

There is no evidence of lymphadenopathy, fever or other any clinical signs of a viral infection during this time.

Throughout the remaining period of SIV infection, the peripheral blood CD4+ T cell counts remain stable in African natural hosts, and there is a paucity of a chronic T cell activation [43,51,52] (Figure 2.2 and Table 2.1).

TABLE 2.1   Similarities and differences between pathogenic HIV/SIVmac infections and SIV infections in natural hosts*

		Pathogenic infections		Natural hosts	
		Acute phase	Chronic phase	Acute phase	Chronic phase
Virus mutation rate *in vivo*		+	+	+	+
Viral load	*Blood*	+	+	+	+
	LN	+	+	+	+/−
	Gut	+	+	+	+
Virus cytopathicity		+	+	+	+
SIV-susceptibility of central memory CD4+ T cell		+	+	nd	−
T cell activation	*Blood*	+	+	+	−
	LN	+	+	+/−	−
	Gut	+	+	+	−
CD4+ T cell apoptosis		+	+	−	−
Pro-inflammatory profiles	IFN-α	+	+	+	nd
	IFN-γ, IL-1β, IL-8, IL-18, MIP-1α, MIP-1β, MIP-3α, TNF-α, Rantes	+	+	+	−
Anti-inflammatory profiles	IL-10, TGF-β	+	+	+	−
ISG expression levels	*Blood*	+	+	+	−
	LN	+	+	+	−
	Gut	+	+	+	−
Microbial translocation		+	+	−	−

* Parameters are presented as qualitative: +, increase as compared to the baseline before infection; −, no major change; nd, not determined.

Thus, natural hosts for SIV generally do not show any signs of chronic T cell activation despite chronically sustained levels of viral replication [53].

HOST CELL TARGETS AND VIRAL LOAD

Cell Targets

In both natural hosts and pathogenic HIV/SIV infections, the main cell type supporting virus replication appears to be a population of short-lived, activated CD4+ T cells [49,53−55]. Of note, CD4+ T cell counts in peripheral blood of uninfected AGMs vary to a great extent according to age and individual. Indeed, the CD4+ T cell count decreases with age. Young AGMs (1.4−3.5 years old) display between 800 and 2,900 CD4+ T cells/µl (with a median of 1,400 CD4+ T cells/µl). CD4+ T cell counts decrease by about 50 cells per year both in healthy and in SIV-infected AGMs. Similar observations have been made in healthy SMs [56]. Some adult AGMs have only 100 or less CD4+ T cells/µl in peripheral blood, a lymphocyte count associated with opportunistic infections and AIDS in humans while AGMs stay healthy [53,57].

The SIVs, like HIV, use CD4 as a major receptor. The coreceptors have been defined as principally being CCR5, Bonzo and Bob, and, more rarely, CXCR4 [53,58−60]. Lower frequencies of CCR5+ CD4+ T cells have been observed in SMs, AGMs, mandrills, sun-tailed monkeys and chimpanzees [54,60,61]. SIVsmm and SIVagm, which use CCR5 as a coreceptor, still induce high viremia in the context of these low levels. Thus, either the levels of CCR5+ expressing cells may still be sufficient to allow infection, or the SIVs use additional coreceptors in vivo. Indeed, a recent report showed that SMs lacking a functional CCR5 still had robust plasma viral loads [60]. Thus, even though the level of CCR5+ CD4+ T cells is a major difference between natural hosts and macaques/humans, it does not appear to impact viral load levels.

A brief leukopenia is observed following primary SIV infection of natural hosts which affects a large number of cell subsets, including CD4+ T cells. Experiments on in vivo CD4+ cell depletion in SMs led to a transient decrease of the viremia and showed that the number of activated CD4+ T cells is the main determinant of viremia in SIV-infected SMs [62]. Concomitant with the early leukopenia around the peak of viremia (Figure 2.2), a transient decrease in CD4+ T cell frequency has also been occasionally observed in the LNs of AGMs and mandrills [43,51]. Even though SIV infection has a measurable impact on CD4+ T cell counts in acute infection, SIV-infected natural hosts tend to maintain close to normal levels of peripheral blood CD4+ T cell counts in chronic infection. SIV-infected SMs and AGMs also experience an early dramatic depletion of mucosal CD4+ T cells. This is particularly true for memory CD4+ T cell subsets that are the primary target cells for HIV/SIV infection in the gut [63,64]. Partial restoration of CD4+ T cells is observed after 1 year post-infection in AGMs

(35 to 75 percent of the pre-infection values), and in SMs this recovery was complete following suppressive antiretroviral therapy [32,65].

An extreme CD4+ T cell depletion is sometimes observed in SMs infected with dual-tropic SIV. SIV infection in SMs is indeed, in rare cases, associated with a decline in CD4+ T cells in the chronic phase [66,67]. It has recently been shown in these animals that a population of double-negative T cells partially compensates for CD4+ T cell function [68]. Indeed, recent observations have suggested that the CD4 molecule becomes downregulated in AGM CD4+ T cells as these cells are activated [69,70]. The functional properties usually associated with memory CD4+ T cells are then assumed by these CD4-negative T cells. However, the exact molecular pathways regarding how this is accomplished are still unknown.

An increase in activated CD8+ T cells, and to a lesser extent CD4+ T cells, is observed in the peripheral blood of natural hosts during primary SIV infection [32,51,65,71]. After the acute infection, these levels return to normal. SIVmac-infected RMs show higher T cell activation levels during the primary phase, and these remain above normal levels during the chronic phase of SIV infection. RMs with rapid disease progression have much more subdued T cell function, and relatively low levels of Ki-67 expression may be observed. Rapidly progressing RMs can demonstrate the contra-intuitive finding that CD4+ T cell numbers in peripheral blood may eventually reach levels seen prior to infection. However, flow cytometry phenotyping has revealed a drastically changed ratio of memory to naive CD4+ T cells (most of the cells are of naive phenotype), possibly indicating a complete inability to refill the memory pool and a pathologic redistribution of CD4+ T cells from tissues to peripheral blood [72,73].

Careful flow-cytometry investigations have shown that the low frequencies of CCR5+ CD4+ T cells are not characteristic for the total CD4+ T cell population. In fact, their reduced level is rather due to a change in the relative distribution of memory-associated CD4+ T cell subsets. While naive CD4+ T cells and central memory CD4+ T cells basically do not express CCR5 in humans and NHPs, this molecule is found on transitional and effector memory CD4+ T cells. However, these two latter CD4+ T cell subsets are either significantly reduced in numbers (transitional CD4+ T cells) or completely absent in AGMs (effector memory CD4+ T cells) (R.C. Zahn *et al.*, unpublished observation). As these subsets are reduced or completely absent from AGMs, the number of CCR5+ CD4+ T cells is also significantly reduced. Nevertheless, a reduction of CCR5+ target cells certainly appears to be a beneficial trait that natural hosts must have acquired during their fight to cope with SIV infection. Interestingly, this observation is not true for CD8+ T cells; all memory-associated T cell subsets are present in AGMs, which correlates with the observation that there is no reduction of CCR5+ CD8+ T cells.

Although the bulk of viral replication *in vivo* is supported by CD4+ T cells, SIVs have also the potential to infect macrophages in the lung [74]. Some SIVs, such as SIVagm.gri, replicate well in macrophages. Moreover, SIVagm strains isolated from the brain of infected AGMs are macrophage-tropic, while those isolated from the LNs of the same animals were more restricted to T cells [49]. However, no SIV-infected macrophages are detectable in the gut [32].

The susceptibility of dendritic cells (DCs) to SIV infection in natural hosts is not known, but it has been shown that these cells have the ability to efficiently attach and transmit the virus through DC-SIGN [75].

Viral Load

Studies in AGMs have shown that SIVagm acquires mutations *in vivo* as rapidly as RMs (Table 2.1). Thus, it has the same potential capacity to escape the immune responses as HIV and SIVmac. The high mutation rate of SIVagm was the first indirect demonstration of an uncontrolled replication *in vivo* [29]. Similar to HIV-1/SIV-infected humans and macaques, naturally or experimentally infected natural hosts indeed show high viremia levels with plasmatic viral RNA levels persisting at levels similar to or higher than those associated with pathogenic progression (Figure 2.2) [53].

The mucosal immune system plays a central role in both transmission of HIV infection and AIDS pathogenesis. Seventy percent of CD4+ T cells are located in the gut, the majority of which have an activated or memory phenotype. In line with this, the major site of HIV-1/SIVmac replication is the gut. Similar to SIVmac, SIVagm also replicates at high levels in the gut, both in the acute and the chronic phases of infection [76]. The infected cells are localized in the lamina propria and Peyer's patches [32,74]. Moreover, the distribution of the virus in other tissues (e.g., thymus, cerebrospinal fluid, lung, etc.) is similar to HIV-1/SIVmac [49,74,76].

While the number of productively infected cells in LNs during acute SIVagm and SIVsmm infections is similar to that in SIVmac infection, this number is very low during the chronic phase, with a slightly higher viral load in SMs than AGMs [36,47,77–81]. The proviral load in AGMs LNs is also very low during the chronic phase as compared to blood and gut [42,49,77]. This contrasts with humans infected with HIV-1 and macaques infected with SIVmac, which both show a 5- to 10-times more extensive proviral burden in the LNs than in blood cells [82]. The mechanism of lower viral load in LN of natural hosts is not known, but is likely to be multifactorial. This might be correlated to the fact that AGMs have fewer activated T cells in LNs than macaques during acute infection [50]. A recent study demonstrated that central memory CD4+ T cells of SMs are less susceptible to SIV infection compared to RMs [83]. Since memory CD4+ T cells in the LN are predominantly of the central memory phenotype, this might in part be an additional explanation for the lower viral load in LNs. The reasons for this higher resistance of central memory T cells to SIV infection in natural hosts are unknown so far. Lower viral load in LN may also be related to a more rapid immune clearance of virus from lymphoid tissue in natural hosts [81].

IMMUNE RESPONSES

Inflammation

In contrast to HIV-infected humans and SIV-infected macaques, natural hosts of SIV do not show evidence of chronic immune activation despite the presence of ongoing viral replication and high levels of viremia (Figure 2.2 and Table 2.1). In humans and macaques, chronic immune activation is considered today as the driving force of CD4+ T cell dysfunction and depletion leading to AIDS [84–86]. This generalized immune activation state is reflected in high levels of T cell activation. Even patients with undetectable viremia (HAART-treated patients and HIV controllers) still show higher T cell activation levels as compared to healthy controls [87,88]. The degree of T cell activation around seroconversion is predictive of the risk of progression towards AIDS [84,89]. The absence of aberrant immune activation during chronic SIV infection in natural hosts is manifested by normal lymphocyte turnover and an absence of lymphoid tissue immunopathology. LNs show a normal architecture, no lymphadenopathy, and thus no increased trafficking or sequestration of lymphocytes. They display no major follicular hyperplasia, no infiltration of CD8+ T cells into germinal centers, no virus trapping on follicular dendritic cells and less upregulation of gene expressions in LNs as compared to blood and gut [47,53,66,74,77,90–95].

The absence of chronic immune activation has major implications, and is likely the single most important factor contributing to the lack of disease progression in natural hosts. The mechanisms by which natural hosts avoid immunopathology despite persistent SIV replication remain largely unknown. Unlike chronic persistent viral infection such as LCMV where immunopathology is associated with an intact cellular immune response, this is not the case in SIV-infected SMs. In both chronic and acute SIV infections, SMs mount a cellular immune response that is comparable in magnitude to that mounted by SIV-infected RMs (Table 2.2) [71,81,96].

In order to understand how the immune activation is controlled in natural hosts, the study of the innate immune response is necessary. The study of early events following experimental SIV infection of SMs and AGMs has conclusively shown that the absence of chronic immune activation is a result of active down-modulation of inflammation rather than the failure to respond to SIV infection.

Indeed, natural hosts mount an innate immune response post-SIV infection manifested by the rapid and robust upregulation of type I interferon-stimulated genes (ISG) and an increase in some pro-inflammatory cytokines and chemokines, such as IP-10 (Table 2.1). IL-2, IL-6, IFN-γ and MCP-1 have been shown to increase similarly in SMs and RMs during the first 2 weeks following SIV infection [71]. AGMs did not show an increase in some of the pro-inflammatory cytokines, such as TNF-α and IL-6, while IFN-γ was induced transiently as compared to RMs [51,90]. In RMs, the sustained and non-specific

TABLE 2.2 Antiviral host responses

		AGM	SM	Macaque
Innate immunity	ADCC/NK	nd	nd	+
	PDC IFN-α	+	+	+
SIV-specific CD4 T cells		+/−	+	+
SIV-specific CD8 T cells		+	+	+
Anti-SIV IgG		+	+	+
Anti-Env antibodies		+	+	+
Anti-p27 antibodies		(−)	(−)	+

IFN-γ production might drive inflammation [97]. Only a weak increase of IL-8 and IL-18 has been observed in AGMs in comparison to RMs [98]. IL-8 was also not detected in SMs. Beta-chemokines can be increased to the same extent as in pathogenic SIV infection (Table 2.1); however, this production is only transient. There is no persistent increase of pro-inflammatory cytokines during the chronic phase in natural hosts [35,51,71,90,92,93,98−101].

After the robust acute immune activation there is an active early down-modulation of immune activation in natural hosts which is lacking in pathogenic SIV infection. Thus, the transcriptional profile in the chronic phase of infection differed significantly between natural hosts and macaques. In RMs, chronic infection is characterized not only by persistent expression of ISGs, but also by increased expression of markers associated with cell activation and proliferation (e.g., Ki-67, CD38, chemokines, cell-cycling genes) and CD8+ T cell exhaustion (e.g., lymphocyte-activation gene 3 [LAG3], T cell immunoglobulin mucin 3 [TIM3]) [90,92,102]. The processes inducing this down-modulation are currently a major field of investigation.

Another distinguishing feature of non-progressive SIV infection is the absence of microbial translocation [32,103]. Elevated plasma LPS levels are absent in both chronically SIVsmm-infected SMs and SIVagm-infected AGMs. T helper 17 cells (Th17) and the balance between Th17 and Tregs are preserved, maintaining mucosal integrity [35,104]. Thus, the preservation of the epithelial barrier and the lack of microbial translocation very likely contribute to the maintenance of a non-inflammatory environment and to the absence of chronic immune activation in natural hosts.

The overall picture appears to be that natural hosts mount an early and robust immune response which may be more effective than pathogenic hosts in clearing virus from secondary lymphoid tissue and avoiding LN damage [81].

Then there is an active dampening of inflammation. During the chronic phase, immune functions are intact and mucosal integrity is maintained. Moreover, there is no aberrant inflammation and no hyperactivation in response to chronic virus replication.

Dendritic Cells

The study of DCs is important to understand the regulation of immune activation. DCs play a pivotal role in linking innate and adaptive immune responses. They are the only cells capable of activating naive T cells. They recognize viruses or microbial components through TLRs or other pattern recognition receptors (PRR). In response to stimuli, they migrate to secondary lymphoid organs [105] and interact with NK cells, monocytes, T cells and B cells to orchestrate the early immune response [106–110]. There are two major subsets of DC in the blood: myeloid DCs (MDCs) and plasmacytoid DCs (PDCs). *In vivo*, both in SIV-infected natural hosts and in pathogenic HIV/SIVmac infections, PDCs are the first cells mobilized (increasing in blood during the first week). They are among the first cells to recognize the virus. It has been shown in SIVmac-infected RMs that PDCs are recruited to the infection site within 2 hours in response to MIP-3α production. They contribute to inflammation by secreting interferon-alpha (IFN-α) and other cytokines. They also migrate to inflamed tissues, such as the gut, during SIV infection [111]. PDCs and MDCs then decline in blood during the acute phase. Afterwards, their frequency in blood returns to baseline levels in natural hosts while it continues to decline in pathogenic infections with disease progression [112,113]. These cells seem to be transiently recruited to inflamed LNs in natural hosts [99], while in macaques they seem to be constantly recruited concomitantly to an increase of their susceptibility to apoptosis [114–116]. In rapid progressors there is a decrease of PDCs in LNs, probably due to their massive apoptosis [107,117,118].

MDCs are essential innate immune system cells that are characterized by their ability to secrete large amounts of IL-12 and other cytokines such as IL-15. IL-12 allows the induction of T helper 1 (Th1) cells, which subsequently activate the cytotoxic T lymphocyte (CTL) responses to clear virus-infected cells [119]. IL-12 and IL-15 activate NK cells. In SIVmac infection, it seems that there is a chronic recruitment, activation and death of MDCs within LNs [118]. Little is known about the role of MDC in SIV-infected natural hosts. It has been shown that AGM MDCs express the same markers as human and macaque MDCs [120]. *In vitro* they are unable to undergo a complete maturation process and are therefore weak T cell stimulators, in contrast to MDCs cultured from macaques and humans [120]. Studies need to be done to explore MDC maturation profiles *in vivo*.

PDCs express TLR7 and TLR9, and are therefore able to be sensors of viral RNA and DNA. They secrete up to 1,000 times more type I interferon (IFN-α and -β) than other cells in response to viral infection [121]. Other cells also express PRRs that are capable of sensoring viruses, but HIV/SIV signals mainly through TLR7, although signaling by HIV-1 through TLR9 is not excluded [101,119,122]. It has been suggested that intra-cytoplasmic receptors are potentially able to recognize HIV, but this recognition does not generally seem to be active [123]. HIV-1-infected cells induce better IFN-α production by PDCs than cell free-virus [123]. Human PDC stimulation by HIV-1 results in the production of different cytokines, such as IL-12, TNF-α and IFN-α. MDCs do not mature upon exposure to HIV-1. Of note, TNF-α and IFN-α produced by HIV-1-stimulated PDCs are sufficient to induce bystander maturation of MDCs. SIVsmm and SIVmac signal through TLR7 and TLR9 [101]. *In vitro* stimulation experiments of natural hosts' PDCs showed controversial results, with the IFN-α production in response to TLR7 or TLR9 agonists being either similar or smaller than that observed with macaques' PDCs [98,99,101,116]. These studies used different stimuli, such as synthetic TLR ligands, viruses not related to HIV/SIV (HSV, influenza), or SIVmac. Only one study used species-specific SIVs and showed that the levels of IFN-α produced were similar between AGMs and RMs before and during chronic infection [90]. During acute infection, it has been shown in AGMs that PDCs displayed increased IFN-α production ability in response to a TLR9 ligand, HSV [99,116,117]. The PDCs' responses to TLR7 agonists or species-specific SIVs during the primary infection have not been studied in natural hosts. Further studies of these cells in natural host infection are therefore needed.

IFN-α is detected in significant levels in AGM plasma during primary infection [35,90,99]. Moreover, CD123+ IFN-α+ cells are easily detected in AGM and SM LNs during acute infection. The magnitude of plasma IFN-α and LN IFN-α mRNA seems to be lower in AGMs than in macaques [98,99]; however, only limited data are available. Plasma IFN-α concentrations correlate with ISG expression levels in acute infection. As described earlier, a rapid and strong upregulation of the expression of ISGs occurs in AGMs and SMs during the primary phase of SIV infection, which denotes the *in vivo* activity of IFN-I (Table 2.1) [90,92,93]. Interestingly, the ISG response is downregulated quickly and reaches baseline levels shortly after the end of the acute infection, highlighting that efficient regulation mechanisms are acting in natural hosts. On the contrary, this response is sustained in RMs, in which the failure to control the innate response is associated with pathogenesis. An additional difference has been observed between the innate responses in AGMs and RMs. This concerns the LNs where the control of ISG expression in AGMs, was stronger than in blood [90,91]. This is in line with previously reported major differences in LNs of AGMs as compared to RMs [53,90,91].

Thus, natural hosts mount a robust type-I IFN response to acute SIV infection, and have functional IFN-α/β-producing PDCs *in vivo* [93]. However, in contrast to pathogenic infection of RMs, SIV-infected SMs and AGMs resolve these innate immune responses before or during the transition to chronic infection.

NK Cells

Natural killer (NK) cells are an important component of the innate immune system. They have been implicated in the control of several viral infections. Compelling genetic evidence based on HLA and KIR polymorphisms has shown NK cells to be an important determinant of HIV disease progression [124]. Perturbations of NK cell phenotype and function are characteristic of chronic pathogenic HIV/SIV infection in humans and RMs, and include a decline in the cytokine-producing CD56+ CD16− subset and an increase in the cytolytic CD16+ subset of circulating NK cells [125,126]. A marked increase in activated and Ki-67-positive proliferating NK cells is seen during acute pathogenic SIV in RMs [127,128]. There are limited data on perturbations of NK cells in natural hosts (Table 2.2). A recent cross-sectional study showed that NK cell subsets based on CD16 and CD56 co-expression were similar in SMs and RMs [129]. Unlike SIV-infected RMs, SIV-infected SMs showed no decline in the frequency and function of NK cells. On the contrary, cytolytic activity of SM NK cells was increased following SIV infection, and was higher than that of SIV-negative and SIV-infected RMs [129]. Furthermore, during acute infection an increase in NK cell number is seen in both RMs and SMs; however, there are differences in the kinetics of expansion [129]. Thus, SMs display a significantly lower increase in NK cell activation during acute infection compared to RMs [81].

In summary, NK cells have been studied in SMs. In acute infection, they are activated and seem to display an increased cytolytic activity. They might contribute to the decline of viremia at the end of the acute phase. This needs, however, to be confirmed by further studies. No decline in the number and function has been described, in contrast to pathogenic infection. However, only few markers have been studied for SM NK cells, and no studies of NK cells of other natural hosts have been performed so far. Moreover, the cross-talk between DCs and NK cells has not yet been addressed in natural hosts.

NKT Lymphocytes

Natural killer T (NKT) lymphocytes are a small subset of T lymphocytes that are rapid responders of the innate immune system and mediate potent immunoregulatory and effector functions in a variety of disease settings [130]. NKT lymphocytes recognize antigen presented by the non-polymorphic MHC class-I-like CD1d molecules, and are characterized by a restricted TCR repertoire. Classic NKT cells are characterized by an invariant TCR α-chain and restricted TCR Vβ usage. Invariant NKT cells consist of a Vα24−Jα18 chain preferentially paired with Vβ11 in humans, and a Vα14−Jα18 chain paired with Vβ8.2, Vβ7 or Vβ2 in mice. NKT cells can rapidly respond to glycolipid antigens presented by the MHC class-I-like non-polymorphic CD1d molecule, resulting in potent production of IL-10, TGF-β, and several Th1 and T helper 2 (Th2) cytokines. Although they represent a very small fraction of T lymphocytes,

NKT cells can modulate immune responses by rapid production of a wide array of cytokines, thereby influencing other innate and adaptive arms of the immune system, such as DCs, NK cells, macrophages, CD4+ and CD8+ T lymphocytes, and B lymphocytes.

The precise role of NKT lymphocytes in HIV/SIV infection remains unresolved. CD4+ NKT lymphocytes in humans and macaques express CCR5 and are highly susceptible to HIV/SIV infection *in vitro*. A selective and rapid loss of both CD4+ and CD4− NKT lymphocytes has been observed in the peripheral blood of HIV-infected humans with variable reconstitution after antiretroviral therapy [131−134]. A similar decline of CD4+ NKT lymphocytes was reported in SIVmac-infected pig-tailed macaques [135]. Although the consequences of NKT lymphocyte depletion in HIV infection are not known, it is speculated that loss of NKT lymphocytes might result in increased susceptibility to opportunistic infections, as well as contributing to increased immune activation in pathogenic HIV/SIV infection. This has raised interest in investigating NKT lymphocytes in natural hosts of SIV. Two recent reports have provided a detailed characterization of NKT lymphocytes in SMs and provided some interesting findings [136,137]. In contrast to published reports of NKT lymphocytes in Asian macaques, CD1d-restricted invariant NKT lymphocytes in SMs do not express CD4 or CCR5, thus rendering them potentially resistant to depletion by SIV infection. Consistent with this, naturally SIV-infected SMs have similar frequency and phenotype of circulating NKT lymphocytes compared to SIV-negative SMs. SM NKT lymphocytes are a heterogeneous population comprised chiefly of CD8+ and double-negative T lymphocyte subsets with a CXCR3-positive memory phenotype, and expression of NKG2D and CD161 as the prominent NK cell markers. Functionally, SM NKT lymphocytes show robust production of Th1 and Th2 cytokines, including IL-10, and undergo degranulation on NKT ligand-specific activation, indicating that they have both effector and immunoregulatory functional capabilities. The IL-10 cytokine-secreting profile of SM NKT lymphocytes along with their preservation in naturally SIV-infected SMs raises the possibility that NKT lymphocytes play an important role in downregulating immune activation during natural SIV infection.

γδ T Cells

γδ T cells are a minor group of T lymphocytes that are composed of two predominant subsets based on the differential expression of Vδ1 and Vδ2 genes. They can expand during bacterial infections. Alterations of γδ T-cell subsets have been described during progressive HIV infection and SIVmac infections of RMs [138]. Specifically, the Vδ1 subset, which is usually localized to the mucosal tissues but not the periphery, becomes prevalent in the peripheral blood relative to the Vδ2 subset [139,140]. In natural host infection, no such perturbation in γδ T-cell subsets is observed [139]. Additionally, contrary to pathogenic infection, $\gamma\delta$ T cells from SIV-infected SMs retain their ability to express Th1 cytokines. Moreover, they may play a role in the maintenance of an intact mucosal epithelium [138].

For all the innate cell subsets studied so far, a similar pattern in terms of preserved immune function in SIV-infected natural hosts was observed, contrasting with the depletion/dysfunction of these cells observed in pathogenic SIV infection. The cause and effect in relation to the absence of disease progression remain unknown. Whether this is merely a reflection of the absence of chronic immune activation and thereby a global preservation of immune functions, or whether these innate immune cells also play a role in active down-modulation of immune activation, remains to be determined.

T Cell Responses to SIV in Natural Hosts

Th Profiles in SIV-Infected Natural Hosts

The transcription factors *t-bet* and *gata3* are essential for the induction of Th1 and Th2 responses, respectively. Their expression has been quantified in AGMs in acute infection. In the peripheral blood mononuclear cells (PBMCs) of both AGMs and RMs, *gata3* expression was upregulated [141]. However, only RMs presented an upregulation of *t-bet*, whereas AGMs did not. This is in agreement with the weak induction of pro-inflammatory cytokines observed in this species. A tendency towards Th2 cells has also been reported in chronically infected SMs [94,142].

One of the major findings in RMs was the observation that IL-17-secreting (Th17) cells are lost following SIV infection. This is important, as Th17 cells might account for a breakdown in mucosal immunity and an increase in microbial translocation across the gastrointestinal mucosa [143]. Of note, Th17 cells are preserved in natural hosts [35,143].

SIV-Specific CD4+ T Cell Responses

The question arises as to whether natural hosts present a SIV-specific T cell response. In HIV-1/SIVmac infection, loss of SIV-specific CD4+ T cell responses is associated with disease progression. *In vitro* stimulation with SIVagm antigens showed that there are few SIV-specific CD4+ T cells in AGMs (Table 2.2) [144,145]. This might be due to the loss of CD4 expression on stimulated cells. SIV-specific CD4+ T cell responses are more easily detected in SIVsmm-infected SMs [96,146]. In one study on acute SIVsmm infection, the early anti-SIV response consisted of both CD4 and CD8 responses in SMs. Interestingly, the CD4 responses were equivalent to the CD8 responses [81]. In one study on the chronic phase, the CD8 anti-SIV responses in naturally SIV-infected SMs dominated over the CD4 responses [96]. This latter finding is consistent with what is seen in chronic SIVagm and SIVmac infections.

SIV-Specific CD8+ T Cell Responses

AGMs and SMs display high numbers of CD8+ T cells. In order to evaluate whether adaptive immune responses contribute to the maintenance of a disease-free course of SIV infection in natural hosts, or whether SIV infection in natural hosts would alter differentially the adaptive response, several labs have studied the breadth and magnitude of CD8+ T cell responses. In RMs, CD8+ T cell responses are quite diverse and the magnitude depends on the expression of certain MHC class I alleles that may support very strong responses (i.e., Mamu-A01, -B08, B17, and others). Due to a paucity of knowledge regarding different MHC class I alleles in AGMs, such detailed investigations have so far not been conducted in this species. However, investigations using peptide pools either in intracytoplasmic cytokine staining detected by flow cytometry or by ELISPOT assays have shown that CD8+ T cell responses are elicited following SIVagm infection [144,147].

SMs show several key similarities to the cellular immune response mounted in HIV-infected humans and SIV-infected RMs. A detailed analysis of the SIV-specific cellular immune response against the entire SIV proteome has been conducted in SMs both during chronic infection [96,146] and during acute infection [81]. In AGMs, SIV-specific CD8+ T cell responses tend to be slightly lower than in RMs, while SMs seem to have quite comparable responses when compared to pathogenic SIV-infected RMs.

An early report on experimental infection of SMs with the macaque-passaged SIVmac239 virus showed an induction of a robust SIV-specific CTL response in SMs with CTL escape [148,149]. However, SIVmac239 infection was atypical of natural infection because primary viremia was rapidly controlled to near undetectable levels [149]. More recently it was reported that in the setting of experimental infection with the primary SIVsmm isolate, SIVsmE041, which reproduced the set-point viremia levels seen in natural SIV infection, SMs mounted an acute SIV-specific cellular immune response that was comparable in magnitude to that in RMs infected with SIVmac239 or SIVsmE041 [71,81].

Kinetic analysis of the cellular immune response in the first 6 months post-SIV infection showed comparable magnitude, breadth and specificity of the SIV-specific IFN-γ ELISPOT response in SMs and RMs. However, SMs showed a higher frequency of polyfunctional Gag-specific CD8+ T lymphocytes in the first 10 weeks following SIV infection, a greater reduction in peak plasma viremia, and a more rapid disappearance of productively SIV-infected cells from the LNs compared to SIVmac239-infected RMs. These data suggest that qualitative differences in the early SIV-specific cellular immune response might contribute to faster viral load reduction and absence of chronic immunopathology in lymphoid tissues of SIV-infected SMs [81].

In RMs, the proof for a role of CD8 cells in viral containment was obtained when CD8+ lymphocytes were depleted *in vivo* by an antibody. Thus, a number of studies showed that SIV viremia was significantly increased when CD8+ lymphocyte responses were temporally inhibited [150,151]. A significant increase in plasma viremia was also observed in naturally-infected SMs following CD8+ lymphocyte depletion (A. Kaur, unpublished data). CD8+ lymphocyte depletion during primary SIV infection in RMs consistently resulted in a more rapid disease progression in this species. When a similar treatment in AGMs was performed, an increased viremia was also observed, indicating that CD8 lymphocytes participate in partial viral suppression in these animals [147,152,153]. However, while such treatment results in rapid disease progression in RMs, no signs of SIV-induced illness or death in AGMs have been seen. Therefore, these data suggest that even though CD8 responses contribute to viral suppression in natural hosts, they may not play a significant role in the non-pathogenic course of infection. However, it is also possible that the elimination of CD8+ lymphocytes needs to be performed for a much longer duration to induce disease progression. This cannot be achieved with currently available reagents.

Regulatory T Cells

Regulatory T cells (Treg) can suppress antigen-specific CD4 and CD8 responses, and also control inappropriate or exaggerated immune activation induced by pathogens [154]. In HIV/SIV infection, CD25+ FoxP3+ Treg cells have been shown to accumulate in the gut and LNs [155,156]. However, the ramifications of these observations on HIV/SIV disease progression are still unknown [157,158].

SIV-infected AGMs showed an early induction of IL-10, TGF-β, FoxP3 and PD1, raising the possibility that early induction of Treg in natural hosts rapidly dampens acute inflammation and prevents immunopathology [51,79]. A population of CD25+ FoxP3+ Treg cells has indeed been identified after infection in AGMs and SMs [35,159]. In contrast to pathogenic infections, the balance between Th17 and Treg cells is maintained. So far, there is no clear indication, though, that they play a major role in the downregulation of immune activation in natural hosts. Additional suppressive T cell populations, including Tr1 and Th3, have not been studied in natural hosts.

B Cell Responses

Leukopenia typically seen in primary infection in both non-natural hosts and natural hosts also affects B cells in peripheral blood. However, within a relatively short period of time these cells reappear in peripheral blood of AGMs. B cell areas in lymphatic tissues of HIV/SIV-infected humans and RMs undergo characteristic pathogenic changes. Germinal centers become hyper-inflated, and it may eventually become difficult to determine the physiological anatomic components as germinal centers may even fuse into each other. Relatively early in infection, HIV-1 and SIVmac virus particles can be found in large quantities on the extracellular surfaces of follicular dendritic cells, appearing as a diffuse staining in *in situ* hybridization. While most T cells in germinal centers from healthy individuals express the CD4 molecule, a huge influx of CD8+ T cells can regularly be observed following HIV-1 and SIVmac infections. As the disease progresses, follicular dendritic cells are lost and germinal centers disappear. During the initial phase of the pathogenic infection, B cells, similarly to T cells, are hyperactivated and produce a large amount of virus-specific antibodies. Subsequently, progression towards AIDS can lead to a loss of memory B cells. All of these pathogenic sequelae of AIDS virus infection on B cells in non-natural hosts are not observed in natural hosts. In fact, in AGMs there is no lymphadenopathy and thus probably no major trafficking and sequestration of lymphocytes into LNs. There is also generally no significant B cell hyperplasia. No infiltration of CD8+ T cells into germinal centers is observed [53]. For unknown reasons, the deposition of virus antigen is almost never detected on follicular dendritic cells in germinal centers of natural hosts [42,77,80].

The kinetic of seroconversion is similar in non-natural and natural hosts [42]. However, seroconversion in natural hosts is characterized by low titers of total SIV-specific antibodies and the development of neutralizing antibodies with a weak neutralizing activity. Antibodies against Env are always detected, while there is a selective paucity of an anti-P27 antibody response in most natural hosts (Table 2.2) [42,149,160,161]. The task of humoral immune responses in any virus infection is to elicit high titer neutralizing antibodies. For very complex reasons that are beyond the scope of this chapter, most antibodies generated following HIV or SIV infection in non-pathogenic hosts are directed against type-specific epitopes. Similarly, virus-specific antibody responses in non-natural hosts are tremendously inefficient. The major problem in developing effective high-affinity antibodies in pathogenic infection is in part due to the escape of the virus. Similarly, it is quite likely that this problem occurs in natural hosts too, as its virus is also undergoing rapid sequence mutations.

To obtain more direct proof for the role of humoral immune responses, CD20+ B cells have temporally been eliminated *in vivo*. These types of investigation showed in RMs that B cell responses have very little impact on primary viremia. Long-term depletion of B cells in RMs has shown that virus replication was significantly increased during chronic infection. However, B cell depletion in SIVmac251-infected RMs also affected the maintenance of memory CD8+ T cell responses. Thus, the role of humoral immune responses during chronically SIV-infected RMs could not be easily determined. In contrast to these observations in a non-natural host NHP, B cell depletion had very little effect on viremia in SIV-infected AGMs, and no signs of an AIDS-like disease were observed [152].

It is, however, possible that secondary functions, like Fc-γ receptor-mediated functions, are assisting antibodies to eliminate the virus. With regard to antibody assays, many more detailed and elaborate studies have been performed in non-natural hosts than in natural hosts.

In summary, there is clear evidence that natural hosts also mount a neutralizing antibody response [162]. However, this is not more efficient than in non-natural hosts, which is in line with the high viremia levels. Also, the reasons why they produce less anti-p27 antibody are unknown, and it is unclear whether this has any relation to the lower immune activation.

HYPOTHESES OF NON-PATHOGENICITY

In AIDS, immunodeficiency is a complex phenomenon that is initially triggered by the virus but very rapidly related to interplay with the host responses. Immune activation control is a key element in the lack of disease progression in natural hosts. This observation has contributed to the increased attention given to the role of immune activation in HIV infection. Today, chronic immune activation is considered to be the crucial factor that drives pathogenesis. Several hypotheses, which are not mutually exclusive, have been proposed to explain the lack of chronic immune activation in natural hosts [53,163–165].

The role that some of the viral factors, such as the Env and Nef proteins, might play is explained in Chapter 1 [166,167].

In natural hosts, the function of the T cell regenerative compartment (i.e., bone marrow, thymus and LNs) is preserved [94]. CD4+ T cell proliferation in bone marrow seems even to be increased in chronically infected SMs. A few SMs have shown slightly higher immune activation levels in chronic infection. This is correlated with a higher expression of CD95 on CD4+ T cells [94].

In HIV/SIV infections, increased apoptosis of both infected and uninfected CD4+ and CD8+ T cells accompanying the chronic immune activation has been observed [168]. In the 1990s, Ameisen and colleagues observed that the largest level of T cell apoptosis in peripheral blood can be found in CD8+ T cells [169,170]. This is likely due to a higher proliferation of CD8+ than CD4+ T cells to attempt to expand the AIDS virus-specific CD8+ T cell pool in an effort to combat virus-infected cells. However, many CD4+ T cells undergo apoptosis as well. Interestingly, most of them are not infected. Studies in RMs have shown that the levels of apoptosis during primary infection are predictive of the rate of disease progression to AIDS [78]. A little susceptibility to apoptosis is occasionally seen in CD8+ T cell subsets of natural hosts [71,94,170]. However, they never show an increased level of apoptosis in CD4+ T cells [71,170,171].

Several mechanisms have been suggested for the induction of apoptosis in pathogenic infection. TRAIL is a death ligand induced by type I IFN. It may stimulate apoptosis of uninfected CD4+ T lymphocytes, as it is upregulated in HIV-1/SIVmac infections [71,172]. The soluble form of TRAIL is increased in the plasma of HIV-1-infected humans or SIVmac-infected RMs during the acute phase, but not detected in acute SIV infection of natural hosts [71,173]. Moreover, the gene expression of *TRAIL* is different in the LNs of AGMs and RMs, as it was only increased in RM LN CD4+ cells [90]. Since *in vitro* IFN-α stimulated AGM PBMCs upregulate *TRAIL* expression, AGMs seem to control *TRAIL* expression *in vivo* by an as yet unknown mechanism [90]. A possible role for IL-18, which is induced by caspase-1 but not upregulated in AGMs in contrast to RMs, has also been suggested [98].

In natural hosts, it is thus probably easier to maintain homeostasis, since there is no need to compensate for a loss of non-infected CD4+ T cells dying by bystander cell death. It is unclear so far whether the lack of CD4+ T cell apoptosis is directly implicated in protection against AIDS.

Other hypotheses for non-pathogenicity involve host determinants. In natural hosts, only a low fraction of CD4+ T cells express CCR5. SM CD4+ T cells fail to upregulate CCR5, and this phenomenon is more pronounced in central memory CD4+ T cells. Importantly, central memory CD4+ T cells seem to be relatively spared from SIVsmm infection. Indeed, the ratio of infected central memory T cells *versus* effector memory T cells is inversed as compared to SIVmac infection. The preservation of central memory T cell homeostasis might be a key factor in protection against AIDS. In pathogenic SIV and HIV infections, the progressive depletion of central memory CD4+ T cells is critical to the irreversible loss of the total CD4+ T cells and the size of the latent CD4+ T cell reservoir. It will be interesting to find out the reason for this relative protection of central memory CD4+ T cells in SMs, and whether it also exists in other natural hosts.

Central memory CD4+ T cells are temporarily lost in the gut during acute infection, but then partially recover. Th17 cells are always preserved in natural hosts. This might contribute to the lack of microbial translocation and systemic immune activation [32,163].

Kinetic studies on innate and adaptive immune responses have shown that the lack of chronic immune activation is indeed not due to a lack of immune response to viral infection, but clearly to an active downregulation. It is important to decipher and understand the early phase of infection. Significant levels of type I IFN were detected during the acute phase in natural hosts, and subsequently many ISGs were concomitantly induced [90–92,99,174]. However, contrary to RMs, AGMs and SMs were able to downregulate ISG expression at the onset of chronic infection despite persistently high levels of viral replication [90–92]. Moreover, the control of ISG expression was even stronger in AGM LNs [90,91,174]. The control of immune activation might indeed be particularly crucial at the LN level, as these are the sites where the T cell responses are induced. Interestingly, some of the ISGs that were regulated differently in LNs between AGMs and RMs are directly involved in cell trafficking [90,100]. For instance, the expression of *CXCL9*, *CXCL10* and *CXCL11*, the ligands of CXCR3, was chronically upregulated only in RMs. CXCR3-ligands are responsible for the recruitment of circulating activated immune cells (dendritic cells, Th1-type T cells, etc.) to LNs and inflammatory sites [175,176]. Although essential for effective host defense against infection, the enhanced and continuous recruitment of activated cells to LNs may play a key role in the induction and/or exacerbation of chronic inflammation. In contrast, natural hosts are characterized by a lack of lymphadenopathy and the preservation of LN architecture and function, suggesting a lack of sustained immune cell trafficking to LNs [46,51,53,71,79,101,177]. This reduced trafficking in AGMs could be related to differences in receptor expression (CXCR3, CCR5, CCR7) or production of their ligands. Moreover, the lower levels of CCR5 and the fact that it is not upregulated on memory CD4+ T cells might reduce the homing of these CD4+ T cells to inflamed tissues [54,60,68,69]. Less trafficking or less infection of central memory T cells could explain the lower viral load that has been observed during chronic infection in AGM LNs.

CONCLUSION

In conclusion, the inflammatory response that is induced in acute infection might be necessary for the establishment of a persistent infection [178] and the induction of moderate antiviral immune responses, responsible for the reduction of the viremia peak to set-point levels, while its subsequent control might be essential for protection of the host against the collateral damage of chronic immune activation. Preservation of central memory T cells' homeostasis and immunoregulation at the LN level might be particularly crucial, as these are the sites where the T cell responses are induced.

Future studies are needed to further investigate, in natural hosts:

- what the virus determinants for protection against AIDS are
- to what levels antiviral immune responses are involved in protection
- why the inflammation is only transient, and what causes its downregulation
- why there is no disruption of the intestinal epithelial cell barrier
- why central memory T cells are protected against infection
- whether the lower viral load in LNs is the result of low immune activation or the opposite.

The mechanisms may be linked to each other. The answers to these questions will help to identify factors necessary for protection against AIDS.

REFERENCES

[1] Hirsch VM, Olmsted RA, Murphey-Corb M, Purcell RH, Johnson PR. An African primate lentivirus (SIVsm) closely related to HIV-2. Nature 1989;339:389−92.

[2] Keele BF, Van Heuverswyn F, Li Y, Bailes E, Takehisa J, Santiago ML, et al. Chimpanzee reservoirs of pandemic and nonpandemic HIV-1. Science 2006;313:523−6.

[3] Van Heuverswyn F, Li Y, Neel C, Bailes E, Keele BF, Liu W, et al. Human immunodeficiency viruses: SIV infection in wild gorillas. Nature 2006;444:164.

[4] Hahn BH, Shaw GM, De Cock KM, Sharp PM. AIDS as a zoonosis: Scientific and public health implications. Science 2000;287:607−14.

[5] VandeWoude S, Apetrei C. Going wild: Lessons from naturally occurring T-lymphotropic lentiviruses. Clin Microbiol Rev 2006;19:728−62.

[6] Van Heuverswyn F, Peeters M. The origins of HIV and implications for the global epidemic. Curr Infect Dis Rep 2007;9:338.

[7] Keele BF, Jones JH, Terio KA, Estes JD, Rudicell RS, Wilson ML, et al. Increased mortality and AIDS-like immunopathology in wild chimpanzees infected with SIVcpz. Nature 2009;460:515.

[8] Ling B, Apetrei C, Pandrea I, Veazey RS, Lackner AA, Gormus B, et al. Classic AIDS in a sooty mangabey after an 18-year natural infection. J Virol 2004;78:8902—8.

[9] Pandrea I, Onanga R, Rouquet P, Bourry O, Ngari P, Wickings EJ, et al. Chronic SIV infection ultimately causes immunodeficiency in African non-human primates. AIDS 2001;15:2461—2.

[10] Traina-Dorge V, Blanchard J, Martin L, Murphey-Corb M. Immunodeficiency and lymphoproliferative disease in an African green monkey dually infected with SIV and STLV-I. AIDS Res Hum Retroviruses 1992;8:97—100.

[11] Chahroudi A, Meeker T, Lawson B, Ratcliffe S, Else J, Silvestri G. Mother-to-infant transmission of simian immunodeficiency virus is rare in sooty mangabeys and is associated with low viremia. J Virol 2011;85:5757—63.

[12] Jolly C, Phillips-Conroy JE, Turner TR, Broussard S, Allan JS. SIVagm incidence over two decades in a natural population of Ethiopian grivet monkeys (*Cercopithecus aethiops aethiops*). J Med Primatol 1996;25:78—83.

[13] Müller MC, Barre-Sinoussi F. SIVagm: Genetic and biological features associated with replication. Front Biosci 2003;8:d1170.

[14] Nerrienet E, Amouretti X, Müller-Trutwin MC, Poaty-Mavoungou V, Bedjebaga I, Nguyen HT, et al. Phylogenetic analysis of SIV and STLV type I in mandrills (*Mandrillus sphinx*): Indications that intracolony transmissions are predominantly the result of male-to-male aggressive contacts. AIDS Res Hum Retroviruses 1998;14:785—96.

[15] Fultz PN, Gordon TP, Anderson DC, McClure HM. Prevalence of natural infection with simian immunodeficiency virus and simian T-cell leukemia virus type I in a breeding colony of sooty mangabey monkeys. AIDS 1990;4:619—25.

[16] Lackner AA, Veazey RS. Current concepts in AIDS pathogenesis: Insights from the SIV/macaque model. Annu Rev Med 2007;58:461.

[17] Souquiere S, Bibollet-Ruche F, Robertson DL, Makuwa M, Apetrei C, Onanga R, et al. Wild *Mandrillus sphinx* are carriers of two types of lentivirus. J Virol 2001;75:7086—96.

[18] Müller MC, Saksena NK, Nerrienet E, Chappey C, Herve VM, Durand JP, et al. Simian immunodeficiency viruses from central and western Africa: Evidence for a new species-specific lentivirus in tantalus monkeys. J Virol 1993;67:1227—35.

[19] Pandrea I, Apetrei C, Dufour J, Dillon N, Barbercheck J, Metzger M, et al. Simian immunodeficiency virus SIVagm.sab infection of Caribbean African green monkeys: A new model for the study of SIV pathogenesis in natural hosts. J Virol 2006;80:4858—67.

[20] Otsyula MG, Gettie A, Suleman M, Tarara R, Mohamed I, Marx P. Apparent lack of vertical transmission of simian immunodeficiency virus (SIV) in naturally infected African green monkeys, *Cercopithecus aethiops*. Ann Trop Med Parasitol 1995;89:573—6.

[21] Santiago ML, Rodenburg CM, Kamenya S, Bibollet-Ruche F, Gao F, Bailes E, et al. SIVcpz in wild chimpanzees. Science 2002;295:465.

[22] Sharp PM, Shaw GM, Hahn BH. Simian immunodeficiency virus infection of chimpanzees. J Virol 2005;79:3891.

[23] Rudicell RS, Holland Jones J, Wroblewski EE, Learn GH, Li Y, Robertson JD, et al. Impact of simian immunodeficiency virus infection on chimpanzee population dynamics. PLoS Pathog 2010;6:e1001116.

[24] Bibollet-Ruche F, Decker JM, Li Y, Easlick JL, Kutsch O, Keele BF, et al. A chimpanzee CD4 glycosylation site polymorphism governs susceptibility to SIVcpz infection. Whistler, British Columbia, Canada: Paper presented at the Keystone Symposia: HIV Evolution, Genomics and Pathogenesis; 2011.

[25] Corbet S, Müller-Trutwin MC, Versmisse P, Delarue S, Ayouba A, Lewis J, et al. env sequences of simian immunodeficiency viruses from chimpanzees in Cameroon are strongly related to those of human immunodeficiency virus group N from the same geographic area. J Virol 2000;74:529−34.

[26] Bibollet-Ruche F, Galat-Luong A, Cuny G, Sarni-Manchado P, Galat G, Durand JP, et al. Simian immunodeficiency virus infection in a patas monkey (*Erythrocebus patas*): evidence for cross-species transmission from African green monkeys (*Cercopithecus aethiops sabaeus*) in the wild. J Gen Virol 1996;77:773−81.

[27] Jin MJ, Rogers J, Phillips-Conroy JE, Allan JS, Desrosiers RC, Shaw GM, et al. Infection of a yellow baboon with simian immunodeficiency virus from African green monkeys: Evidence for cross-species transmission in the wild. J Virol 1994;68:8454−60.

[28] van Rensburg EJ, Engelbrecht S, Mwenda J, Laten JD, Robson BA, Stander T, et al. Simian immunodeficiency viruses (SIVs) from eastern and southern Africa: Detection of a SIVagm variant from a chacma baboon. J Gen Virol 1998;79:1809−14.

[29] Müller-Trutwin MC, Corbet S, Tavares MD, Herve VM, Nerrienet E, Georges-Courbot MC, et al. The evolutionary rate of nonpathogenic simian immunodeficiency virus (SIVagm) is in agreement with a rapid and continuous replication *in vivo*. Virology 1996;223:89−102.

[30] Apetrei C, Gaufin T, Gautam R, Vinton C, Hirsch V, Lewis M, et al. Pattern of SIVagm infection in patas monkeys suggests that host adaptation to simian immunodeficiency virus infection may result in resistance to infection and virus extinction. J Infect Dis 2010;202(Suppl. 3):S371−6.

[31] Barnett SW, Murthy KK, Herndier BG, Levy JA. An AIDS-like condition induced in baboons by HIV-2. Science 1994;266:642−6.

[32] Pandrea I, Gautam R, Ribeiro R, Brenchley JM, Butler IF, Pattison M, et al. Acute loss of intestinal CD4+ T cells is not predictive of SIV virulence. J Immunol 2007;179:3035−46.

[33] Beer BE, Brown CR, Whitted S, Goldstein S, Goeken R, Plishka R, et al. Immunodeficiency in the absence of high viral load in pig-tailed macaques infected with simian immunodeficiency virus SIVsun or SIVlhoest. J Virol 2005;79:14044−56.

[34] Hirsch VM, Dapolito G, Johnson PR, Elkins WR, London WT, Montali RJ, et al. Induction of AIDS by simian immunodeficiency virus from an African green monkey: Species-specific variation in pathogenicity correlates with the extent of *in vivo* replication. J Virol 1995;69:955−67.

[35] Favre D, Lederer S, Kanwar B, Ma ZM, Proll S, Kasakow Z, et al. Critical loss of the balance between Th17 and T regulatory cell populations in pathogenic SIV infection. PLoS Pathog 2009;5:e1000295.

[36] Goldstein S, Ourmanov I, Brown CR, Plishka R, Buckler-White A, Byrum R, et al. Plateau levels of viremia correlate with the degree of CD4+-T-cell loss in simian immunodeficiency virus SIVagm-infected pigtailed macaques: Variable pathogenicity of natural SIVagm isolates. J Virol 2005;79:5153−62.

[37] Gautam R, Carter AC, Katz N, Butler IF, Barnes M, Hasegawa A, et al. *In vitro* characterization of primary SIVsmm isolates belonging to different lineages. *In vitro* growth on rhesus macaque cells is not predictive for *in vivo* replication in rhesus macaques. Virology 2007;362:257.

[38] Apetrei C, Kaur A, Lerche NW, Metzger M, Pandrea I, Hardcastle J, et al. Molecular epidemiology of simian immunodeficiency virus SIVsm in US Primate Centers unravels the origin of SIVmac and SIVstm.J. Virol 2005;79:8991−9005.

[39] Valli PJ, Goudsmit J. Structured-tree topology and adaptive evolution of the simian immunodeficiency virus SIVsm envelope during serial passage in rhesus macaques according to likelihood mapping and quartet puzzling. J Virol 1998;72:3673.

[40] Apetrei C, Lerche NW, Pandrea I, Gormus B, Silvestri G, Kaur A, et al. Kuru experiments triggered the emergence of pathogenic SIVmac. AIDS 2006;20:317−21.

[41] Apetrei C, Gautam R, Sumpter B, Carter AC, Gaufin T, Staprans SI, et al. Virus subtype-specific features of natural simian immunodeficiency virus SIVsmm infection in sooty mangabeys. J Virol 2007;81:7913−23.

[42] Diop OM, Gueye A, Dias-Tavares M, Kornfeld C, Faye A, Ave P, et al. High levels of viral replication during primary simian immunodeficiency virus SIVagm infection are rapidly and strongly controlled in African green monkeys. J Virol 2000;74:7538−47.

[43] Onanga R, Kornfeld C, Pandrea I, Estaquier J, Souquiere S, Rouquet P, et al. High levels of viral replication contrast with only transient changes in CD4(+) and CD8(+) cell numbers during the early phase of experimental infection with simian immunodeficiency virus SIVmnd-1 in *Mandrillus sphinx*. J Virol 2002;76:10256−63.

[44] Reimann KA, Tenner-Racz K, Racz P, Montefiori DC, Yasutomi Y, Lin W, et al. Immunopathogenic events in acute infection of rhesus monkeys with simian immunodeficiency virus of macaques. J Virol 1994;68:2362−70.

[45] Pandrea I, Silvestri G, Onanga R, Veazey RS, Marx PA, Hirsch V, et al. Simian immunodeficiency viruses replication dynamics in African non-human primate hosts: Common patterns and species-specific differences. J Med Primatol 2006;35:194−201.

[46] Onanga R, Souquiere S, Makuwa M, Mouinga-Ondeme A, Simon F, Apetrei C, et al. Primary simian immunodeficiency virus SIVmnd-2 infection in mandrills (*Mandrillus sphinx*). J Virol 2006;80:3301−9.

[47] Rey-Cuille MA, Berthier JL, Bomsel-Demontoy MC, Chaduc Y, Montagnier L, Hovanessian AG, et al. Simian immunodeficiency virus replicates to high levels in sooty mangabeys without inducing disease. J Virol 1998;72:3872−86.

[48] ten Haaft P, Murthy K, Salas M, McClure H, Dubbes R, Koornstra W, et al. Differences in early virus loads with different phenotypic variants of HIV-1 and SIV(cpz) in chimpanzees. AIDS 2001;15:2085−92.

[49] Broussard SR, Staprans SI, White R, Whitehead EM, Feinberg MB, Allan JS. Simian immunodeficiency virus replicates to high levels in naturally infected African green monkeys without inducing immunologic or neurologic disease. J Virol 2001;75:2262−75.

[50] Goldstein S, Brown CR, Ourmanov I, Pandrea I, Buckler-White A, Erb C, et al. Comparison of simian immunodeficiency virus SIVagmVer replication and CD4+ T-cell dynamics in vervet and sabaeus African green monkeys. J Virol 2006;80:4868−77.

[51] Kornfeld C, Ploquin MJ, Pandrea I, Faye A, Onanga R, Apetrei C, et al. Antiinflammatory profiles during primary SIV infection in African green monkeys are associated with protection against AIDS. J Clin Invest 2005;115:1082−91.

[52] Pandrea I, Kornfeld C, Ploquin MJ, Apetrei C, Faye A, Rouquet P, et al. Impact of viral factors on very early *in vivo* replication profiles in simian immunodeficiency virus SIVagm-infected African green monkeys. J Virol 2005;79:6249−59.

[53] Liovat AS, Jacquelin B, Ploquin MJ, Barre-Sinoussi F, Müller-Trutwin MC. African non human primates infected by SIV—why don't they get sick? Lessons from studies on the early phase of non-pathogenic SIV infection. Curr HIV Res 2009;7:39−50.

[54] Pandrea I, Apetrei C, Gordon S, Barbercheck J, Dufour J, Bohm R, et al. Paucity of CD4+CCR5+ T cells is a typical feature of natural SIV hosts. Blood 2007;109:1069−76.

[55] Gordon SN, Dunham RM, Engram JC, Estes J, Wang Z, Klatt NR, et al. Short-lived infected cells support virus replication in sooty mangabeys naturally infected with simian immunodeficiency virus: Implications for AIDS pathogenesis. J Virol 2008;82: 3725−35.

[56] Chakrabarti LA, Lewin SR, Zhang L, Gettie A, Luckay A, Martin LN, et al. Age-dependent changes in T cell homeostasis and SIV load in sooty mangabeys. J Med Primatol 2000; 29:158−65.

[57] Beer B, Denner J, Brown CR, Norley S, zur Megede J, Coulibaly C, et al. Simian immunodeficiency virus of African green monkeys is apathogenic in the newborn natural host. J Acquir Immune Defic Syndr Hum Retrovirol 1998;18:210−20.

[58] Chen Z, Gettie A, Ho DD, Marx PA. Primary SIVsm isolates use the CCR5 coreceptor from sooty mangabeys naturally infected in west Africa: A comparison of coreceptor usage of primary SIVsm, HIV-2, and SIVmac. Virology 1998;246:113−24.

[59] Deng HK, Unutmaz D, KewalRamani VN, Littman DR. Expression cloning of new receptors used by simian and human immunodeficiency viruses. Nature 1997;388: 296−300.

[60] Riddick NE, Hermann EA, Loftin LM, Elliott ST, Wey WC, Cervasi B, et al. A novel CCR5 mutation common in sooty mangabeys reveals SIVsmm infection of CCR5-null natural hosts and efficient alternative coreceptor use *in vivo*. PLoS Pathog 2010;6:e1001064.

[61] Pandrea I, Onanga R, Souquiere S, Mouinga−Ondeme A, Bourry O, Makuwa M, et al. Paucity of CD4+ CCR5+ T cells may prevent transmission of simian immunodeficiency virus in natural nonhuman primate hosts by breast-feeding. J Virol 2008;82:5501−9.

[62] Klatt NR, Villinger F, Bostik P, Gordon SN, Pereira L, Engram JC, et al. Availability of activated CD4+ T cells dictates the level of viremia in naturally SIV-infected sooty mangabeys. J Clin Invest 2008;118:2039.

[63] Veazey RS, Lackner AA. HIV swiftly guts the immune system. Nat Med 2005;11:469.

[64] Zeitz M, Ullrich R, Schneider T, Kewenig S, Riecken E. Mucosal immunodeficiency in HIV/SIV infection. Pathobiology 1998;66:151−7.

[65] Gordon SN, Klatt NR, Bosinger SE, Brenchley JM, Milush JM, Engram JC, et al. Severe depletion of mucosal CD4+ T cells in AIDS-free simian immunodeficiency virus-infected sooty mangabeys. J Immunol 2007;179:3026−34.

[66] Chakrabarti LA, Lewin SR, Zhang L, Gettie A, Luckay A, Martin LN, et al. Normal T-cell turnover in sooty mangabeys harboring active simian immunodeficiency virus infection. J Virol 2000;74:1209−23.

[67] Milush JM, Reeves JD, Gordon SN, Zhou D, Muthukumar A, Kosub DA, et al. Virally induced CD4+ T cell depletion is not sufficient to induce AIDS in a natural host. J Immunol 2007;179:3047−56.

[68] Milush JM, Mir KD, Sundaravaradan V, Gordon SN, Engram J, Cano CA, et al. Lack of clinical AIDS in SIV-infected sooty mangabeys with significant CD4+ T cell loss is associated with double-negative T cells. J Clin Invest 2011: in press.

[69] Beaumier CM, Harris LD, Goldstein S, Klatt NR, Whitted S, McGinty J, et al. CD4 downregulation by memory CD4+ T cells *in vivo* renders African green monkeys resistant to progressive SIVagm infection. Nat Med 2009;15:879.

[70] Murayama Mukai, Inoue M, Yoshikawa. An African green monkey lacking peripheral CD4 lymphocytes that retains helper T cell activity and coexists with SIVagm. Clin Exp Immunol 1999;117:504.

[71] Meythaler M, Martinot A, Wang Z, Pryputniewicz S, Kasheta M, Ling B, et al. Differential CD4+ T-lymphocyte apoptosis and bystander T-cell activation in rhesus macaques and sooty mangabeys during acute simian immunodeficiency virus infection. J Virol 2009;83:572−83.

[72] Monceaux V, Viollet L, Petit F, Cumont MC, Kaufmann GR, Aubertin AM, et al. CD4+ CCR5+ T-cell dynamics during simian immunodeficiency virus infection of Chinese rhesus macaques. J Virol 2007;81:13865−75.

[73] Okoye A, Meier-Schellersheim M, Brenchley JM, Hagen SI, Walker JM, Rohankhedkar M, et al. Progressive CD4+ central memory T cell decline results in CD4+ effector memory insufficiency and overt disease in chronic SIV infection. J Exp Med 2007;204:2171−85.

[74] Goldstein S, Ourmanov I, Brown CR, Beer BE, Elkins WR, Plishka R, et al. Wide range of viral load in healthy African green monkeys naturally infected with simian immunodeficiency virus. J Virol 2000;74:11744−53.

[75] Ploquin MJ, Diop OM, Sol-Foulon N, Mortara L, Faye A, Soares MA, et al. DC-SIGN from African green monkeys is expressed in lymph nodes and mediates infection in *trans* of simian immunodeficiency virus SIVagm. J Virol 2004;78:798−810.

[76] Gueye A, Diop OM, Ploquin MJ, Kornfeld C, Faye A, Cumont MC, et al. Viral load in tissues during the early and chronic phase of non-pathogenic SIVagm infection. J Med Primatol 2004;33:83−97.

[77] Beer B, Scherer J, Megede JZ, Norley S, Baier M, Kurth R. Lack of dichotomy between virus load of peripheral blood and lymph nodes during long-term simian immunodeficiency virus infection of African green monkeys. Virology 1996;219:367.

[78] Cumont MC, Diop O, Vaslin B, Elbim C, Viollet L, Monceaux V, et al. Early divergence in lymphoid tissue apoptosis between pathogenic and nonpathogenic simian immunodeficiency virus infections of nonhuman primates. J Virol 2008;82:1175−84.

[79] Estes JD, Gordon SN, Zeng M, Chahroudi AM, Dunham RM, Staprans SI, et al. Early resolution of acute immune activation and induction of PD-1 in SIV-infected sooty mangabeys distinguishes nonpathogenic from pathogenic infection in rhesus macaques. J Immunol 2008;180:6798−807.

[80] Chakrabarti L, Cumont MC, Montagnier L, Hurtrel B. Variable course of primary simian immunodeficiency virus infection in lymph nodes: Relation to disease progression. J Virol 1994;68:6634−43.

[81] Meythaler M, Wang Z, Martinot A, Pryputniewicz S, Kasheta M, McClure HM, et al. Early induction of polyfunctional simian immunodeficiency virus (SIV)-specific T lymphocytes and rapid disappearance of SIV from lymph nodes of sooty mangabeys during primary infection. J Immunol 2011;186:5151−61.

[82] Pantaleo G, Graziosi C, Demarest JF, Butini L, Montroni M, Fox CH, et al. HIV infection is active and progressive in lymphoid tissue during the clinically latent stage of disease. Nature 1993;362:355−8.

[83] Paiardini M, Cervasi B, Reyes-Aviles E, Micci L, Ortiz AM, Chahroudi A, et al. Low levels of SIV infection in sooty mangabey central memory CD4+ T cells are associated with limited CCR5 expression. Nat Med 2011;17:830.

[84] Deeks SG, Kitchen CM, Liu L, Guo H, Gascon R, Narvaez AB, et al. Immune activation set point during early HIV infection predicts subsequent CD4+ T-cell changes independent of viral load. Blood 2004;104:942−7.

[85] Hazenberg MD, Otto SA, van Benthem BH, Roos MT, Coutinho RA, Lange JM, et al. Persistent immune activation in HIV-1 infection is associated with progression to AIDS. AIDS 2003;17:1881−8.

[86] McMichael AJ, Borrow P, Tomaras GD, Goonetilleke N, Haynes BF. The immune response during acute HIV-1 infection: Clues for vaccine development. Nat Rev Immunol 2010;10:11−23.

[87] Hunt PW, Brenchley J, Sinclair E, McCune Joseph M, Roland M, Page-Shafer K, et al. Relationship between T cell activation and CD4+ T cell count in HIV-seropositive individuals with undetectable plasma HIV RNA levels in the absence of therapy. J Infect Dis 2008;197:126−33.

[88] Ensoli B, Bellino S, Tripiciano A, Longo O, Francavilla V, Marcotullio S, et al. Therapeutic immunization with HIV-1 Tat reduces immune activation and loss of regulatory T-cells and improves immune function in subjects on HAART. PLoS One 2010;5:e13540.

[89] van Asten L, Danisman F, Otto SA, Borghans JA, Hazenberg MD, Coutinho RA, et al. Pre-seroconversion immune status predicts the rate of CD4 T cell decline following HIV infection. AIDS 2004;18:1885−93.

[90] Jacquelin B, Mayau V, Targat B, Liovat AS, Kunkel D, Petitjean G, et al. Nonpathogenic SIV infection of African green monkeys induces a strong but rapidly controlled type I IFN response. J Clin Invest 2009;119:3544−55.

[91] Lederer S, Favre D, Walters KA, Proll S, Kanwar B, Kasakow Z, et al. Transcriptional profiling in pathogenic and non-pathogenic SIV infections reveals significant distinctions in kinetics and tissue compartmentalization. PLoS Pathog 2009;5:e1000296.

[92] Bosinger SE, Li Q, Gordon SN, Klatt NR, Duan L, Xu L, et al. Global genomic analysis reveals rapid control of a robust innate response in SIV-infected sooty mangabeys. J Clin Invest 2009;119:3556−72.

[93] Harris LD, Tabb B, Sodora DL, Paiardini M, Klatt NR, Douek DC, et al. Downregulation of robust acute type I interferon responses distinguishes nonpathogenic simian immunodeficiency virus (SIV) infection of natural hosts from pathogenic SIV infection of rhesus macaques. J Virol 2010;84:7886−91.

[94] Silvestri G, Sodora DL, Koup RA, Paiardini M, O'Neil SP, McClure HM, et al. Nonpathogenic SIV infection of sooty mangabeys is characterized by limited bystander immunopathology despite chronic high-level viremia. Immunity 2003;18:441.

[95] Kaur A, Di Mascio M, Barabasz A, Rosenzweig M, McClure HM, Perelson AS, et al. Dynamics of T- and B-lymphocyte turnover in a natural host of simian immunodeficiency virus. J Virol 2008;82:1084−93.

[96] Wang Z, Metcalf B, Ribeiro RM, McClure H, Kaur A. Th-1-type cytotoxic CD8+ T-lymphocyte responses to simian immunodeficiency virus (SIV) are a consistent feature of natural SIV infection in sooty mangabeys. J Virol 2006;80:2771−83.

[97] Abel K, La Franco-Scheuch L, Rourke T, Ma Z-M, de Silva V, Fallert B, et al. Gamma interferon-mediated inflammation is associated with lack of protection from intravaginal simian immunodeficiency virus SIVmac239 challenge in simian−human immunodeficiency virus 89.6-immunized rhesus macaques. J Virol 2004;78:841−54.

[98] Campillo-Gimenez L, Laforge M, Fay M, Brussel A, Cumont MC, Monceaux V, et al. Nonpathogenesis of simian immunodeficiency virus infection is associated with reduced inflammation and recruitment of plasmacytoid dendritic cells to lymph nodes, not to lack of an interferon type I response, during the acute phase. J Virol 2010;84:1838−46.

[99] Diop OM, Ploquin MJ, Mortara L, Faye A, Jacquelin B, Kunkel D, et al. Plasmacytoid dendritic cell dynamics and alpha interferon production during simian immunodeficiency virus infection with a nonpathogenic outcome. J Virol 2008;82:5145−52.

[100] Durudas A, Milush JM, Chen HL, Engram JC, Silvestri G, Sodora DL. Elevated levels of innate immune modulators in lymph nodes and blood are associated with more-rapid

disease progression in simian immunodeficiency virus-infected monkeys. J Virol 2009;83:12229–40.

[101] Mandl JN, Barry AP, Vanderford TH, Kozyr N, Chavan R, Klucking S, et al. Divergent TLR7 and TLR9 signaling and type I interferon production distinguish pathogenic and nonpathogenic AIDS virus infections. Nat Med 2008;14:1077.

[102] Manches O, Bhardwaj N. Resolution of immune activation defines nonpathogenic SIV infection. J Clin Invest 2009;119:3512.

[103] Brenchley JM, Price DA, Schacker TW, Asher TE, Silvestri G, Rao S, et al. Microbial translocation is a cause of systemic immune activation in chronic HIV infection. Nat Med 2006;12:1365.

[104] Estes JD, Harris LD, Klatt NR, Tabb B, Pittaluga S, Paiardini M, et al. Damaged intestinal epithelial integrity linked to microbial translocation in pathogenic simian immunodeficiency virus infections. PLoS Pathog 2010;6:e1001052.

[105] Cella M, Jarrossay D, Facchetti F, Alebardi O, Nakajima H, Lanzavecchia A, et al. Plasmacytoid monocytes migrate to inflamed lymph nodes and produce large amounts of type I interferon. Nat Med 1999;5:919.

[106] Colonna M, Trinchieri G, Liu Y-J. Plasmacytoid dendritic cells in immunity. Nat Immunol 2004;5:1219.

[107] Fonteneau J-F, Larsson M, Beignon A-S, McKenna K, Dasilva I, Amara A, et al. Human immunodeficiency virus type 1 activates plasmacytoid dendritic cells and concomitantly induces the bystander maturation of myeloid dendritic cells. J Virol 2004;78:5223–32.

[108] Jaehn PS, Zaenker KS, Schmitz J, Dzionek A. Functional dichotomy of plasmacytoid dendritic cells: Antigen-specific activation of T cells versus production of type I interferon. Eur J Immunol 2008;38:1822–32.

[109] McKenna K, Beignon A-S, Bhardwaj N. Plasmacytoid dendritic cells: Linking innate and adaptive immunity. J Virol 2005;79:17.

[110] Siegal FP, Kadowaki N, Shodell M, Fitzgerald-Bocarsly PA, Shah K, Ho S, et al. The nature of the principal type 1 interferon-producing cells in human blood. Science 1999;284: 1835–7.

[111] Ansari AA, Reimann KA, Mayne AE, Takahashi Y, Stephenson ST, Wang R, et al. Blocking of α4-β7 gut-homing integrin during acute infection leads to decreased plasma and gastrointestinal tissue viral loads in simian immunodeficiency virus-infected rhesus macaques. J Immunol 2011;186:1044–59.

[112] Grassi F, Hosmalin A, McIlroy D, Calvez V, Debre P, Autran B. Depletion in blood CD11c-positive dendritic cells from HIV-infected patients. AIDS 1999;13:759–66.

[113] Soumelis V, Scott I, Gheyas F, Bouhour D, Cozon G, Cotte L, et al. Depletion of circulating natural type 1 interferon-producing cells in HIV-infected AIDS patients. Blood 2001;98: 906–12.

[114] Lore K, Sonnerborg A, Brostrom C, Goh LE, Perrin L, McDade H, et al. Accumulation of DC-SIGN+CD40+ dendritic cells with reduced CD80 and CD86 expression in lymphoid tissue during acute HIV-1 infection. AIDS 2002;16:683–92.

[115] Zimmer MI, Larregina AT, Castillo CM, Capuano III S, Falo Jr LD, Murphey-Corb M, et al. Disrupted homeostasis of Langerhans cells and interdigitating dendritic cells in monkeys with AIDS. Blood 2002;99:2859–68.

[116] Malleret B, Maneglier B, Karlsson I, Lebon P, Nascimbeni M, Perie L, et al. Primary infection with simian immunodeficiency virus: Plasmacytoid dendritic cell homing to lymph nodes, type I interferon, and immune suppression. Blood 2008;112:4598–608.

[117] Brown KN, Wijewardana V, Liu X, Barratt-Boyes SM. Rapid influx and death of plasmacytoid dendritic cells in lymph nodes mediate depletion in acute simian immunodeficiency virus infection. PLoS Pathog 2009;5:e1000413.

[118] Wijewardana V, Soloff AC, Liu X, Brown KN, Barratt-Boyes SM. Early myeloid dendritic cell dysregulation is predictive of disease progression in simian immunodeficiency virus infection. PLoS Pathog 2010;6:e1001235.

[119] Altfeld M, Fadda L, Frleta D, Bhardwaj N. DCs and NK cells: Critical effectors in the immune response to HIV-1. Nat Rev Immunol 2011;11:176−86.

[120] Mortara L, Ploquin MJY, Faye A, Scott-Algara D, Vaslin B, Butor C, et al. Phenotype and function of myeloid dendritic cells derived from African green monkey blood monocytes. J Immunol Methods 2006;308:138.

[121] Liu YJ. IPC: Professional type 1 interferon-producing cells and plasmacytoid dendritic cell precursors. Annu Rev Immunol 2005;23:275.

[122] Beignon AS, McKenna K, Skoberne M, Manches O, DaSilva I, Kavanagh DG, et al. Endocytosis of HIV-1 activates plasmacytoid dendritic cells via Toll-like receptor−viral RNA interactions. J Clin Invest 2005;115:3265−75.

[123] Lepelley A, Louis S, Sourisseau M, Law HK, Pothlichet J, Schilte C, et al. Innate sensing of HIV-infected cells. PLoS Pathog 2011;7:e1001284.

[124] Kulkarni S, Martin MP, Carrington M. The Yin and Yang of HLA and KIR in human disease. Sem Immunol 2008;20:343.

[125] Alter G, Teigen N, Davis BT, Addo MM, Suscovich TJ, Waring MT, et al. Sequential deregulation of NK cell subset distribution and function starting in acute HIV-1 infection. Blood 2005;106:3366−9.

[126] Reeves RK, Gillis J, Wong FE, Yu Y, Connole M, Johnson RP. CD16- natural killer cells: Enrichment in mucosal and secondary lymphoid tissues and altered function during chronic SIV infection. Blood 2010;115:4439−46.

[127] Giavedoni LD, Velasquillo MC, Parodi LM, Hubbard GB, Hodara VL. Cytokine expression, natural killer cell activation, and phenotypic changes in lymphoid cells from rhesus macaques during acute infection with pathogenic simian immunodeficiency virus. J Virol 2000;74:1648−57.

[128] Kaur A, Hale CL, Ramanujan S, Jain RK, Johnson RP. Differential dynamics of CD4(+) and CD8(+) T-lymphocyte proliferation and activation in acute simian immunodeficiency virus infection. J Virol 2000;74:8413−24.

[129] Pereira LE, Johnson RP, Ansari AA. Sooty mangabeys and rhesus macaques exhibit significant divergent natural killer cell responses during both acute and chronic phases of SIV infection. Cell Immunol 2008;254:10.

[130] Bendelac A, Savage PB, Teyton L. The biology of NKT cells. Annu Rev Immunol 2007;25:297.

[131] Motsinger A, Haas DW, Stanic AK, Van Kaer L, Joyce S, Unutmaz D. CD1d-restricted human natural killer T cells are highly susceptible to human immunodeficiency virus 1 infection. J Exp Med 2002;195:869−79.

[132] Fleuridor R, Wilson B, Hou R, Landay A, Kessler H, Al-Harthi L. CD1d-restricted natural killer T cells are potent targets for human immunodeficiency virus infection. Immunology 2003;108:3.

[133] Motsinger A, Azimzadeh A, Stanic AK, Johnson RP, Van Kaer L, Joyce S, et al. Identification and simian immunodeficiency virus infection of CD1d-restricted macaque natural killer T cells. J Virol 2003;77:8153−8.

[134] Sandberg JK, Fast NM, Palacios EH, Fennelly G, Dobroszycki J, Palumbo P, et al. Selective loss of innate CD4+ Vα24 natural killer T cells in human immunodeficiency virus infection. J Virol 2002;76:7528−34.

[135] Fernandez CS, Chan AC, Kyparissoudis K, De Rose R, Godfrey DI, Kent SJ. Peripheral NKT cells in simian immunodeficiency virus-infected macaques. J Virol 2009;83:1617−24.

[136] Rout N, Else JG, Yue S, Connole M, Exley MA, Kaur A. Heterogeneity in phenotype and function of CD8+ and CD4/CD8 double-negative natural killer T cell subsets in sooty mangabeys. J Med Primatol 2010;39:224−34.

[137] Rout N, Else JG, Yue S, Connole M, Exley MA, Kaur A. Paucity of CD4+ natural killer T (NKT) lymphocytes in sooty mangabeys is associated with lack of NKT cell depletion after SIV infection. PLoS One 2010;5:e9787.

[138] Kosub DA, Lehrman G, Milush JM, Zhou D, Chacko E, Leone A, et al. Gamma/delta T-cell functional responses differ after pathogenic human immunodeficiency virus and nonpathogenic simian immunodeficiency virus infections. J Virol 2008;82: 1155−65.

[139] Harris LD, Klatt NR, Vinton C, Briant JA, Tabb B, Ladell K, et al. Mechanisms underlying gamma/delta T-cell subset perturbations in SIV-infected Asian rhesus macaques. Blood 2010;116:4148−57.

[140] Boullier S, Dadaglio G, Lafeuillade A, Debord T, Gougeon ML. V delta 1 T cells expanded in the blood throughout HIV infection display a cytotoxic activity and are primed for TNF-alpha and IFN-gamma production but are not selected in lymph nodes. J Immunol 1997;159:3629−37.

[141] Ploquin MJ, Desoutter JF, Santos PR, Pandrea I, Diop OM, Hosmalin A, et al. Distinct expression profiles of TGF-beta1 signaling mediators in pathogenic SIVmac and non-pathogenic SIVagm infections. Retrovirology 2006;3:37.

[142] Bostik P, Watkins M, Villinger F, Ansari AA. Genetic analysis of cytokine promoters in nonhuman primates: Implications for Th1/Th2 profile characteristics and SIV disease pathogenesis. Clin Dev Immunol 2004;11:35−44.

[143] Brenchley JM, Paiardini M, Knox KS, Asher AI, Cervasi B, Asher TE, et al. Differential Th17 CD4 T-cell depletion in pathogenic and nonpathogenic lentiviral infections. Blood 2008;112:2826−35.

[144] Lozano Reina JM, Favre D, Kasakow Z, Mayau V, Nugeyre MT, Ka T, et al. Gag p27-specific B- and T-cell responses in simian immunodeficiency virus SIVagm-infected African green monkeys. J Virol 2009;83:2770−7.

[145] Zahn RC, Rett MD, Korioth-Schmitz B, Sun Y, Buzby AP, Goldstein S, et al. Simian immunodeficiency virus (SIV)-specific CD8+ T-cell responses in vervet African green monkeys chronically infected with SIVagm. J Virol 2008;82:11577−88.

[146] Dunham R, Pagliardini P, Gordon S, Sumpter B, Engram J, Moanna A, et al. The AIDS-resistance of naturally SIV-infected sooty mangabeys is independent of cellular immunity to the virus. Blood 2006;108:209−17.

[147] Zahn RC, Rett MD, Li M, Tang H, Korioth-Schmitz B, Balachandran H, et al. Suppression of adaptive immune responses during primary SIV infection of sabaeus African green monkeys delays partial containment of viremia but does not induce disease. Blood 2010;115:3070−8.

[148] Kaur A, Alexander L, Staprans SI, Denekamp L, Hale CL, McClure HM, et al. Emergence of cytotoxic T lymphocyte escape mutations in nonpathogenic simian immunodeficiency virus infection. Eur J Immunol 2001;31:3207−17.

[149] Kaur A, Grant RM, Means RE, McClure H, Feinberg M, Johnson RP. Diverse host responses and outcomes following simian immunodeficiency virus SIVmac239 infection in sooty mangabeys and rhesus macaques. J Virol 1998;72:9597−611.

[150] Schmitz JE, Kuroda MJ, Santra S, Sasseville VG, Simon MA, Lifton MA, et al. Control of viremia in simian immunodeficiency virus infection by CD8+ lymphocytes. Science 1999;283:857−60.

[151] Jin X, Bauer DE, Tuttleton SE, Lewin S, Gettie A, Blanchard J, et al. Dramatic rise in plasma viremia after CD8+ T cell depletion in simian immunodeficiency virus-infected macaques. J Exp Med 1999;189:991−8.

[152] Schmitz JE, Zahn RC, Brown CR, Rett MD, Li M, Tang H, et al. Inhibition of adaptive immune responses leads to a fatal clinical outcome in SIV-infected pigtailed macaques but not vervet African green monkeys. PLoS Pathog 2009;5:e1000691.

[153] Gaufin T, Ribeiro R, Gautam R, Dufour J, Mandell D, Apetrei C, et al. Experimental depletion of CD8+ cells in acutely SIVagm-infected African green monkeys results in increased viral replication. Retrovirology 2010;7:42.

[154] Belkaid Y, Rouse BT. Natural regulatory T cells in infectious disease. Nat Immunol 2005;6:353.

[155] Epple HJ, Loddenkemper C, Kunkel D, Troeger H, Maul J, Moos V, et al. Mucosal but not peripheral FOXP3+ regulatory T cells are highly increased in untreated HIV infection and normalize after suppressive HAART. Blood 2006;108:3072−8.

[156] Estes JD, Li Q, Reynolds, Matthew R, Wietgrefe S, Duan L, Schacker T, et al. Premature induction of an immunosuppressive regulatory T cell response during acute simian immunodeficiency virus infection. J Infect Dis 2006;193:703−12.

[157] Karlsson I, Malleret B, Brochard P, Delache B, Calvo J, Le Grand R, et al. Suppressive activity of regulatory T cells correlates with high CD4+ T-cell counts and low T-cell activation during chronic simian immunodeficiency virus infection. AIDS 2011;25:585−93.

[158] Li L, Liu Y, Bao Z, Chen L, Wang Z, Li T, et al. Analysis of CD4+CD25+Foxp3+ regulatory T cells in HIV-exposed seronegative persons and HIV-infected persons with different disease progressions. Viral Immunol 2011;24:57−60.

[159] Pereira LE, Villinger F, Onlamoon N, Bryan P, Cardona A, Pattanapanyasat K, et al. Simian immunodeficiency virus (SIV) infection influences the level and function of regulatory T cells in SIV-infected rhesus macaques but not SIV-infected sooty mangabeys. J Virol 2007;81:4445−56.

[160] Fultz PN, Stricker RB, McClure HM, Anderson DC, Switzer WM, Horaist C. Humoral response to SIV/SMM infection in macaque and mangabey monkeys. J Acquir Immune Defic Syndr 1990;3:319−29.

[161] Norley SG, Kraus G, Ennen J, Bonilla J, Konig H, Kurth R. Immunological studies of the basis for the apathogenicity of simian immunodeficiency virus from African green monkeys. Proc Natl Acad Sci USA 1990;87:9067−71.

[162] Li B, Stefano-Cole K, Kuhrt DM, Gordon SN, Else JG, Mulenga J, et al. Nonpathogenic simian immunodeficiency virus infection of sooty mangabeys is not associated with high levels of autologous neutralizing antibodies. J Virol 2010;84:6248−53.

[163] Brenchley JM, Silvestri G, Douek DC. Nonprogressive and progressive primate immunodeficiency lentivirus infections. Immunity 2010;32:737.

[164] Sodora DL, Allan JS, Apetrei C, Brenchley JM, Douek DC, Else JG, et al. Toward an AIDS vaccine: lessons from natural simian immunodeficiency virus infections of African nonhuman primate hosts. Nat Med 2009;15:861−5.

[165] d'Ettorre G, Paiardini M, Ceccarelli G, Silvestri G, Vullo V. HIV-associated immune activation: From bench to bedside. AIDS Res Hum Retroviruses 2011;27.

[166] Schindler M, Münch J, Kutsch O, Li H, Santiago ML, Bibollet-Ruche F, et al. Nef-mediated suppression of T cell activation was lost in a lentiviral lineage that gave rise to HIV-1. Cell 2006;125:1055.

[167] Schindler M, Schmökel J, Specht A, Li H, Münch J, Khalid M, et al. Inefficient Nef-mediated downmodulation of CD3 and MHC-I correlates with loss of CD4+ T cells in natural SIV infection. PLoS Pathog 2008;4:e1000107.

[168] Meythaler M, Pryputniewicz S, Kaur A. Kinetics of T lymphocyte apoptosis and the cellular immune response in SIVmac239-infected rhesus macaques. J Med Primatol 2008;37:33.

[169] Ameisen J, Capron A. Cell dysfunction and depletion in AIDS: The programmed cell death hypothesis. Immunol Today 1991;12:102.

[170] Estaquier J, Idziorek T, de Bels F, Barre-Sinoussi F, Hurtrel B, Aubertin AM, et al. Programmed cell death and AIDS: Significance of T-cell apoptosis in pathogenic and nonpathogenic primate lentiviral infections. Proc Natl Acad Sci USA 1994;91:9431–5.

[171] Gougeon ML, Garcia S, Heeney J, Tschopp R, Lecoeur H, Guetard D, et al. Programmed cell death in AIDS-related HIV and SIV infections. AIDS Res Hum Retroviruses 1993;9:553–63.

[172] Herbeuval J-P, Shearer GM. HIV-1 immunopathogenesis: How good interferon turns bad. Clin Immunol 2007;123:121.

[173] Gasper-Smith N, Crossman DM, Whitesides JF, Mensali N, Ottinger JS, Plonk SG, et al. Induction of plasma (TRAIL), TNFR-2, fas ligand, and plasma microparticles after human immunodeficiency virus type 1 (HIV-1) transmission: Implications for HIV-1 vaccine design. J Virol 2008;82:7700–10.

[174] Harris LD, Tabb B, Sodora DL, Paiardini M, Klatt NR, Douek DC, et al. Downregulation of robust acute type I interferon responses distinguishes nonpathogenic simian immunodeficiency virus (SIV) infection of natural hosts from pathogenic SIV infection of rhesus macaques. J Virol 2010;84:7886–91.

[175] Foley JF, Yu C-R, Solow R, Yacobucci M, Peden KWC, Farber JM. Roles for CXC chemokine ligands 10 and 11 in recruiting CD4+ T cells to HIV-1-infected monocyte-derived macrophages, dendritic cells, and lymph nodes. J Immunol 2005;174:4892–900.

[176] Lacotte S, Brun S, Muller S, Dumortier H. CXCR3, inflammation, and autoimmune diseases. Ann NY Acad Sci 2009;1173:310–7.

[177] Stacey AR, Norris PJ, Qin L, Haygreen EA, Taylor E, Heitman J, et al. Induction of a striking systemic cytokine cascade prior to peak viraemia in acute human immunodeficiency virus type 1 infection, in contrast to more modest and delayed responses in acute hepatitis B and C virus infections. J Virol 2009;3719–33.

[178] Li Q, Skinner PJ, Ha S-J, Duan L, Mattila TL, Hage A, et al. Visualizing antigen-specific and infected cells *in situ* predicts outcomes in early viral infection. Science 2009;323:1726–9.

[179] Beer BE, Bailes E, Goeken R, Dapolito G, Coulibaly C, Norley SG, et al. Simian immunodeficiency virus (SIV) from sun-tailed monkeys (*Cercopithecus solatus*): Evidence for host-dependent evolution of SIV within the C. *l'hoesti* superspecies. J Virol 1999;73:7734–44.

[180] Lernould J. Classification and geographical distribution of guenons: A review. In: Gautier-Hion A, Boulière F, Gautier J, Kingdon J, editors. A Primate Radiation: Evolutionary Biology of the African Guenons. Cambridge: Cambridge University Press; 1988. p. 78.

[181] Sharp PM, Hahn BH. The evolution of HIV-1 and the origin of AIDS. Phil Trans R Soc B Biol Sci 2010;365:2487.

Chapter 3

Implications for Therapy

Ivona Pandrea [1] and Alan L. Landay [2]

[1] *Department of Pathology, Center for Vaccine Research, University of Pittsburgh, Pittsburgh, Pennsylvania, USA,* [2] *Department of Immunology/Microbiology, Rush University Medical Center, Chicago, Illinois, USA*

Chapter Outline

Models of Protection Against HIV/SIV. DOI: 10.1016/B978-0-12-387715-4.00003-4

INTRODUCTION

Simian immunodeficiency viruses (SIVs) are a large group of lentiviruses that naturally infect more than 40 African non-human primate (NHP) species (monkeys and apes) [1,2]. SIV prevalence in the wild ranges from 2 percent to over 80 percent in different species [1,3]. SIVs belong to the genus *Lentivirus* of the family *Retroviridae*. Lentiviruses infect the equine, ovine, bovine and feline families, in addition to simian species and humans [4]. The majority of lentiviruses are known to be macrophage-tropic. The two exceptions are SIVs/HIVs and the feline immunodeficiency viruses (FIVs), which are lymphotropic [1]. Infection with the lymphotropic viruses may be associated with immunodeficiency [1].

Scientific interest in the study of SIVs is due to the observations that both HIV-1 and HIV-2, the two viruses causing AIDS in humans, emerged as a result of cross-species transmissions of SIVs from chimpanzees/gorillas and sooty mangabeys (SMs), respectively [1,2,5,6]. In addition, accidental transmission of SIVsmm, which naturally infects SMs, to different species of Asian macaques resulted in progressive infections in the new macaque hosts [7,8]. In spite of being named by analogy with HIV, infections with SIVs in natural hosts generally do not progress to AIDS [9,10].

The study of the lack of disease progression of SIV infection in natural hosts provides an instructive model for HIV infection, particularly related to evaluating therapeutic approaches aimed at controlling HIV disease progression. The benign coexistence of SIVs and their African NHP hosts has resulted from their interactions over millennia [1], and a long-term adaptation of the primate hosts to prevent the deleterious consequences of lentiviral infection. Although the mechanisms through which non-pathogenicity was achieved are still under investigation, this adaptation has resulted in a pattern of chronic, persistent, life-lasting infection with an incubation period that normally exceeds the lifespan of the species [11,12]. Because this is also the target of current therapeutic approaches in HIV infection, the study of SIV infection in natural hosts can provide invaluable clues with regard to which aspects of HIV pathogenesis have to be manipulated to successfully control disease progression.

NATURAL HOSTS OF SIVS: SPECIES-SPECIFIC VIRUSES, PRIMATE LENTIVIRUS EVOLUTION, CROSS-SPECIES TRANSMISSIONS IN THE WILD AND CAPTIVITY, AND THEIR IMPACT ON THE EMERGENCE OF PATHOGENIC LENTIVIRUSES

Classification and Taxonomy

The simian lentiviruses form one of the five serogroups of the *Lentiviridae* genus consisting of three species: human immunodeficiency virus 1 (HIV-1), human immunodeficiency virus 2 (HIV-2) and simian immunodeficiency virus (SIV). Although only 10 SIVs naturally found in African non-human primates (NHPs) are recognized by ICTV, SIV infection has been described in 42 simian species and subspecies (Figure 3.1). Partial or complete viral sequences are available for 36 species, and 6 additional species have been reported to harbor SIV-specific antibodies [1]. The SIVs from naturally infected NHPs of African origin hosts are designated by a three-letter abbreviation of the host primate species (e.g., SIVagm) [1].

SIV and Primate Species Radiation: Arguments for a Host-Dependent Evolution of SIVs

Since SIVs are only present in non-human primates of African origin, while Asian species of Old World monkeys, such as the colobines and macaques, are not naturally infected with SIV, it is considered that the last common ancestors of the catarrhines (all Old World monkeys and apes) were not infected by SIV 25 million years ago [13,14]. Therefore, it has been suggested that SIV emergence occurred after radiation by these species, possibly from a non-primate source [15].

Phylogenetic analyses of SIV have identified a starburst phylogenetic pattern, which suggests SIVs' evolution from a single ancestor [1]. The phylogenetic distances among the major SIV lineages generally match the phylogenetic relationships among their hosts, which is highly suggestive of host-dependent evolution. In this scenario, SIV ancestors were already infecting NHP ancestors at the time of their speciation, millions of years ago. However, several NHP species are currently infected with SIVs that emerged through

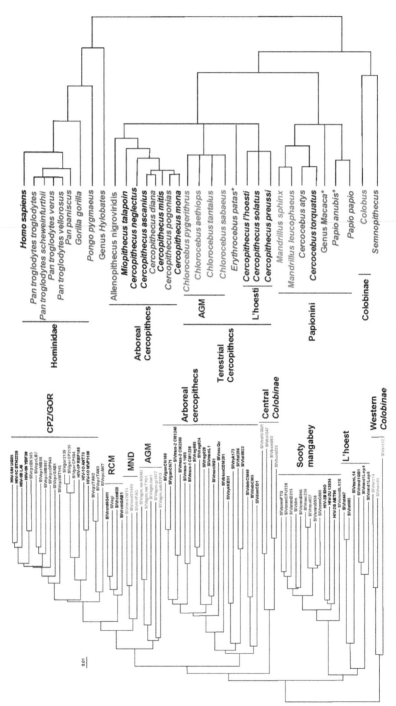

FIGURE 3.1 SIV phylogeny generally overlaps non-human primate phylogeny. Cross-species transmissions and recombination between SIVs infecting different non-human primate hosts altered this pattern. *Adapted from Vande Woude and Apetrei (2006) [1].*

recombination between highly divergent SIVs [16], or through cross-species transmissions [17].

There are six major genetic lineages of SIVs (Figure 3.1):

1. SIVs from arboreal guenons. This cluster is formed by nine distinct SIVs: SIVsyk (sykes monkey) [18,19], SIVblu (blue monkey) [19], SIVgsn (greater spot-nosed guenon) [20,21], SIVdeb (deBrazza monkey) [19], SIV-mon (mona monkey) [20], SIVden (Dent's mona) [22], SIVmus (mustached monkey) [20,23], SIVasc (ascanius monkey) [24] and SIVtal (talapoin monkey) [25,26]. Partial SIVbkm sequences from the black mangabey cluster in this lineage [27]. This SIV lineage is of particular importance because it contains one of the two ancestral viruses of SIVcpz [16], the immediate ancestor of HIV-1.

2. SIV from sooty mangabeys. SIVsmm naturally infects sooty mangabeys (*Cercocebus atys*). SMs from the Ivory Coast harbor SIVsmm strains related to the epidemic HIV-2 groups A and B; SMs in Sierra Leone and Liberia are the sources of the very rare HIV-2 groups C—H and of the viruses that have been accidentally transmitted to macaques [28—30].

3. SIVs from the four species of African green monkeys (AGMs). Four different but closely related SIVagm have been described for each of four species in the *Chlorocebus* genus: SIVver from the vervet, SIVtan from the tantalus monkey, SIVgri from the grivet monkey and SIVsab from the sabeus monkey [21—36]. SIVsab resulted from a recombination event between a SIVagm ancestor and a SIVrcm-like virus [27].

4. SIVs from the l'Hoest supergroup (*Cercopithecus l'hoesti, C. solatus, C. preusi*) and mandrill (*Mandrillus sphinx*): SIVlhoest, SIVsun, SIVpre, and SIVmnd-1 [28—43]. SIVmnd-1 emerged following a cross-species transmission from the solatus monkeys to mandrills [42].

5. SIVs from other papionini monkeys: SIVrcm from red-capped mangabeys [44,45], SIVmnd-2 from mandrills and SIVdrl from drills (*Mandrillus leucophaeus*). The origin of SIVmnd-2 is from a recombination between a SIVrcm-like virus and SIVmnd-1 [46]; SIVrcm is likely an ancestor of the SIVcpz recombinant [27].

6. SIVcol from the mantled colobus [47]. This virus was the first SIV isolated from the Colobinae family; other viruses from the Western colobus species do not cluster with SIVcol [48,49].

SIVs that infect apes contain the *vpu* gene, whereas papionini-infecting SIVs contain a *vpx* gene [50,51]. Three of eight guenon species have been shown to harbor *vpu*-containing viruses (*Cercopithecus mona, C. mitis* and *C. cephus* groups). *Chlorocebus, C. l'hoesti* supergroup and *Miopithecus* monkeys have an eight-gene organization. This points to the Cercopithecini as the origin of SIVs, and also as ancestors of HIV-1 lineage.

Cross-Species Transmission and its Role in the Emergence of SIVs and HIVs

Clear evidence of the cross-species transmission potential of SIVagm has been observed in the wild, where this virus has been isolated from a yellow baboon (*Papio cynocephalus*) [52], chacma baboon (*Papio ursinus*) [53] and patas monkey (*Erythrocebus patas*) [17]. In captivity, in Kenya, SIVagm.ver was transmitted to a white-crowned mangabey (*Cercocebus lunulatus*) housed at the same primate center [54]. It is noteworthy that none of these species has, to date, been reported to carry a specific SIV. Systematic prevalence studies have not yet been carried out to determine whether SIVagm is established as an endemic virus in these species, or if the isolation of these strains is the result of unique, accidental transmissions. SIVagm experimentally-infected patas did not progress to AIDS [55]; however, there is no long-term follow-up from animals infected in the wild or experimentally to conclude that SIVagm is pathogenic in African NHP species following cross-species transmission. There is strong evidence to suggest that recombination between ancestral SIVs found in greater spot-nosed, mustached or mona monkeys with the ones naturally infecting either red-capped mangabeys or mandrills is the source of SIVcpz [20,56]. Four scenarios describing SIVcpz occurrence and emergence are as follows [16]: (i) chimpanzees acquired ancestral viruses through hunting resulting in exposure to more than one SIV type [57,58], which then recombined in the new host; (ii) the two SIVs that generated SIVcpz were transmitted independently to different chimpanzees and then each spread separately in the new host population until co-infection occurred, resulting in SIVcpz; (iii) an ancestral SIV established itself as a chimpanzee virus and, following superinfection with a new SIV, evolved into SIVcpz present today; and (iv) the recombinant virus was generated in another monkey host species yet to be identified, and was subsequently transmitted to chimpanzees.

The most important cross-species transmissions involved transmission of SIVcpz/gor and SIVsmm to humans to become HIV-1 and HIV-2, respectively. Following the discovery in 1986 of HIV-2 [59], which was closely related to the SIVsmm [60], the simian origin of human AIDS was rapidly established [61,62]. The discovery of SIVcpz in the area of HIV-1 epidemic emergence pointed to a simian source for HIV-1 as well [63,64]. In 1998, HIV-1 group N was identified as the closest human counterpart of SIVcpz [65]. HIV-1 group N clearly clusters with SIVcpz from Cameroon in parts of the genome, reinforcing the hypothesis that SIVcpz was the ancestor of HIV-1 [65–67]. Recent large-scale non-invasive surveys of chimps in Cameroon identified SIVcpz strains closely related to HIV-1 group M [68]. Finally, the newly described HIV-1 group P appears to have originated following a cross-species transmission of SIVgor to humans [6]. Altogether these seminal studies have solved the origin of HIV-1 and HIV-2, but the mechanism(s) of the emergence of HIV-1 and HIV-2 in the human population as pathogenic agents is still under debate.

Cross-species transmission is probably not the only requirement for the emergence of HIV, and additional events, such as viral adaptation through serial passages to bypass the intrinsic host restriction factors, may have contributed to successful lentiviral adaptation into new host species [69−71].

In conclusion, naturally occurring cross-species transmissions of SIV demonstrate that successful infection is a rare event. While evidence points to cross-species transmission events leading to emerging lentiviral diseases in primates, including man, the reasons for the success of these infections, and the factors responsible for pathogenicity, have not been clearly delineated. Further studies of natural SIV infections may provide answers to these questions.

Experimental Cross-Species Transmission of SIVs to Macaque Species and the Generation of the Animal Models for AIDS Research

Accidental transmission of SIVsmm from its natural host, the sooty mangabey, to different species of macaques occurred in the early 1970s in different Primate Centers in the USA. The common denominator of these accidental transmissions is co-localization of sooty mangabeys at the same site and performance of concomitant experiments involving multiple species. The circumstances of SIVsmm epizootic occurrences in macaques are now well characterized, and sources have been traced to SMs in different colonies in US Primate Centers [7,72,73]. Over the past 25 years, several SIVsmm strains have been selected for use in macaques for pathogenesis and vaccine studies:

1. In the early 1980s, leprosy experiments were carried out in the Tulane National Primate Research Center (TNPRC) in sooty mangabeys (SMs), with blood and tissues from a leprous SM being serially passaged in rhesus macaques (RMs) [74]. An increasing incidence of AIDS in the recipient RMs was recorded with each passage [74]. This series of experiments generated the reference strain B670 (which was isolated from an animal in the second passage of these experiments) and the strains E660/E543-3, which were generated following additional passages [74−76].
2. Full-length SIVmac/mne sequences form a tight cluster in the HIV-2/ SIVsmm/SIVmac phylogenetic trees that match viral strains from infected captive SMs from the California National Primate Research Center (CNPRC) [7]. SIVstm could also be traced to stump-tailed macaques (STMs) and SMs from CNPRC [77,78]. These isolates define the original source of SIVmac251/mne and SIVstm [7].
3. SIVmac251, the widely used pathogenic virus associated with simian AIDS, was isolated in 1984 at the New England Primate Research Center (NEPRC) [79,80]. The history and derivation of the various SIVmac isolates at the NEPRC revealed that SIVmac251, SIVmac239 and their descendants are all derived from a single SIV-infected RM shipped from CNPRC in 1970

[73], concurrent with an epizootic of lymphomas in RMs [81]. SIVmac infection has been retrospectively documented in RMs from CNPRC [73]. At the NEPRC, the virus circulated undetected in the 1970s [73,82]. At least five serial passages could be documented for SIVmac251, whereas SIVmac239 resulted from four additional serial passages of SIVmac251 [73]. SIVmne also originated at the CNPRC, and is closely related to SIVmac251 and SIVmac239, but is significantly less pathogenic [83]. The fact that SIVmne was passaged through RMs fewer times than SIVmac further supports the serial-passage pathogenicity hypothesis [84]. The emergence of SIVmac at CNPRC may have occurred following kuru experiments carried out in the 1960s at the CNPRC [72].

4. SIVsmmPBj14 is perhaps the most acutely pathogenic strain of SIV for PTM; this isolate was selected during intentional serial passage to develop a highly virulent SIV. A PTM was inoculated with tissues from a naturally infected SIVsmm, and demonstrated symptoms of AIDS after 14 months of incubation [85]. Reinoculation of peripheral blood mononuclear cells (PBMCs) from this animal into PTMs induced lethal disease in 1−2 weeks. Interestingly, SIVsmmPBj14 is also pathogenic in SM [85,86], which is not typically a feature of other macaque passaged SIVsmm strains [87].

Experimental cross-species transmission of SIVagm to different species of Asian macaques demonstrates variable pathogenic outcomes. SIVagm is controlled by the RM host after replicating to high levels during the primary infection [88], whereas SIVagm infection of PTMs was reported to progress to AIDS [89,90]. Overall, PTMs seem to be more susceptible to virulent cross-species SIV infections, as illustrated by progression to AIDS of PTMs infected with SIVlhoest and SIVsun [40,91].

ANIMAL MODELS

Although the number of SIVs naturally infecting different African NHP species is high, there are major intrinsic limitations to the development of animal models in the different species of African NHP hosts [1]: (i) numerous SIVs are only known from sequences, therefore they cannot be used in pathogenesis/treatment studies; (ii) numerous African NHPs that are natural hosts of SIVs are extremely endangered (i.e., suntailed monkeys, diana monkeys, white-crowned mangabeys), which generally precludes invasive studies in these hosts; and (iii) there are no currently available colonies for most of the African NHPs. Therefore, to date, only three models for natural SIV infection have been developed and studied to derive the features of SIV infection in natural hosts: SIVagm-infected African green monkeys [92−95]; SIVsmm-infected sooty mangabeys [8,86,87,96]; and SIVmnd-infected mandrills [29,46,97,98]. As detailed below, studies thus far have not identified major differences in the pathogenesis of SIV infection between the available models, suggesting that any of these models are appropriate for SIV studies.

However, each of these models has advantages and disadvantages over the others, as follows:

1. Both sooty mangabeys and mandrills (which belong to the Papionini tribe) are more closely genetically related to the existing animal models of pathogenic SIV infection, the macaques (as the macaques belong to the same Papionini tribe) [1]. However, both sooty mangabeys and mandrills are endangered species; conversely, African green monkeys are widespread and non-endangered, so invasive studies are permitted in the latter species.

2. SIVsmm, the virus naturally infecting sooty mangabeys, is the direct ancestor of HIV-2, which potentially implies that the study of the pathogenic features of SIVsmm in natural and non-natural hosts is directly informative for the pathogenesis of HIV/AIDS infection [62].

3. Similar to humans, which are infected with two different viruses (HIV-1 and HIV-2) that have different origins, genetic structure and pathogenic potential, mandrills are infected with SIVmnd-1 and SIVmnd-2 [46]; the difference is that, based on existing data, it appears that the SIVmnd types have a similar pathogenicity in their mandrill host [99].

4. Different from mangabeys and mandrills, whose only habitats are in West Africa and in Central Africa, respectively, one of the AGM species (the sabaeus monkey) was naturalized to the Caribbean islands of St Kitts and Barbados approximately 300 years ago [1]. The only difference between the current West-African sabaeus and the Caribbean sabaeus is that the Caribbean population is free of SIV (most likely because this population was formed by young/juvenile pet monkeys during the slave trade, and SIV prevalence in these age groups is generally very low) [100]. We have previously reported that SIVagm.sab infection in Caribbean AGMs faithfully reproduces the pathogenesis of SIVagm infection in African sabaeus monkeys, and therefore Caribbean AGMs are an appropriate model for natural SIV infection [92]. The existence of this Caribbean population of sabaeus monkeys is key to overcoming the current shortage of AGMs, when research on natural hosts of SIVs is expanding and NHP importation from Africa is very difficult.

One of the major goals of the study of SIV infection in natural hosts is to compare and contrast it with pathogenic infections, in order to identify the correlates of the lack of disease progression in the natural host and to manipulate different parameters of pathogenic infection towards a non-pathogenic outcome. To accomplish this goal, pathogenic counterparts of each of the animal models of natural SIV infection have been developed: SIVsmm-infected rhesus macaques and SIVagm-infected pigtailed macaques. The observation that rhesus macaques infected with SIV develop a clinical syndrome which is very similar to AIDS in humans (simian AIDS) was made very soon after the recognition of AIDS [80]. The initial manipulations of the pathogenesis of SIVsmm/mac in rhesus macaques might have seriously altered the intrinsic pathogenicity of the virus and selected strains unadapted for physiological transmission [72]. Thus, SIVmac239, the reference strain for pathogenesis and vaccine studies, resulted from seven *in vivo* passages of SIVsmm and was at least passaged out *in vitro* on human PBMCs, which may have induced alterations in the envelope. As a result, this strain is highly resistant to neutralization and virtually impossible to control through vaccination or through antiretroviral drugs. Other reference strains were submitted to fewer serial passages, and more closely model the pathogenesis of HIV in RMs. The recent discovery of a large array of new SIVsmm strains that were not altered in any respect [7] may provide the opportunity to re-derive strains for use in the RM model that more closely reproduce the pathogenesis of HIV-1 and model the extraordinary diversity of HIV-1 group M, which is currently a major obstacle for developing an effective vaccine against AIDS.

Cross-species transmission of SIVagm to pigtailed macaque also results in a relevant pathogenic model. Upon the direct passage of the virus to pigtailed macaques, the outcome of infection can vary widely, outcomes being rapid progression, normal progression or control. However, upon a single passage of the virus sampled at the time of AIDS the infection is more consistently pathogenic, with a relatively uniform progression to AIDS recorded in all infected animals [101]. One of the advantages of the SIVagm model is that, in addition to this pathogenic model, SIVagm can be used as a model of elite-controlled infection. Indeed, cross-species transmission of SIVagm to rhesus macaques results in an infection that is controlled in 100 percent of cases [88,102]. Thus, using a single SIVagm.sab strain, we can induce a persistent non-progressive ("non-pathogenic") infection in AGMs, a pathogenic infection in pigtailed macaques, and a controlled infection in rhesus macaques.

To date, a consistent pathogenic counterpart for the mandrill infection with the SIVmnd-1 and SIVmnd-2 has not been developed. SIVmnd-1 infection of cynomolgous monkeys is controlled, while RM infection with SIVmnd-1 but not SIVmnd-2 was reported to progress to AIDS [99]. However the data are too preliminary to draw any conclusion.

Direct comparisons between progressive and non-progressive models allow for identification of key parameters of SIV infection that might be crucial for the different clinical outcomes of lentiviral infection in these species. The next section will summarize the most important findings resulting from these comparisons that may impact the treatment of HIV patients.

NATURAL HISTORY OF SIV INFECTION IN NATURAL HOSTS AND KEY PARAMETERS THAT HAVE POTENTIAL PREDICTIVE VALUE TO ASSESS EFFECTIVE THERAPEUTIC INTERVENTIONS

The study of animal models of natural SIV infection has the potential for being highly informative in assessing new therapeutic interventions aimed at controlling HIV disease progression: (i) during chronic infection, with the exception of a robust viral replication, the majority of the biological parameters tend to reach the baseline levels and are remarkably conserved; and (ii) both of the most-utilized models of natural infection (the AGMs and the sooty mangabeys) have pathogenic counterparts (i.e., pigtailed macaques and RMs, respectively) in which the outcome is disease progression upon infection with the same strains that induce persistent, non-progressive infection in natural hosts (SIVagm and SIVsmm, respectively). Thus, by comparing and contrasting the biological markers between pathogenic and natural SIV infection, assessment of therapeutic interventions can be performed.

Receptor and Coreceptor Usage and Availability of Target Cells in Natural Hosts

CD4 Expression in Natural Hosts

SIVs infecting natural hosts use CD4 as a main receptor for entry, similar to SIVmac and HIV-1/2 [1]. However, comparison between AGMs and progressive hosts showed a significantly lower expression of the CD4 receptor on the lymphocytes in all the lymphoid compartments (blood, lymph nodes and intestine) in AGMs [92]. It was recently demonstrated that in AGMs, many CD4+ T cells downregulate CD4 *in vivo* as they enter in the memory pool and are defined by a low expression of CD8α [103]. This downregulation of CD4 by memory T cells is independent of SIV infection, and the CD4^{neg}CD8α^{low} T cells maintain functions that are normally attributed to CD4+ T cells, including production of IL-2 and IL-17, expression of forkhead box P3 (FoxP3) and expression of CD40 ligand [103]. Furthermore, it was reported that loss of CD4 expression protects these T cells from infection by SIVagm *in vivo*, suggesting that absence of SIV-induced disease progression in natural host species may be partially explained by preservation of a subset of T cells that maintain CD4+ T cell function while being resistant to SIV infection *in vivo* [103]. Another study identified a large number of double-negative CD4− CD8− T cells in AGMs, and showed that this cell subset expresses both regulatory markers (FOX-P3 expression) and markers characteristic for Th17 [104]. Although the CD4^{neg}CD8α^{low} T cells are scarce in sooty mangabeys, in three SIVsmm-infected sooty mangabeys downregulation of CD4+ on T cells was reported to result in an increased number of double-negative T cells, which, as described in AGMs, maintained T helper functions [105].

As previously reported in our studies, uninfected sabaeus monkeys (a subspecies of AGMs), a corollary for both immune phenotypes described above, resulted from CD4 downregulation. Thus, half of sabaeus monkeys have a large percentage of DN T cells and only a small proportion of CD4^{neg}-CD8α^{low} T cells, and the other half have a high proportion of CD4^{neg}CD8α^{low} T cells and no DN T cells [92]. SIVagm.sab infection of a large number of sabaeus monkeys having the two different phenotypes did not reveal differences in viral loads (VLs) or degree of CD4+ T cell depletion [92], showing that downregulation of CD4 is probably equally efficient in preserving the T helper cell pool in animals with both immune phenotypes. We recently showed that complete downregulation of CD4 may have been involved in the extinction of SIV infection in some African non-human primates, such as patas monkeys [55]. Thus, CD4 expression and regulation in natural hosts suggest that therapies aimed at down-modulating or blocking CD4 may be considered in humans to either prevent transmission of HIV or delay disease progression in HIV patients. Such therapies are currently under evaluation in humans.

CCR5 Expression in Natural Hosts

A hallmark of pathogenic primate lentiviral infections is early and persistent depletion of mucosal memory/activated CD4+ CCR5+ T cells [1], and virus coreceptor usage is a key factor in determining which CD4+ T cell subsets are depleted. Most of the SIVs naturally infecting African NHPs are reported to use the same system of receptors as used by HIV-1, i.e., CD4 on the T cell surface as a receptor and a transmembrane chemokine receptor as a coreceptor [56,287]. For HIV-1 replication *in vivo*, the most relevant coreceptors are CCR5 and CXCR4; in 50 percent of cases, progression to AIDS is characterized by a switch in viral tropism from CCR5 to CXCR4 viruses [106]. Most of the SIVs naturally infecting African NHPs use CCR5 as the main coreceptor [107,108]. However, in NHPs no correlation can be established between coreceptor usage and pathogenesis *in vivo*. Thus, SIVmac, the SIV derived from SMs that is highly pathogenic for macaques, is CCR5-tropic in spite of being more virulent than HIV-1 [108,109]. SIVmnd-1, SIVagm.sab and some strains of SIVsmm were reported to use CXCR4 [93,110,111], but no pathologic correlation has been described in these monkey species. Moreover, experimental infection of sabaeus AGMs with the dual-tropic SIVagm.sab does not show a different pattern of viral replication or disease progression compared to other SIV infections in natural NHP hosts [93]. Furthermore, *in vivo*, SIVagm.sab depletes CCR5+ CD4+ T cells and not CXCR4+ CD4+ T cells in both natural and heterologous hosts, such as pigtailed and RMs [88]. SIVrcm uses CCR2b instead of CCR5 or CXCR4 as the coreceptor for viral entry [112]. This finding is host-related in that the CCR5 gene of most red-capped mangabeys contains a 24-base pair deletion in the Env binding region of the CCR5 [45,112]. As such, this may constitute an example of convergent evolution, similar to humans who possess the Δ32 mutation in the CCR5 gene. Transmission of SIVrcm to pigtailed macaques (that harbor functional CCR5) resulted in a rapid expansion of viral tropism to CCR4 and depletion of CD4+ T cells instead of macrophages, which are the major immune cell population expressing CCR2 [113]. Adult, uninfected, natural hosts express lower levels of CCR5 on memory CD4+ T cells from PBMCs and mucosal tissues, compared to disease-susceptible hosts such as macaques, baboons and humans [114]. Moreover, the levels of CCR5 on the CD4+ T cells are significantly lower in babies of natural hosts compared with susceptible species [115]. In contrast to macaques, in which at 6 months of age CCR5 is already at the level reported in adults, in AGMs expression of CCR5 remains very low in animals younger than 2 years. There is a direct correlation between levels of CCR5 on CD4+ T cells and SIV prevalence in wild AGMs. Thus, maternal-to-infant transmission of SIVagm is extremely rare in AGMs, possibly because of the very low levels of CCR5 in infants, while prevalence of SIV infection increases with age and is paralleled by increased expression of the CCR5 coreceptor [115]. Experimental attempts to transmit SIV through breastfeeding from acutely-infected mandrill dams which experienced very high VLs failed, confirming the lack of breastfeeding SIV transmission in natural hosts [115]. Also, we showed that in order to successfully infect AGMs intrarectally, higher doses of virus are necessary compared to pigtailed macaques and RMs, possibly because of the differences in CCR5 expression [116].

Chimpanzees, which are considered a more recent host of SIV and are more susceptible to disease progression, show an intermediate level of CD4+ CCR5+ T cells [114]. All these data suggest that African species with endemic naturally occurring SIVs may be less susceptible to pathogenic disease or to SIV breastfeeding transmission because they have fewer receptor targets for infection, or because fewer cells homed to the mucosal sites [115]. Both circumstances may either allow preservation of key CD4+ T cells subsets or contribute to the low levels of immune activation reported in natural hosts.

These findings support strategies to block CCR5 in humans to prevent HIV transmission or to diminish immune activation and prevent disease progression. Microbicides aimed at blocking CCR5 have already been reported to be successful in both animal models and humans, while CCR5 inhibitors are currently being tested with the aim to reduce the levels of immune activation in chronically HIV-infected patients.

Viral Replication

To determine whether lack of disease progression of SIV infection in natural hosts is due to low levels of viral replication, a series of studies has investigated the dynamics of early and chronic SIV replication by performing experimental SIV infections in natural hosts such as SMs, AGMs and mandrills (MNDs) [88,92–98,115] (Figure 3.2). These studies showed a consistent pattern of SIV viral load dynamics in natural hosts, with a peak of viremia (10^6–10^9 copies/ml of plasma) occurring around days 9–11 post-infection. Peak viremia is followed by a sharp decline (2–3 logs) and attainment of a stable level of viral replication (set point), which is maintained during the chronic phase of infection [117].

Viral loads quantified during the chronic phase of infection in natural SIV hosts are higher than those in HIV-1 chronically-infected asymptomatic patients [117–119]. Longitudinal analyses of the dynamics of plasma viremia

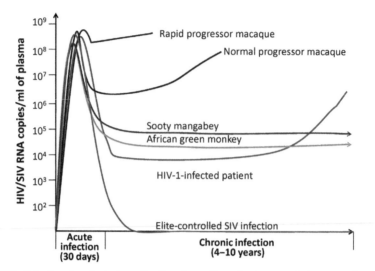

FIGURE 3.2 Levels of viral replication in pathogenic (progressive), non-pathogenic (persistent non-progressive) and elite-controlled lentivirus infection.

in natural SIV infections suggest that the level of viral replication is relatively constant over time [118,119].

Therefore, pathogenesis studies carried out in natural hosts of SIVs have demonstrated that it is possible to avoid disease progression despite very high levels of virus replication.

One may argue that natural hosts are completely atypical from this point of view, because in HIV-infected patients the levels of plasma VLs are the best predictor of disease progression. Asymptomatic patients show low levels of VL, while progression to AIDS in patients resulting from failure of the immune system to control HIV replication, or failure of antiretroviral treatments, is always associated with significant increases in VL [120,121]. However, in the few cases of AIDS described in MNDs and SMs, the quantification of viral replication over 20 years showed that the animals that developed disease had higher VLs starting with the set point of SIV infection, and experienced an increase in VL at the time of disease progression [11]. These reports clearly demonstrate that levels of viremia represent a good predictor for disease progression even in natural hosts. The difference between African NHPs and humans/macaques is that the levels of viremia is maintained constant over decades, as shown by longitudinal studies [117–119]. This is probably possible due to the low levels of immune activation described in natural hosts, which render African NHPs very resilient to high levels of viral replication.

The corollary of these findings is that the goal of the therapeutic approaches in HIV-infected patients should be not only to control virus replication, but also to target immune parameters as described below.

Adaptive Immune Responses

Maintenance of VLs at constant levels in natural hosts for decades suggests that the partial virus control is due to humoral or cellular immune responses. Numerous studies have determined that, in natural hosts, the levels of anti-SIV binding and neutralizing antibodies are either low or in the same range as those reported for HIV-1 infection [1,122]. The potential role of humoral immune responses for the control of viral replication in natural hosts was assessed in AGMs by ablating anti-SIV antibody production through a long-term depletion of B cells [123]. This study demonstrated that humoral immune responses do not play a major role in controlling viral replication in the natural host [123]. This is also true for SIVsmm-infected RMs that did not show significant changes in the levels of viral replication or disease progression when depleted of B cells and infected with a neutralization-sensitive SIVsmm strain [124].

Conversely, cellular immune responses observed in natural hosts seem to be involved in the control of viral replication, with a direct correlation between the levels of cellular immune responses and plasma VLs being reported in SMs [125]. However, cellular immune responses do not appear to be superior to those observed during SIV infection of RMs [125,126].

Recently, several groups have performed experimental *in vivo* CD8+ cell depletion studies in natural hosts and reported that administration of anti-CD8 monoclonal antibodies during both acute and chronic SIV infection resulted in increased virus replication in both AGMs and SMs [127−130]. During acute infection, CD8 cell depletion did not result in a significant increase of peak viremia but in a plateau of high VLs after the peak, which were controlled with the recovery of CD8+ T cells [130]. During chronic SIV infection, CD8 cell depletion *in vivo* also resulted in an increase of viral replication in natural hosts [127,130]. Dual CD8+ and CD20+ cell depletion studies also pointed to cellular immune responses as the main factors involved in the control of viral replication in natural hosts [128,129]. None of the *in vivo* immune cell depletion studies reported any case of disease progression.

These studies suggest that therapies aimed to increase potency of cellular immune responses may be beneficial in HIV-infected patients. However, as these therapies also have the potential to increase the number of target cells by increasing the turnover and the levels of immune activation of CD4+ T cells, they should be applied with caution and tested first in animal models of AIDS.

CD4$^+$ T Cell Dynamics During SIV Infection in Natural Hosts (Figure 3.3)

Acute SIV infection in the natural host induces a massive mucosal CD4+ T cell depletion that is of the same magnitude as in pathogenic HIV/SIV infections [114,131]. However, in spite of persistently high viral replication there is

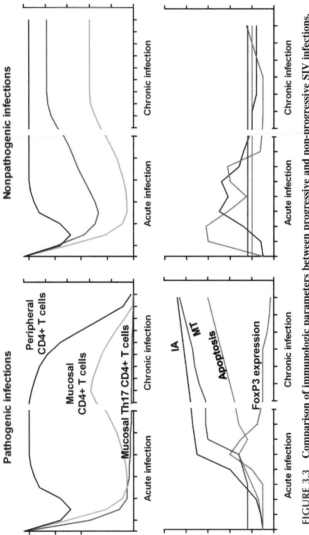

FIGURE 3.3   Comparison of immunologic parameters between progressive and non-progressive SIV infections.

a partial immune restoration of CD4+ T cells in natural hosts during chronic infection, probably due to the normal levels of immune activation and lack of CD4 T cell apoptosis in these species [114]. In marked contrast with HIV infection, in which a failure of the lymphoid regenerative capacity is an important factor in the pathogenesis of the immunodeficiency [132], the regenerative capacity of the CD4+ T cell compartment is fully preserved in natural hosts [133] and may play a key role in determining the lack of disease progression.

These data clearly show that acute mucosal CD4+ T cell depletion is not the determinant of AIDS progression, but recovery of mucosal and peripheral CD4 T cells is a strong prognostic marker for lack of disease progression [10]. Therefore, the therapy of the HIV-infected patient should include strategies that will allow for full peripheral and mucosal CD4+ T cell recovery with maximal viral suppression.

Immune Activation/Inflammation and Bystander Apoptosis during Natural SIV Infections (Figure 3.3)

Studies performed in SMs, AGMs and MNDs indicate that both acute and chronic SIV infection of natural hosts is associated with lower levels of T cell activation, pro-inflammatory responses and immunopathology [88,96−98,119,134,135]. As a result, the levels of bystander apoptosis are significantly lower in natural infection compared to pathogenic HIV/SIV infection [88,136]. During acute infection, the levels of immune activation (defined by markers such CCR5, HLA-DR, CD38, CD69 and Ki-67) and inflammation (defined by the levels of pro-inflammatory cytokine such as IL-6, IFN-α etc.) are only transiently increased in the natural hosts and at lower levels compared to progressive hosts infected with SIVmac [10]. When chronic SIV infection in natural hosts is compared to SIVmac infection in RMs, the differences are even more striking, natural infections showing: (i) normal levels of proliferating CD4+ and CD8+ T cells in the blood and lymph nodes; (ii) normal production of pro-inflammatory cytokines; (iii) a low frequency of apoptotic T cells in the LNs and intestine; and (iv) normal *in vitro* susceptibility to apoptosis [10]. The levels of activation/inflammation return to pre-infection values in the natural hosts despite continuously high viremia in the chronic phase of SIV infection. Also, SIV-infected African NHP hosts display normal lymph-node morphology, without evidence of either hyperplasia or depletion throughout the SIV infection [122]. No fibrosis was detected in lymphoid tissues in SIV-infected natural hosts. In contrast, macaques maintain high levels of immune activation and increased T cell apoptosis (during the chronic infection). Chronically SIV-infected macaques also develop lymphadenopathy with paracortical and follicular hyperplasia [122]. Severe fibrosis develops and disturbs the lymph-node architecture in progressive HIV/SIV infections, which hampers CD4 T cell reconstitution [137]. In the rare cases of AIDS described in natural hosts, increased levels of immune activation were reported in the lymph nodes, and this was associated with severe CD4+ T cell depletion and increased fibrosis [11,138].

These observations support the hypothesis that chronic immune activation is the main determinant of disease progression during HIV and SIV infection by contributing and accelerating the rate of CD4+ T cell depletion and by ultimately determining the general collapse of the immune system due to impairment and exhaustion of all the immune cell subsets [139]. The role of immune activation in the clinical course of HIV infection is supported by the observations that a proportion of HIV patients do not show recovery of the CD4+ T cells despite virological success (complete suppression of viral replication) after HAART (highly active antiretroviral therapy). These patients have higher levels of immune activation and a higher rate of disease progression [139].

All these results provide support for approaches aimed at downregulating T cell activation during HIV infection. Also, maintaining non-harmful levels of immune activation should be considered in vaccine strategies as well as in adjuvant usage. Conversely, induction of immune activation during chronic infection may result in disease progression in natural hosts, and thus such models can be employed for proof-of-concept research aimed at studying the potential of different chemical agents (i.e., adjuvants or other stimulants of the immune system) to influence disease progression.

Tregs (Regulatory T Cells) (Figure 3.3)

One of the causes of low immune activation levels in AGMs infected with SIVagm may be due to a strong induction of TGF-β1 and FOXP3 immediately after infection (24 h), followed by a significant increase in IL-10 expression which also occurs very early (at day 7 post-infection) in the SIVagm infection [95,140]. Conversely, SIVmac-infected macaques develop these types of responses only later on during infection [95,140]. In HIV-infected humans and SIV-infected rhesus macaques, significant increases of β-chemokine expression have been reported to contribute to non-specific inflammation and immune activation, as well as to high VLs in lymphoid tissues [10]. In sharp contrast to pathogenic lentiviral infections, only a transient increase of IFN-γ expression and no changes in the levels of TNF-α and MIP-1α/β expression were observed in SIVagm-infected AGMs [10]. These results, combined with the finding of an early increase in the levels of CD4+CD25+ T cells, suggest that SIVagm infection of AGMs is associated with the rapid establishment of an anti-inflammatory environment which may prevent the host from developing the aberrant chronic T cell hyperactivation that is correlated with progression to AIDS during HIV-1 infection [133,141]. CD4+CD25+ T cells are maintained in chronically infected AGMs and SMs in contrast to SIVmac-infected macaques [142]. In HIV-infected patients, data regarding

Tregs are contradictory, reporting either an increase in Tregs and suppression of adaptive immune responses, or a decrease in Tregs and strong correlations between the numbers of Tregs and the levels of immune activation [142].

Due to the dual functions of Tregs (decreasing immune activation and suppressing adaptive immune responses), therapies that aim to modulate this T cell subset should be carefully tested in animal models prior to administration to HIV patients.

Th17 (Figure 3.3)

Th17 cells are a recently described lineage of CD4+ T helper cells that are characterized by the production of IL-17 [143]. In particular, the signature cytokines of Th17 cells appear to be critical for antimicrobial immunity due to their involvement in the recruitment, activation and migration of neutrophils, as well as in promoting the production of antimicrobial molecules (i.e., defensins) and stimulating the proliferation of enterocytes and the transcription of tight-junction proteins, such as claudins [144]. As a result, it is considered that Th17 cells confer protection against various extracellular pathogens [144]. In keeping with the role of Th17 cells in mucosal immunity, and the observed differences in mucosal barrier integrity during pathogenic and non-pathogenic HIV and SIV infection, the dynamics of Th17 cells differ between natural and non-natural hosts of SIV [104,145]. Thus, in pathogenic HIV and SIV infections mucosal Th17 cells are lost, while they are preserved in the non-pathogenic SIV infection of natural hosts [104,145]. The natural host thus represents an attractive system to directly test the role of Th17 in SIV pathogenesis, through experimental depletion of these cells. In chronically HIV-infected patients Th17 cell depletion was specific for the gastrointestinal tract, since Th17 cells were maintained at healthy frequencies in the blood and bronchoalveolar lavage [104,145,146]. To date, there has been no interventional study to directly determine the role of Th17 cells in SIV/HIV pathogenesis.

The observation that natural hosts for SIV evolved to preserve Th17 cells suggests that therapies aimed to protect this T cell subset may be beneficial for HIV-infected patients. However, due to the fact that TH17 cells are also a potent pro-inflammatory cell subset, and there is no general consensus regarding Th17 loss during HIV infection, these therapies should be carefully applied and thoroughly tested in animal models.

Dendritic Cells

In progressive SIV/HIV infection, dendritic cells play an important role by increasing both transmission and disease progression through production of large amounts of pro-inflammatory cytokines, and induction and maintenance of increased activation of the adaptive immune system. It was recently suggested that the lack of immune activation in natural hosts is due to the inability of the dendritic cells to produce IFN-α when stimulated with TLR7/9 [147]. Several reports, however, have shown that IFN RNA as well the genes stimulated by interferon are increased in natural hosts during acute infection [133,141,148]. Plasma interferon is also transiently increased in SIVagm-infected AGMs during acute infection, at levels that are lower than in SIVmac-infected macaques [95]. During chronic infection there is a significant downregulation of IFN production in natural hosts [149] compared to progressive ones, in which IFN remains increased and probably contributes to the generalized increased levels of immune activation/inflammation that ultimately lead to disease progression.

These results indicate that therapies aimed at inhibiting TLR 7/9 ligands or IFN may be useful in controlling immune activation in HIV-infected patients.

Microbial Translocation (Figure 3.3)

It has been reported that one of the mechanisms of excessive immune activation observed in pathogenic SIV/HIV infection is through damage of the mucosal barrier inflicted as a consequence of massive viral replication, especially during acute infection, and of massive mucosal CD4+ T cell depletion through either direct viral killing or bystander apoptosis [150]. This immunologic and structural damage to the mucosal barrier will eventually lead to a "leaky gut" and microbial translocation from the gut lumen into the systemic circulation, which contributes to chronic immune activation and progression to AIDS [151]. This hypothesis is strongly supported by the observation that, in stark contrast to pathogenic infections, African NHPs are able to maintain their intestinal barrier integrity [88,131], perhaps through the suppression of inflammation and better epithelial preservation due to the lack of excessive apoptosis and Th17 depletion. Thus the natural host does not develop enteropathy in the initial stages of the chronic infection, despite significant mucosal CD4+ T cell depletion, in contrast to progressive hosts. As a result of maintenance of the integrity of the mucosal barrier, natural hosts maintain normal levels of T cell activation and apoptosis and show significant recovery of mucosal CD4+ T cells during chronic infection despite high levels of viral replication.

These results strongly suggest that therapies aimed to reduce the levels of microbial translocation should be considered in HIV patients, with the aim to reduce immune activation and inflammation and allow a better response (CD4 T cell reconstitution) when combined with ART.

TREATMENT

Suppression of HIV replication through HAART has significantly improved the clinical outcome and survival of HIV patients during the past two decades. It became very clear that, besides the issues related to drug resistance, ART is not always efficient in normalizing the levels of immune activation and inflammation, even in patients in which suppression of viral replication below the limit of detection of conventional commercial assays is achieved through HAART. In patients that maintain increased levels of immune activation/ inflammation despite virologic suppression, the immune reconstitution is suboptimal. Furthermore, some ART regimens have the potential to induce significant metabolic abnormalities that may enhance inflammation and cardiovascular risk, thus diminishing the benefits of reducing VLs and increasing CD4+ T cell counts. The question raised by these observations is whether or not adjuvant immune therapies may normalize the levels of immune activation/inflammation and improve immune reconstitution in HIV patients. The following section will review such therapeutical attempts applied to HIV patients and/or to NHP models of AIDS (Figure 3.4).

Strategies to Regenerate T Cell Compartments after Depletion during HIV/SIV Infection

IL-2

The rationale for IL-2 administration was that this cytokine, which is essential for growth, survival and differentiation of numerous immune cell subsets and for clonal expansion of Ag-selected cells is deficient in HIV-1 infection [152]. Moreover, central and effector CD4+ T memory cells isolated from SIV-infected macaques show a decreased expression of IL-2 during progression to AIDS [153]. *In vitro*, exogenous IL-2 administration corrects the cell cycle

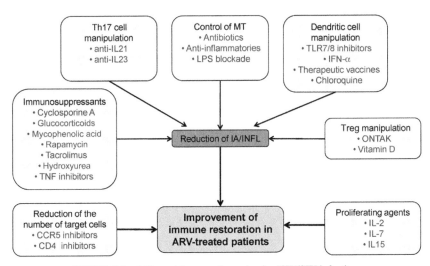

FIGURE 3.4   Adjuvant immunotherapies for HIV/SIV infection.

perturbation of lymphocytes from HIV patients [154]. Therefore, numerous studies using different doses (high *versus* low) and different regimens (continuous *versus* intermittent) of IL-2 have been conducted in ART-treated HIV-infected patients and in non-vaccinated and vaccinated SIVmac-infected macaques. IL-2 approved by the FDA as Proleukin in United States is licensed for the treatment of metastatic melanoma or renal cell carcinoma.

The majority of studies have reported notable sustained increases in CD4+ T cell counts in patients treated with IL-2 and ART compared to patients treated with ART alone [152]. However, IL-2 treatment of HIV patients did not confer immunological control of viral replication at cessation of ART, and IL-2 treatment alone did not increase virus-specific responses [152]. Low doses of IL-2 administered to vaccinated SIV-infected RMs significantly increased gag-specific CD8+ T cell responses but reduced gag-specific CD4+ T cell responses and expanded the frequency of CD4+CD25+ T cells [155]. Similar reports were published in IL-2-treated HIV patients on ART [156,157]. IL-2 treatment in healthy rhesus macaques was reported to increase the proliferation of transitional (CD28+CCR7^{neg}) CD8+ and CD4+ T cell subsets, but had little effect on fully differentiated CD28^{neg}CCR7^{neg} effector memory cells, which may explain the poor effect of IL-2 on increasing virus-specific responses [158].

Results from two major phase III clinical trials ESPRIT and SILCAAT, that involved more than 5,800 patients with different stages of HIV infection from 25 different countries, clearly established that the CD4+ T cell increases after IL-2 therapy do not translate into reduced risk of opportunistic diseases or death compared with the risk in volunteers who are taking only ART [157]. Furthermore, as previously reported, IL-2 administration was associated with systemic inflammatory syndrome [156,157], disorders of heart and blood vessels, injection site reactions and psychiatric disorders.

IL-15

As HIV/SIV infection targets CD4+ effector memory T cells, resulting in dramatic depletion of CD4+ T cells at mucosal sites, with little or no regeneration during the chronic infection, attempts to improve regeneration of this CD4+ T cell subset are fully justified. IL-15 directs NK and NKT cell development as well as CD8+ memory T cell function and homeostasis [159]. Several *in vitro* studies have demonstrated a major role for IL-15 in regulating the homeostasis of CD8+ memory T cells during HIV infection [160,161] by enhancing their activation and survival *in vitro*, and by enhancing (IFN-γ) production and direct *ex vivo* cytotoxicity of HIV-specific CD8+ T cells. Levels of IL-15 were determined to be predictive for a favorable outcome of structured treatment interruptions (STIs) in patients with chronic HIV infection [162]. Also, *in vitro* treatment of PBMCs isolated from HIV-infected patients with IL-15 resulted in improvement of natural killer function and reduction of the burden of replication-competent HIV in autologous PBMCs [163]. *In vivo* IL-15 administration to SIV-infected rhesus macaques had beneficial effects in increasing the numbers of circulating CD8+ T cells (particularly the effector memory subset) [164]. The pro-proliferative activity of IL-15 in the NHP model is not restricted only to CD8+ T cells, but also extends to the CD4+ T cells that are either effector memory or differentiating toward effector memory phenotype. A reduced capacity of IL-15 to increase the numbers of CD4 effector memory was observed in SIV-infected rhesus with uncontrolled infection, but responsiveness to IL-15 was restored after ART administration which resulted in virologic control and reduction of immune activation levels [158]. These data suggest a possible beneficial effect of IL-15 in improving immune restoration in ARV-treated HIV patients. However, IL-15 treatment during the acute SIVmac infection significantly increased viral set points and accelerated the development of simian AIDS despite increasing numbers of CD8 and NK cells and induction of stronger SIV-specific CD8+ T cell responses [165]. Increased plasma levels of IL-15 during the primary infection are correlated with higher susceptibility of memory CD4+ T cells to SIV [166], and IL-15 administration abrogates the vaccine-induced decrease of the viral set point in SIVmac251-infected macaques [167]. All of these studies have shown that effective application of therapeutic IL-15 in HIV infection is problematic, and highly dependent on target cell availability and responsiveness. Treatment during acute HIV infection, although efficient in increasing the number of effector CD4+ T cells, may be detrimental to the HIV patient by generating increased numbers of target cells, while IL-15 treatment during chronic infection will probably fail to induce proliferation of effector memory CD4+ T cells and thus has few chances to result in immune restoration.

IL-7

The rationale for considering IL-7 as an agent for immune reconstitution is the same as for IL-2 and IL-15. Together with IL-2, IL-4, IL-15 and IL-21, IL-7 regulates the expansion and contraction of adaptive T cell subsets [168,169] by increasing proliferation and preventing apoptosis in naive and central memory T cells in mice, humans and NHPs [170–172]. Administration of IL-7 to NHPs impacted both CD4+ and CD8+ T cell compartments from both periphery and tissues (such as lymph nodes, spleen, gut and lungs) by promoting proliferation of naive, central memory, transitional and effector memory subsets [170,173]. No increases of viral loads were observed in either untreated or ART-treated SIV-infected macaques [173–175], thus supporting the idea that IL-7 may be a successful candidate for immunotherapy in HIV-infected patients. The safety and activity of recombinant human IL-7 (rhIL-7) administration were examined in HIV-infected persons [176,177]. Single-dose as well as multiple-dose treatment with subcutaneous rhIL-7 was well tolerated, with injection-site reactions and transient elevations of liver function tests being the most notable side effects. Transient increases in plasma HIV-RNA levels were observed in IL-7-treated patients, especially in those treated with higher doses of the recombinant cytokine. IL-7 induced CD4+ and CD8+ T cells to enter cell cycle; cell-cycle entry was also confirmed for antigen-specific CD8+ T cells. RhIL-7 increased the numbers of circulating CD4+ and CD8+ T cells, predominantly of naive and central memory phenotype. Surprisingly, IL-7 treatment was not associated with T cell activation [177]. The frequency of CD4+ T cells with a regulatory T cell phenotype (CD25^{high}CD127^{low}) did not change after rhIL-7 administration. Due to its biologic and toxicity profile, rhIL-7 seems to be a potential immunotherapeutic agent for HIV infection in combination with ART [176,177]. A possible limitation for the use of Il-7 in HIV patients might be that this cytokine may enhance HIV replication [176−178], induces a state of virus permissiveness in CD4+ T cells [179] and stimulates transcription and replication of the HIV provirus integrated in mononuclear cells [180]. The pharmacokinetic properties of IL-7 allow intermittent cytokine therapy as an adjuvant of ART. Whether this approach may confer a clinical benefit to the HIV patient remains to be established in large-scale clinical studies.

Strategies to Reduce the Number of Target Cells

Receptor (CD4) and coreceptor (CCR5) blockers were successful in preventing mucosal HIV/SIV transmission in humans and rhesus macaques, and are therefore currently being tested as microbicides [181−183].

Clinical trials with the CCR5 antagonist Maraviroc showed that while the ability of this drug to suppress HIV is no better compared to other ART, its ability to induce CD4+ T cell gains is superior to other antiretroviral drugs [184]. This was true even for patients infected with CXCR4-tropic HIV strains, which did not benefit from viral suppression after Maraviroc treatment [185], thus raising the question of whether CCR5 inhibitors may reduce immune activation and inflammation. Indeed, several clinical trials, such as MERIT, the ACTG 5256 pilot trial and a European study, showed that Maraviroc treatment determined a decrease in the levels of CD4+ and CD8+ T cell activation in peripheral but not at mucosal sites. Levels of IL-6, CRP and D-dimer were found to be decreased after Maraviroc administration [186]. Recently, however, the ACTG 5256 trial reported that the CD4+ T cell gain after CCR5 blockage was not shown to be as significant as in earlier studies (MERIT and MOTIVATE trials). Several studies showed that Maraviroc treatment may also impact CCR5+ cell distribution by downregulating the chemotactic activity of neutrophils, dendritic cells and macrophages. For equivalent HIV RNA declines, CCR5-receptor blockade differentially impacted CD8+ T cell and PDC numbers in the circulation. These results confirm that cell surface CCR5 expression on these cells directs trafficking during HIV infection [187]. In conclusion, due to its capacity to significantly reduce VLs in naive or

ART-experienced (and sometimes resistant) HIV patients, low toxicity and capacity to reduce immune activation/inflammation and to improve immune restoration, the CCR5 blockers should be considered valuable candidates for the treatment of HIV patients.

Therapies aimed to block or genetically modify CCR5 are supported by the case of an HIV patient who underwent stem-cell transplantation for acute myeloid leukemia preceded by intensive chemotherapy and total body irradiation. The graft received by this patient was sampled from a CCR5-$\Delta 32/\Delta 32$ donor (and thus naturally resistant to infection with CCR5-tropic viruses due to absence of CCR5 on the cell surface). After transplantation, virus replication became undetectable in the HIV patient despite discontinuation of anti-retroviral therapy [188]. The 3.5-year follow-up of the patient demonstrated cure of the HIV infection, with complete control of viral replication, complete immune reconstitution in blood and intestine, and seroreversion [189].

An alternative hypothetical new HIV treatment, HIV Immunotoxin Therapy (HIT), has been proposed that includes temporary depletion of all CD4+ cells and elimination of the extracellular reservoir with HIV immunotoxin therapy [190]. A combination of humanized antibodies was suggested to achieve this goal: a humanized antibody against CD4 fused to an apoptosis-inducing toxin to deplete HIV host cells, and a humanized antibody against CD21 to void the extracellular reservoir. Once HIV VL reaches zero, the authors suggest withdrawing the HIT and administering reagents (e.g., IL-2) that accelerate the natural replacement of the CD4+ T cells and macrophages. The authors suggest that this method could provide a mechanism to extinguish HIV, but whether this approach is clinically feasible remains to be determined [190].

Control of Microbial Translocation

Permanent translocation of microbial products through the damaged intestinal mucosa was proposed to be one of the mechanisms of chronic hyperimmune activation in pathogenic SIV and HIV infections [150]. Administration of LPS to non-progressive hosts resulted in increased immune activation/inflammation and increased viral loads [191]. Therefore, a therapeutic strategy to block MT in HIV-infected patients appears to be fully justified to control disease progression. This goal may be achieved through several avenues aimed to: (i) block intestinal inflammation; (ii) reduce the gut microbial flora; or (iii) bind LPS at intestinal level and hamper its translocation into the systemic circulation. In the first category we may consider drugs that are currently used for the treatment of inflammatory bowel diseases (ulcerative colitis and Crohn's disease), which are also characterized by high levels of microbial translocation. Several combinations of antibiotics have been reported to be efficient in reducing the levels of microbial translocation in either HIV-infected patients [150] or in patients with hepatic encephalopathy who also have high levels of microbial translocation. Rifaximin is a semisynthetic derivative of rifampin with broad activity against Gram negatives, Gram positives and anaerobes, and thus significantly decreases the gastrointestinal flora [192]. The lack of rifaximin absorption explains both drug efficacy (low risk of resistance due to negligible plasma levels and thus low exposure to selective pressure [193]) and safety in treating enteric infections. Rifaximin is better and safer than other agents (neomycin, metronidazole and cefotaxime) in improving symptoms and reducing ammonia levels in patients with hepatic encephalopathy (another condition associated with MT) [192]. Rifaximin is currently being tested in both SIV-infected macaques and HIV-infected patients. Finally, there are several drugs that can bind/block LPS in the intestinal lumen and may thus improve the levels of microbial translocation in HIV patients. In these categories, two drugs are currently being tested in pathogenic HIV and SIV infections. Sevelamer, a commonly prescribed non-calcium, non-metal-based phosphate binder in CKD, also possesses anti-inflammatory properties, as its use has been associated with a reduction in systemic markers of inflammation. Emerging studies have provided direct evidence that sevelamer shows *in vitro* LPS-binding properties. Indirect clinical evidence suggests that Sevelamer might also limit translocation of LPS from the intestinal lumen into the bloodstream [194]. Immunolin, a natural immunoglobulin bovine product, preserves gut barrier function, neutralizes LPS *in vitro* and reduces the levels of LPS or inflammatory cytokines in several animal models of inflammation [195−197]. Immunolin is currently being tested in HIV-infected patients. Results of these studies will indicate whether the agents mentioned above are good candidates for immunotherapy in HIV-infected patients.

Strategies to Modulate T Regulatory Cells

Numerous studies have generated many conflicting results with regard to the role of this T cell subset in HIV/SIV pathogenesis [142]. Strong evidence that Tregs may play a positive role in controlling immune activation in natural hosts comes from a Treg depletion experiment using Ontak, which directly assessed the role of Tregs in SIV pathogenesis [134]. This experiment demonstrated that even after a modest depletion of Tregs the levels of immune activation increased dramatically in chronically SIVagm-infected AGMs, followed by a significant (3 logs) and sustained increase in VLs and CD4+ T cell depletion at mucosal sites [134]. When AGMs are treated with Ontak during acute SIVagm infection, they lose the capacity to control immune activation and viral replication (Pandrea, unpublished results). These findings corroborate recent studies showing that Tregs are able to suppress viral replication in HIV-infected patients [198], and previous experiments showing that blockade of CTLA-4, a immunoregulatory molecule expressed on activated T cells and a subset of regulatory T cells, significantly increases T cell activation and viral replication in primary SIV_{mac251} infection, particularly at mucosal sites [199].

Altogether, these findings suggest that therapies aimed to increase levels of Tregs or anti-inflammatory cytokines may be beneficial in HIV-infected patients. This idea is supported by the results of a clinical trial (ISS OBS T-002) in which virologically-suppressed HAART-treated individuals were immunized with Tat. Immunization was safe, and induced durable immune responses and persistent increases of regulatory T cells associated with a reduced pattern of CD4+ and CD8+ cellular activation (CD38 and HLA-DR) together with reduction of biochemical activation markers. Increase in central and effector memory and reduction in terminally-differentiated effector memory CD4+ and CD8+ T cells were associated with increases of CD4+ and CD8+ T cell responses against Env and recall antigens. Importantly, the more immune-compromised individuals experienced greater therapeutic effects [200]. These findings support therapies that increase numbers of Tregs or Treg function to intensify HAART efficacy by reducing immune activation, and restoration of immune homeostasis. Recently, it has been shown that whole-body irradiation (used in bone marrow transplants and for cancer treatment) increases the percentage of CD4+CD25+ Treg cells in the periphery, making the hosts favorable to tolerance induction [201]. This method may be an option for individuals who are severely immune compromised and who do not respond to ART and other therapies.

Studies in the murine model suggest that one of the compounds that may inhibit the differentiation and migration of Th17 cells is vitamin D [202]. Furthermore, vitamin D (Alfacalcidol) was reported to improve the Th17/Treg imbalance in vitamin D-deficient patients [203] or in patients with early rheumatoid arthritis [204] by inhibiting the IL-17 expression of Th17 cells and increasing the number of Tregs. Vitamin D also increased the capacity of Treg cells to suppress the proliferation of autologous CD4+CD25− cells [203]. Thus, vitamin D seems to be a easier and safer therapeutic avenue to increasing numbers of Tregs in HIV patients, compared to the transfer of engineered Fox-P3-expressing cells through retroviral-mediated ectopic expression of Fox-P3 [205].

However, due to the dual activity of the Tregs, these therapies should be tested in animal models prior to administration to HIV patients.

Strategies to Manipulate Dendritic Cells

IFN production during HIV/SIV infection is an illustration of a Jekyll-and-Hyde type effect. Two rationales were advanced for administering IFN to HIV patients: (i) IFN has antiviral properties (clearly demonstrated for other viral infections such as hepatitis C); and (ii) cells taken from people with AIDS could not be stimulated to produce IFN in the test tube [206]. Initial studies regarding IFN administration in HIV patients conducted one decade ago generated conflicting results reporting either benefits, such as significant decreases of VLs and increased survival [207−210], or lack of effects on viral replication and clinical course of infection [211], or even decreases in CD4+

T cell numbers [212]. More recent studies have reiterated the capacity of IFN to reduce VLs in HIV-infected patients [213].

However, due to the fact that overproduction of IFN is a feature of pathogenic HIV infection but not of the non-pathogenic infections in sooty mangabeys and AGMs, other recent studies have proposed that IFN may be the cause of chronic aberrant immune activation in pathogenic HIV and SIV infections [133,141]. Furthermore, it is known that IFN inhibits the development of white blood cells, platelets and red blood cell precursors, and selectively inhibits the proliferation of the CD4 lymphocyte subset.

These studies suggested that therapies aimed at inhibiting IFN may be useful in controlling immune activation in HIV-infected patients. Surprisingly, IFN administration to sooty mangabeys that have high viral loads but lack immune activation and IFN production during chronic infection resulted in a reduction of VLs and not the expected opposite effect of increasing immune activation and virus replication (Silvestri, personal communication).

As IFN-α is mainly produced by dendritic cells, alternate therapies were considered to stimulate this immune cell subset to produce antiviral factors using TLR ligands. It was indeed demonstrated that stimulating TLR7 or TLR8 either by single-stranded HIV RNA or by synthetic compounds induced changes in the lymphoid microenvironment unfavorable to HIV. Both TLR7 and TLR8 agonists efficiently inhibited HIV replication in lymphoid suspension cells of tonsillar origin [214]. Also, inactivated-virus-pulsed dendritic cells expanded and eradicated HIV *in vitro* [215]. SIVmac-infected macaques and HIV patients immunized with autologous monocyte-derived DCs loaded with autologous inactivated HIV-1 experienced significant decreases in plasma VL levels [216]. The significant decrease in plasma VL induced by DC immunotherapy was associated with either strong, sustained [217] or only moderate HIV-1-specific cellular responses in the NCT00402142 clinical trial [217,218]. However, other clinical trials have only reported a modest virological response after DC immunotherapy, despite the fact that generally it elicited some degree of immunological response [219–223].

Moreover, when TLR7 or TLR9 agonists were applied intravaginally to prevent mucosal SIV transmission the effect was not protection but the opposite, and resulted in increased inflammation, increased rates of mucosal transmission and higher VLs [224]. Furthermore, the use of CpG as a vaccine adjuvant for an aldrithiol-2-inactivated SIV therapeutic AIDS vaccine, although it enhanced SIV-specific antibody responses, did not improve the control of SIV replication after ART. The lack of benefit of this intervention was reported to be related to the high levels of SIV-specific lymphocyte proliferation in the CpG adjuvant group [225].

These studies indicate that reagents that inhibit TLR7 or TLR9 rather than their agonists would be beneficial to control immune activation. Indeed, blocking of IFN-α production using chloroquine, an endosomal inhibitor, was tested in a novel *in vitro* model system with the aim of characterizing the effects of chloroquine on HIV-1-mediated TLR signaling, IFN-α production and T cell activation, and the results indicated that chloroquine blocks TLR-mediated activation of pDC and MyD88 signaling, as shown by decreases in the levels of the downstream signaling molecules IRAK-4 and IRF-7 and by inhibition of IFN-α synthesis [152]. Chloroquine decreased CD8+ T cell activation induced by aldrithiol-2-treated HIV-1 in peripheral blood mononuclear cell cultures. In addition to blocking pDC activation, chloroquine also blocked negative modulators of the T cell response, such as indoleamine 2,3-dioxygenase (IDO) and programmed death ligand 1 (PDL-1) [226]. This study indicates that TLR stimulation and production of IFN-α by pDC contributes to immune activation, and that blocking of these pathways using chloroquine may interfere with events contributing to HIV pathogenesis. These results suggest that a safe, well-tolerated drug such as chloroquine can be proposed as an adjuvant therapeutic candidate along with highly active antiretroviral therapy to control immune activation in HIV-1 infection [226]. These data corroborate clinical studies showing that the frequency of CD38+ HLA-DR+ CD8 T cells, as well as Ki-67 expression in CD8+ and CD4+ T cells, was significantly reduced during chloroquine treatment in HIV patients. These data indicate that *in vivo* treatment with chloroquine reduces systemic T cell immune activation, and thus the use of chloroquine may be beneficial for certain groups of HIV-infected individuals [227,228].

All the data presented so far indicate that therapies aimed to modulate the function of dendritic cells and IFN production should be carefully tested and applied with caution due to possible dual effects.

Strategies to Manipulate Th17 Cells

Previous studies have proposed that loss of Th17 cells in the gut during HIV/SIV pathogenic infections may contribute to loss of preservation of gut epithelial integrity, low resistance against gut flora and increased microbial translocation [104,145,146]. In high contrast, Th17 cells are preserved in non-progressive SIV infection of natural hosts [104,145]. Altogether, these studies suggest that therapies aimed to increase the number of Th17 cells may be beneficial for HIV patients. This may be achieved by administration of adalimumab, an anti-TNF blocker that was shown to increase frequency of Th17 cells as well IL-17 production by peripheral T helper cells in rheumatoid arthritis (RA) patients [229]. Note, however, that the increase in peripheral Th17 cells in RA patients after anti-TNF therapy is accompanied by a decrease in Th17-specific CCR6 expression, which might prevent homing of these potentially pro-inflammatory cells to the tissues where they are needed in order to improve the outcome of the HIV infection [230]. The alternative of increasing Th17 cells by using the anti-CTLA4 blocking antibody tremelimumab (which was shown to increase Th17 cells in the peripheral blood of patients with metastatic melanoma) is not clinically feasible due to high toxicity. However, the relation between increases in Th17 cells and severe autoimmune toxicity after CTLA4 blockade may provide insights into the mechanisms of the anti-CTLA4-induced toxicities [231]. Finally, administration of IL-21 or IL-23 and TGF-β, three cytokines involved in differentiation of Th17 cells, may be an alternative solution to restore the numbers of Th17 cells in HIV-infected patients [232].

Th17 cells also have very strong pro-inflammatory properties [230,233], and therefore they may fuel HIV/SIV infection during early stages by increasing the number of target cells in the gut. Combined with increasing gut inflammation through pro-inflammatory cytokine production, this effect may result in increased damage of the intestinal barrier and translocation of microbes into the circulation, which in turn will contribute to increased immune activation. Moreover, during the chronic phase preserved or even increased numbers of pro-inflammatory Th17 cells from other compartments such as lymph nodes, blood and lung may also contribute to the increased levels of systemic immune activation/inflammation and to both AIDS progression and to non-HIV/SIV related deaths through co-morbidities such as cardiovascular and lung disease. The second scenario is supported by studies that found that HIV-infected patients have a significant increase in IL-17-producing CD4+ T cells compared to seronegative individuals [234]. Finally, recent reports have shown that Th17 cells could potentially enhance viral persistence and inhibit T-cell cytotoxicity in a model of murine chronic virus infection [235]. These data would suggest that reducing Th17 numbers may be an option aimed to reduce immune activation and inflammation in the HIV-infected patient. This aim may be achieved by administration of anti-IL-23 or anti-IL-21 antibodies. Anti-IL-23 antibodies are already successfully used in the treatment of inflammatory bowel disease such as Crohn's disease and ulcerative colitis, as well as in treatment of psoriasis, rheumatoid arthritis and multiple sclerosis— all chronic inflammatory conditions. The efficacy of an anti-IL-23 antibody is currently being tested in SIV-infected NHPs.

Immune-Suppressive Drugs

The natural hosts demonstrated that keeping immune activation/inflammation at bay even in the presence of high viral replication allows immune recovery and prevents disease progression. On the other hand, HIV-infected patients do not achieve normal levels of immune activation even when virally suppressed on HAART. Thus, immunosuppressive drugs may be required for controlling these high levels of immune activation and their deleterious effects during HIV infection. Several classes of drugs have been tested during clinical trials, in association with ART or not [152,236]. The use of immunosuppressive drug therapy in HIV-infected patients has so far not shown major detrimental effects, and some drugs in combination with HAART have even demonstrated possible beneficial effects for specific HIV settings [237].

Cyclosporin A

Cyclosporin A is a calcineurin inhibitor used to prevent rejection after kidney, liver, bone marrow and pancreas transplants [238], as well as in the management of diverse autoimmune disorders such as psoriasis, rheumatoid arthritis, atopic dermatitis, etc. Cyclosporine inhibits T cell activation, proliferation, effector functions (pro-inflammatory cytokine production such as Il-2, IL-4 and TNF-α) and apoptosis [238]. Cyclosporine also upregulates the function of suppressor T cells and the expression of the anti-inflammatory cytokine TGF-β [152,239]. Moreover, cyclosporine can modulate HIV infectivity by forming a complex in the virion core with HIV-Gag protein, disrupting cyclophilin incorporation into virions and blocking nuclear import of HIV-DNA in activated CD4+T cells [240,241].

Increases in the numbers of CD4+ T cells were reported in HIV patients treated with cyclosporine, but the number of T helper cells returned to pretreatment levels at treatment discontinuation [242]. The follow-up of the cyclosporine-treated patients [243] did not show significant improvements in the clinical course of HIV infection. These initial studies were followed by a small-scale study in which HIV patients were treated with cyclosporine and ART during the primary infection for a 8-week period, and compared to patients treated with HAART alone. Viral replication was suppressed at comparable levels in the patients treated with cyclosporine + ART vs ART alone, but CD4+ T cell recovery and the proportion of INF-γ secreting CD4+ T cells were significantly higher in the cyclosporine + ART-treated patients compared to those treated with HAART alone. These data suggested that administration of cyclosporine reduces the levels of immune activation during acute infection and has a beneficial impact on the long course of infection [244]. However, a more recent randomized, clinical trial reported no virologic, immunologic, or clinical benefit of immunosuppression with cyclosporine as an adjunct to ART in patients identified and treated during acute HIV-1 infection. Reduced proliferation of T cells during treatment rules out insufficient drug levels as an explanation for the lack of benefit [245]. Furthermore, a study in chronically infected HIV patients showed no clinical and immunologic benefit, and demonstrated that cyclosporine administration resulted in an increase in viral replication [246]. Altogether, these studies suggest that cyclosporine treatment is not indicated in the management of HIV-1 infection.

Mycophenolic Acid (MPA)

There are several reasons why MPA has been considered as a candidate for therapy in HIV patients. First, MPA selectively inhibits the *de novo* synthesis of purines in T and B lymphocytes, thus preventing proliferation of these lymphocytes [247,248]. Second, it has been shown that MPA suppresses HIV replication *in vitro* and enhances antiviral activity of specific anti-HIV drugs, such as NRTI currently used in ARV combinations such as abacavir [249], didanosine (ddI) and tenofovir (TFV) [250,251]. Finally, MPA is effective *in vitro* both against wild-type and NRTI-resistant HIV strains [250,251].

Initial clinical studies suggested a beneficial effect of MPA in reducing viremia even in patients with late-stage advanced AIDS with multidrug-resistant HIV infection [249]. MPA also decreased the numbers of proliferating CD4+ and CD8+ T cells and the viral load from purified CD4+ T cells [249]. Furthermore, in patients treated with MPA after HAART interruption, a reduced rebound of plasma VL compared with patients who did not receive MPA was observed [249]. The patients who received MPA achieved longer-term control of virus replication (greater than 1 year) compared with the control group after HAART interruption. The conclusion was that HAART interruption along with MPA was safe, and it may prolong the control of virus replication [252]. The results from other clinical studies, however, have failed to show significant decreases in HIV viremia or in the number of latently infected cells [253,254]. Thus, more data are necessary to establish whether mycophenolic acid is a good therapy for HIV patient management.

Glucocorticoids

Glucocorticoids are steroid hormones involved in suppressing inflammation by binding to the glucocoticoid receptor and thus upregulating the expression of anti-inflammatory proteins in the nucleus and repressing the expression of pro-inflammatory proteins (cytokines, enzymes, receptors and adhesion molecules) in the cytoplasm. Glucocorticoids are therefore used to treat diseases caused by a hyperactive immune system, such as rheumatoid arthritis, asthma, inflammatory bowel disease and autoimmune diseases. In many of these circumstances they are the most effective therapy available [255]. Preclinical studies have shown that glucocorticoids rescue CD4+ T cells from activation-induced apoptosis triggered by HIV-1 [256]. Prednisolone given to patients with asymptomatic HIV infection for 1 year resulted in a significant improvement of CD4+ T cell counts as a consequence of reduction of the levels of T cell apoptosis and activation. No modifications in VLs were observed. The drug had only mild side effects [257,258]. Long-term follow-up of the same patients demonstrated that prednisolone delayed CD4+ T cell loss in a VL-dependent manner for a median of 2 years [259].

In a more recent study, the prednisolone-treated patients had a stable CD4 cell count over 3 years. There were no significant differences in VLs between the prednisolone treated and untreated patients. The same results were obtained in patients treated with prednisolone in conjunction with structured treatment interruption [260]. All these results suggest that low-dose glucocorticoids may be beneficial to preserve the CD4+ helper T cells in HIV patients and to reduce the duration of HAART. There are, however, some side effects reported for this type of therapy that should be more thoroughly investigated. Also, the efficacy of corticosteroids should be tested in more prospective randomized trials.

Rapamycin

Rapamycin (Rapamune, Sirolimus) is a macrolide exhibiting potent antitumor and immunosuppressive activity [261,262]. Rapamycin is thus used in clinical settings to prevent rejection in organ transplantation and to treat certain types of cancer. Rapamycin inhibits the response to IL-2, and thereby blocks activation and proliferation of T and B cells [263]. Treatment of human T lymphoid cells with rapamycin resulted in a marked diminution of HIV-1 transcription [264]. In addition, rapamycin synergistically enhances the anti-HIV activity of entry inhibitors such as vicriviroc, aplaviroc and enfuvirtide *in vitro* [265]. It was also shown that rapamycin inhibits HIV-1 replication *in vitro* through other different mechanisms, including downregulation of CCR5 on lymphocytes and monocytes [265,266]. All these effects support the use of rapamycin in addition to ART. Its efficacy remains, however, to be established in clinical trials.

Hydroxyurea

Hydroxyurea, an inhibitor of DNA synthesis, is a drug used in myeloproliferative disorders such as polycythemia vera and essential thrombocythemia. It is also used to reduce the rate of attacks in sickle-cell disease, and in the treatment of psoriasis and systemic mastocytosis. By inhibiting ribonucleotide reductase, hydroxyurea depletes the pool of deoxynucleoside triphosphates, particularly dATP, available for DNA synthesis. *In vitro* experiments have demonstrated control of viral production in activated and resting T cells by hydroxyurea [267–269]. Other activities of hydroxyurea include potentation of the activity of nucleoside reverse transcriptase inhibitors (NRTIs), compensation for resistance to adenosine analogue NRTIs, and potential increased phosphorylation of pyrimidine NRTIs. Beneficial immunomodulatory effects of hydroxyurea, such as decreasing levels of cell proliferation, decreasing activation of CD8+ T cells, increasing levels of naive CD4+ and CD8+ T cells, and preservation of the HIV-1-specific immune response, were also reported [268]. Thus, hydroxyurea has been used in clinical trials for the treatment of HIV patients in combination with nucleoside analogs. The results of these initial studies are variable, and indicate either that hydroxyurea is safe and augments suppression of HIV-1 replication when used in combination with didanosine, stavudine and lamivudine [270–275], or shows severe side effects and no beneficial effect on plasma VL or CD4+ T cell numbers [276–278]. More recent clinical trials reported that the side effects of hydroxyurea overwhelmed the beneficial effects on VL, immune reconstitution and levels of immune activation [279]. Additional studies showed that addition of hydroxyurea to ART (ABC/EFV/ddI) blunted the CD4+ cell response, did not appear to enhance antiviral activity, and resulted in more treatment-limiting adverse events [280].

Increase Cellular Immune Responses

Anti-PD-1

Based on the observation that in HIV infection the level of expression of co-inhibitory receptor programmed death-1 (PD-1) on T cells correlates with increased VLs, decreased CD4+ T cell counts and decreased HIV-specific T cell function [281], an anti-PD-1 is considered a promising immunotherapy for HIV [282]. PD-1 blockade in SIV-infected rhesus macaques, however, resulted in conflicting results. On one hand, PD-1 blockade using an antibody to PD-1 resulted in rapid expansion of virus-specific CD8+ T cells with improved functional quality in both blood and gut. PD-1 blockade also resulted in proliferation of memory B cells and increases in SIV envelope-specific antibody. These improved immune responses were associated with significant reductions in plasma VL and also prolonged survival of SIV-infected macaques [283]. In another study, consistent improvements in VLs were not observed after anti-PD-1 administration. In this study, the impact of PD-1 blockade on the magnitude and function of SIV-specific T cell responses was evaluated, but no significant differences were observed. In terms of CD4+ T cell counts, PD-1 blockade resulted only in transient increases [284].

Thus, the efficacy of anti-PD-1 reagents should be more extensively tested to establish their real benefit. Also, it should be noted that PD-1 may play an important role in switching off potentially harmful T cell responses that target body tissues thus causing autoimmune disease, which may have a severe negative effect on HIV patients.

CONCLUSIONS

Studies in natural hosts of SIVs have demonstrated that controlling immune activation prevents disease progression even in the context of high VLs over long periods of time. Currently, ARV therapies do not completely control immune activation/inflammation in HIV patients, resulting in incomplete immune reconstitution, non-HIV co-morbidities (cardiovascular diseases) and premature aging. It is generally agreed that management of the HIV-infected patient should include strategies to keep reducing immune activation/inflammation. The numerous studies carried out thus far have established significant milestones in this area of investigation. These trials, however, have been unsuccessful or shown opposing results, with the same agents being reported to have either beneficial effects or harmful consequences in different trials. This can be explained by the complexity of the mechanisms responsible for aberrant immune activation in progressive HIV/SIV infections, and by the differences in the severity and the causes of immune activation at different time points during infection. Immune activation being determined by multiple factors will make it very difficult to find a single agent, or to fine-tune a combination of agents, that may normalize it. Also, such drug combinations should probably be tailored to patients that are acutely *versus* chronically infected, to address the factors that are critical in inducing immune activation. Testing immunotherapies in HIV patients at different stages of infection, undergoing different regimens of ART and having different lifestyle risk factors for increasing IA/INFL and co-morbidities may hide the effects (either positive or negative) of these therapies or may result in opposite and thus confusing results in different clinical trials.

The animal models of HIV/AIDS offer an opportunity for testing immunotherapeutic agents during different stages of infection (which can be thoroughly defined by immunologic and virologic parameters), in the presence or absence of ART and in the absence of lifestyle risk factors such as alcohol consumption, smoking and diet. These models may be thus very useful for preclinical studies that test the safety and efficacy of immunomodulatory agents.

Efforts in developing, testing and combining immunomodulatory drugs are only in their infancy, and research in this area should continue in order to develop therapies that will improve HIV patients' survival, in the same way that ART did a decade ago.

REFERENCES

[1] VandeWoude S, Apetrei C. Going wild: Lessons from T-lymphotropic naturally occurring lentiviruses. Clin Microbiol Rev 2006;19:728−62.

[2] Hahn BH, Shaw GM, De Cock KM, Sharp PM. AIDS as a zoonosis: Scientific and public health implications. Science 2000;287:607−14.

[3] Aghokeng AF, Ayouba A, Mpoudi-Ngole E, Loul S, Liegeois F, Delaporte E, et al. Extensive survey on the prevalence and genetic diversity of SIVs in primate bushmeat provides insights into risks for potential new cross-species transmissions. Infect Genet Evol 2009;10:386−96.

[4] Miller RJ, Cairns JS, Bridges S, Sarver N. Human immunodeficiency virus and AIDS: Insights from animal lentiviruses. J Virol 2000;74:7187−95.

[5] Van Heuverswyn F, Li Y, Neel C, Bailes E, Keele BF, Liu W, et al. Human immunodeficiency viruses: SIV infection in wild gorillas. Nature 2006;444:164.

[6] Plantier JC, Leoz M, Dickerson JE, De Oliveira F, Cordonnier F, Lemee V, et al. A new human immunodeficiency virus derived from gorillas. Nat Med 2009;15:871−2.

[7] Apetrei C, Kaur A, Lerche NW, Metzger M, Pandrea I, Hardcastle J, et al. Molecular epidemiology of simian immunodeficiency virus SIVsm in US Primate Centers unravels the origin of SIVmac and SIVstm. J Virol 2005;79:8991−9005.

[8] Murphey-Corb M, Martin LN, Rangan SR, Baskin GB, Gormus BJ, Wolf RH, et al. Isolation of an HTLV-III-related retrovirus from macaques with simian AIDS and its possible origin in asymptomatic mangabeys. Nature 1986;321:435−7.

[9] Pandrea I, Apetrei C. Where the wild things are: Pathogenesis of SIV infection in African nonhuman primate hosts. Curr HIV/AIDS Rep 2010;7:28−36.

[10] Pandrea I, Sodora DL, Silvestri G, Apetrei C. Into the wild: Simian immunodeficiency virus (SIV) infection in natural hosts. Trends Immunol 2008;29:419−28.

[11] Pandrea I, Silvestri G, Apetrei C. AIDS in African nonhuman primate hosts of SIVs: A new paradigm of SIV infection. Curr HIV Res 2009;6:57−72.

[12] Pandrea I, Onanga R, Rouquet P, Bourry O, Ngari P, Wickings EJ, et al. Chronic SIV infection ultimately causes immunodeficiency in African non-human primates. AIDS 2001;15:2461−2.

[13] Beer BE, Bailes E, Sharp PM, Hirsch VM. Diversity and evolution of primate lentiviruses. In: Kuiken CL, Foley B, Hahn B, Korber B, McCutchan F, Marx PA, et al., editors. Human Retroviruses and AIDS. Los Alamos, NM: Los Alamos National Laboratory; 1999. p. 460−74.

[14] Gordon S, Pandrea I, Dunham R, Apetrei C, Silvestri G. The call of the wild: What can be learned from studies of SIV infection of natural hosts? In: Leitner T, Foley B, Hahn B, Marx P, McCutchan F, Mellors J, et al., editors. HIV Sequence Compendium 2004. Los Alamos, NM: Theoretical Biology and Biophysics Group, Los Alamos National Laboratory; 2005. p. 2−29.

[15] Sharp PM, Bailes E, Gao F, Beer BE, Hirsch VM, Hahn BH. Origins and evolution of AIDS viruses: Estimating the time-scale. Biochem Soc Trans 2000;28:275−82.

[16] Sharp PM, Shaw GM, Hahn BH. Simian immunodeficiency virus infection of chimpanzees. J Virol 2005;79:3891−902.

[17] Bibollet-Ruche F, Galat-Luong A, Cuny G, Sarni-Manchado P, Galat G, Durand JP, et al. Simian immunodeficiency virus infection in a patas monkey (*Erythrocebus patas*): evidence for cross-species transmission from African green monkeys (*Cercopithecus aethiops sabaeus*) in the wild. J Gen Virol 1996;77:773−81.

[18] Hirsch VM, Dapolito GA, Goldstein S, McClure H, Emau P, Fultz PN, et al. A distinct African lentivirus from Sykes' monkeys. J Virol 1993;67:1517−28.

[19] Bibollet-Ruche F, Bailes E, Gao F, Pourrut X, Barlow KL, Clewley J, et al. A new simian immunodeficiency virus lineage (SIVdeb) infecting de Brazza's monkeys (*Cercopithecus neglectus*): Evidence for a *Cercopithecus* monkey virus clade. J Virol 2004;78:7748−62.

[20] Courgnaud V, Abela B, Pourrut X, Mpoudi-Ngole E, Loul S, Delaporte E, et al. Identification of a new simian immunodeficiency virus lineage with a *vpu* gene present among different *Cercopithecus* monkeys (*C. mona, C. cephus,* and *C. nictitans*) from Cameroon. J Virol 2003;77:12523−34.

[21] Courgnaud V, Salemi M, Pourrut X, Mpoudi-Ngole E, Abela B, Auzel P, et al. Characterization of a novel simian immunodeficiency virus with a *vpu* gene from greater spot-nosed monkeys (*Cercopithecus nictitans*) provides new insights into simian/human immunodeficiency virus phylogeny. J Virol 2002;76:8298−309.

[22] Dazza MC, Ekwalanga M, Nende M, Bin Shamamba K, Bitshi P, Saragosti S. Characterization of novel simian immunodeficiency virus from *Cercopithecus mona denti* (SIVden) from the Democratic Republic of Congo. J Virol 2005;79: 8560−71.

[23] Aghokeng AF, Bailes E, Loul S, Courgnaud V, Mpoudi-Ngolle E, Sharp PM, et al. Full-length sequence analysis of SIVmus in wild populations of mustached monkeys (*Cercopithecus cephus*) from Cameroon provides evidence for two co-circulating SIVmus lineages. Virology 2007;360:407−18.

[24] Verschoor EJ, Fagrouch Z, Bontjer I, Niphuis H, Heeney JL. A novel simian immunodeficiency virus isolated from a Schmidt's guenon (*Cercopithecus ascanius schmidti*). J Gen Virol 2004;85:21−4.

[25] Osterhaus AD, Pedersen N, van Amerongen G, Frankenhuis MT, Marthas M, Reay E, et al. Isolation and partial characterization of a lentivirus from talapoin monkeys (*Myopithecus talapoin*). Virology 1999;260:116−24.

[26] Liegeois F, Courgnaud V, Switzer WM, Murphy HW, Loul S, Aghokeng A, et al. Molecular characterization of a novel simian immunodeficiency virus lineage (SIVtal) from northern talapoins (*Miopithecus ogouensis*). Virology 2006;349:55−65.

[27] Takemura T, Ekwalanga M, Bikandou B, Ido E, Yamaguchi-Kabata Y, Ohkura S, et al. A novel simian immunodeficiency virus from black mangabey (*Lophocebus aterrimus*) in the Democratic Republic of Congo. J Gen Virol 2005;86:1967−71.

[28] Apetrei C, Metzger MJ, Richardson D, Ling B, Telfer PT, Reed P, et al. Detection and partial characterization of simian immunodeficiency virus SIVsm strains from bush meat samples from rural Sierra Leone. J Virol 2005;79:2631−6.

[29] Damond F, Apetrei C, Robertson DL, Souquiere S, Lepretre A, Matheron S, et al. Variability of human immunodeficiency virus type 2 (HIV-2) infecting patients living in France. Virology 2001;280:19−30.

[30] Damond F, Worobey M, Campa P, Farfara I, Colin G, Matheron S, et al. Identification of a highly divergent HIV type 2 and proposal for a change in HIV type 2 classification. AIDS Res Hum Retroviruses 2004;20:666−72.

[31] Allan JS, Short M, Taylor ME, Su S, Hirsch VM, Johnson PR, et al. Species-specific diversity among simian immunodeficiency viruses from African green monkeys. J Virol 1991;65:2816−28.

[32] Jin MJ, Hui H, Robertson DL, Muller MC, Barre-Sinoussi F, Hirsch VM, et al. Mosaic genome structure of simian immunodeficiency virus from west African green monkeys. EMBO J 1994;13:2935−47.

[33] Hirsch VM, McGann C, Dapolito G, Goldstein S, Ogen-Odoi A, Biryawaho B, et al. Identification of a new subgroup of SIVagm in tantalus monkeys. Virology 1993;197: 426−30.

[34] Fomsgaard A, Allan J, Gravell M, London WT, Hirsch VM, Johnson PR. Molecular characterization of simian lentiviruses from east African green monkeys. J Med Primatol 1990;19:295−303.

[35] Muller MC, Saksena NK, Nerrienet E, Chappey C, Herve VM, Durand JP, et al. Simian immunodeficiency viruses from central and western Africa: Evidence for a new species-specific lentivirus in tantalus monkeys. J Virol 1993;67:1227−35.

[36] Fukasawa M, Miura T, Hasegawa A, Morikawa S, Tsujimoto H, Miki K, et al. Sequence of simian immunodeficiency virus from African green monkey, a new member of the HIV/SIV group. Nature 1988;333:457−61.

[37] Bailes E, Gao F, Bibollet-Ruche F, Courgnaud V, Peeters M, Marx PA, et al. Hybrid origin of SIV in chimpanzees. Science 2003;300:1713.

[38] Tsujimoto H, Cooper RW, Kodama T, Fukasawa M, Miura T, Ohta Y, et al. Isolation and characterization of simian immunodeficiency virus from mandrills in Africa and its relationship to other human and simian immunodeficiency viruses. J Virol 1988;62:4044−50.

[39] Tsujimoto H, Hasegawa A, Maki N, Fukasawa M, Miura T, Speidel S, et al. Sequence of a novel simian immunodeficiency virus from a wild-caught African mandrill. Nature 1989;341:539−41.

[40] Hirsch VM, Campbell BJ, Bailes E, Goeken R, Brown C, Elkins WR, et al. Characterization of a novel simian immunodeficiency virus (SIV) from l'Hoest monkeys (*Cercopithecus l'hoesti*): Implications for the origins of SIVmnd and other primate lentiviruses. J Virol 1999;73:1036−45.

[41] Beer BE, Bailes E, Dapolito G, Campbell BJ, Goeken RM, Axthelm MK, et al. Patterns of genomic sequence diversity among their simian immunodeficiency viruses suggest that l'Hoest monkeys (*Cercopithecus l'hoesti*) are a natural lentivirus reservoir. J Virol 2000;74:3892−8.

[42] Beer BE, Bailes E, Goeken R, Dapolito G, Coulibaly C, Norley SG, et al. Simian immunodeficiency virus (SIV) from sun-tailed monkeys (*Cercopithecus solatus*): Evidence for host-dependent evolution of SIV within the *C. l'hoesti* superspecies. J Virol 1999;73:7734—44.

[43] Worobey M, Telfer P, Souquiere S, Hunter M, Coleman CA, Metzger MJ, et al. Island biogeography reveals the deep history of SIV. Science 329:1487.

[44] Georges-Courbot MC, Lu CY, Makuwa M, Telfer P, Onanga R, Dubreuil G, et al. Natural infection of a household pet red-capped mangabey (*Cercocebus torquatus torquatus*) with a new simian immunodeficiency virus. J Virol 1998;72:600—8.

[45] Beer BE, Foley BT, Kuiken CL, Tooze Z, Goeken RM, Brown CR, et al. Characterization of novel simian immunodeficiency viruses from red-capped mangabeys from Nigeria (SIVrcmNG409 and -NG411). J Virol 2001;75:12014—27.

[46] Souquiere S, Bibollet-Ruche F, Robertson DL, Makuwa M, Apetrei C, Onanga R, et al. Wild *Mandrillus sphinx* are carriers of two types of lentivirus. J Virol 2001;75:7086—96.

[47] Courgnaud V, Pourrut X, Bibollet-Ruche F, Mpoudi-Ngole E, Bourgeois A, Delaporte E, et al. Characterization of a novel simian immunodeficiency virus from guereza colobus monkeys (*Colobus guereza*) in Cameroon: A new lineage in the nonhuman primate lentivirus family. J Virol 2001;75:857—66.

[48] Courgnaud V, Formenty P, Akoua-Koffi C, Noe R, Boesch C, Delaporte E, et al. Partial molecular characterization of two simian immunodeficiency viruses (SIV) from African colobids: SIVwrc from Western red colobus (*Piliocolobus badius*) and SIVolc from olive colobus (*Procolobus verus*). J Virol 2003;77:744—8.

[49] Locatelli S, Lafay B, Liegeois F, Ting N, Delaporte E, Peeters M. Full molecular characterization of a simian immunodeficiency virus, SIVwrcpbt from Temminck's red colobus (*Piliocolobus badius temminckii*) from Abuko Nature Reserve, The Gambia. Virology 2008;376:90—100.

[50] Apetrei C, Marx PA. African lentiviruses related to HIV. J Neurovirol 2005;11(Suppl. 1):33—49.

[51] Apetrei C, Robertson DL, Marx PA. The history of SIVs and AIDS: Epidemiology, phylogeny and biology of isolates from naturally SIV infected non-human primates (NHP) in Africa. Front Biosci 2004;9:225—54.

[52] Jin MJ, Rogers J, Phillips-Conroy JE, Allan JS, Desrosiers RC, Shaw GM, et al. Infection of a yellow baboon with simian immunodeficiency virus from African green monkeys: Evidence for cross-species transmission in the wild. J Virol 1994;68:8454—60.

[53] van Rensburg EJ, Engelbrecht S, Mwenda J, Laten JD, Robson BA, Stander T, et al. Simian immunodeficiency viruses (SIVs) from eastern and southern Africa: Detection of a SIVagm variant from a chacma baboon. J Gen Virol 1998;79:1809—14.

[54] Tomonaga K, Katahira J, Fukasawa M, Hassan MA, Kawamura M, Akari H, et al. Isolation and characterization of simian immunodeficiency virus from African white-crowned mangabey monkeys (*Cercocebus torquatus lunulatus*). Arch Virol 1993;129:77—92.

[55] Apetrei C, Gaufin T, Gautam R, Vinton C, Hirsch V, Lewis M, et al. Pattern of SIVagm infection in patas monkeys suggests that host adaptation to simian immunodeficiency virus infection may result in resistance to infection and virus extinction. J Infect Dis 2010;202(Suppl. 3):S371—376.

[56] Barlow KL, Ajao AO, Clewley JP. Characterization of a novel simian immunodeficiency virus (SIVmonNG1) genome sequence from a mona monkey (*Cercopithecus mona*). J Virol 2003;77:6879—88.

[57] Mitani JC, Watts DP. Demographic influences on the hunting behavior of chimpanzees. Am J Phys Anthropol 1999;109:439—54.

[58] Watts DP, Mitani JC. Hunting behaviour of chimpanzees at Ngogo, Kibale national Park, Uganda. Intl J Primatol 2002;23:1−28.

[59] Clavel F, Guetard D, Brun-Vezinet F, Chamaret S, Rey MA, Santos-Ferreira MO, et al. Isolation of a new human retrovirus from West African patients with AIDS. Science 1986;233:343−6.

[60] Clavel F, Guyader M, Guetard D, Salle M, Montagnier L, Alizon M. Molecular cloning and polymorphism of the human immune deficiency virus type 2. Nature 1986;324: 691−5.

[61] Chen Z, Luckay A, Sodora DL, Telfer P, Reed P, Gettie A, et al. Human immunodeficiency virus type 2 (HIV-2) seroprevalence and characterization of a distinct HIV-2 genetic subtype from the natural range of simian immunodeficiency virus-infected sooty mangabeys. J Virol 1997;71:3953−60.

[62] Gao F, Yue L, Robertson DL, Hill SC, Hui H, Biggar RJ, et al. Genetic diversity of human immunodeficiency virus type 2: Evidence for distinct sequence subtypes with differences in virus biology. J Virol 1994;68:7433−47.

[63] Gao F, Bailes E, Robertson DL, Chen Y, Rodenburg CM, Michael SF, et al. Origin of HIV-1 in the chimpanzee *Pan troglodytes troglodytes*. Nature 1999;397:436−41.

[64] Peeters M, Honore C, Huet T, Bedjabaga L, Ossari S, Bussi P, et al. Isolation and partial characterization of an HIV-related virus occurring naturally in chimpanzees in Gabon. AIDS 1989;3:625−30.

[65] Simon F, Mauclere P, Roques P, Loussert-Ajaka I, Muller-Trutwin MC, Saragosti S, et al. Identification of a new human immunodeficiency virus type 1 distinct from group M and group O. Nat Med 1998;4:1032−7.

[66] Roques P, Robertson DL, Souquiere S, Apetrei C, Nerrienet E, Barre-Sinoussi F, et al. Phylogenetic characteristics of three new HIV-1 N strains and implications for the origin of group N. AIDS 2004;18:1371−81.

[67] Muller-Trutwin MC, Corbet S, Souquiere S, Roques P, Versmisse P, Ayouba A, et al. SIVcpz from a naturally infected Cameroonian chimpanzee: Biological and genetic comparison with HIV-1 N. J Med Primatol 2000;29:166−72.

[68] Keele BF, Van Heuverswyn F, Li Y, Bailes E, Takehisa J, Santiago ML, et al. Chimpanzee reservoirs of pandemic and nonpandemic HIV-1. Science 2006;313:523−6.

[69] Apetrei C, Marx PA. Simian retroviral infections in human beings. Lancet 2004;364:137−8.

[70] Marx PA, Apetrei C, Drucker E. AIDS as a zoonosis? Confusion over the origin of the virus and the origin of the epidemics. J Med Primatol 2004;33:220−6.

[71] Drucker E, Alcabes PG, Marx PA. The injection century: Massive unsterile injections and the emergence of human pathogens. Lancet 2001;358:1989−92.

[72] Apetrei C, Lerche NW, Pandrea I, Gormus B, Metzger M, Silvestri G, et al. Kuru experiments triggered the emergence of pathogenic SIVmac. AIDS 2006;20:317−21.

[73] Mansfield KG, Lerche NW, Gardner MB, Lackner AA. Origins of simian immunodeficiency virus infection in macaques at the New England Regional Primate Research Center. J Med Primatol 1995;24:116−22.

[74] Gormus BJ, Martin LN, Baskin GB. A brief history of the discovery of natural simian immunodeficiency virus (SIV) infections in captive sooty mangabey monkeys. Front Biosci 2004;9:216−24.

[75] Hirsch VM, Dapolito G, Goeken R, Campbell BJ. Phylogeny and natural history of the primate lentiviruses, SIV and HIV. Curr Opin Genet Dev 1995;5:798−806.

[76] Hirsch VM, Johnson PR. Pathogenic diversity of simian immunodeficiency viruses. Virus Res 1994;32:183−203.

[77] Khan AS, Galvin TA, Lowenstine LJ, Jennings MB, Gardner MB, Buckler CE. A highly divergent simian immunodeficiency virus (SIVstm) recovered from stored stump-tailed macaque tissues. J Virol 1991;65:7061−5.

[78] Lowenstine LJ, Lerche NW, Yee JL, Uyeda A, Jennings MB, Munn RJ, et al. Evidence for a lentiviral etiology in an epizootic of immune deficiency and lymphoma in stump-tailed macaques (*Macaca arctoides*). J Med Primatol 1992;21:1−14.

[79] Daniel MD, Letvin NL, King NW, Kannagi M, Sehgal PK, Hunt RD, et al. Isolation of T-cell tropic HTLV-III-like retrovirus from macaques. Science 1985;228:1201−4.

[80] Letvin NL, Daniel MD, Sehgal PK, Desrosiers RC, Hunt RD, Waldron LM, et al. Induction of AIDS-like disease in macaque monkeys with T-cell tropic retrovirus STLV-III. Science 1985;230:71−3.

[81] Gardner MB. The history of simian AIDS. J Med Primatol 1996;25:148−57.

[82] Hunt RD, Blake BJ, Chalifoux LV, Sehgal PK, King NW, Letvin NL. Transmission of naturally occurring lymphoma in macaque monkeys. Proc Natl Acad Sci USA 1983;80:5085−9.

[83] Benveniste RE, Arthur LO, Tsai CC, Sowder R, Copeland TD, Henderson LE, et al. Isolation of a lentivirus from a macaque with lymphoma: Comparison with HTLV-III/LAV and other lentiviruses. J Virol 1986;60:483−90.

[84] Morton WR, Kuller L, Benveniste RE, Clark EA, Tsai CC, Gale MJ, et al. Transmission of the simian immunodeficiency virus SIVmne in macaques and baboons. J Med Primatol 1989;18:237−45.

[85] Fultz PN, Zack PM. Unique lentivirus−host interactions: SIVsmmPBj14 infection of macaques. Virus Res 1994;32:205−25.

[86] Fultz PN, McClure HM, Anderson DC, Switzer WM. Identification and biologic characterization of an acutely lethal variant of simian immunodeficiency virus from sooty mangabeys (SIV/SMM). AIDS Res Hum Retroviruses 1989;5:397−409.

[87] Kaur A, Grant RM, Means RE, McClure H, Feinberg M, Johnson RP. Diverse host responses and outcomes following simian immunodeficiency virus SIVmac239 infection in sooty mangabeys and rhesus macaques. J Virol 1998;72:9597−611.

[88] Pandrea IV, Gautam R, Ribeiro RM, Brenchley JM, Butler IF, Pattison M, et al. Acute loss of intestinal CD4+ T cells is not predictive of simian immunodeficiency virus virulence. J Immunol 2007;179:3035−46.

[89] Goldstein S, Ourmanov I, Brown CR, Plishka R, Buckler-White A, Byrum R, et al. Plateau levels of viremia correlate with the degree of CD4+ T-cell loss in simian immunodeficiency virus SIVagm-infected pigtailed macaques: Variable pathogenicity of natural SIVagm isolates. J Virol 2005;79:5153−62.

[90] Hirsch VM, Dapolito G, Johnson PR, Elkins WR, London WT, Montali RJ, et al. Induction of AIDS by simian immunodeficiency virus from an African green monkey: Species-specific variation in pathogenicity correlates with the extent of *in vivo* replication. J Virol 1995;69:955−67.

[91] Beer BE, Brown CR, Whitted S, Goldstein S, Goeken R, Plishka R, et al. Immunodeficiency in the absence of high viral load in pig-tailed macaques infected with simian immunodeficiency virus SIVsun and SIVlhoest. J Virol 2005;79:14044−56.

[92] Pandrea I, Apetrei C, Dufour J, Dillon N, Barbercheck J, Metzger M, et al. Simian immunodeficiency virus (SIV) SIVagm.sab infection of Caribbean African green monkeys: New model of the study of SIV pathogenesis in natural hosts. J Virol 2006;80:4858−67.

[93] Pandrea I, Kornfeld C, Ploquin MJ-I, Apetrei C, Faye A, Rouquet P, et al. Impact of viral factors on very early *in vivo* replication profiles in SIVagm-infected African green monkeys. J Virol 2005;79:6249−59.

[94] Diop OM, Gueye A, Dias-Tavares M, Kornfeld C, Faye A, Ave P, et al. High levels of viral replication during primary simian immunodeficiency virus SIVagm infection are rapidly and strongly controlled in African green monkeys. J Virol 2000;74:7538−47.

[95] Kornfeld C, Ploquin MJ, Pandrea I, Faye A, Onanga R, Apetrei C, et al. Antiinflammatory profiles during primary SIV infection in African green monkeys are associated with protection against AIDS. J Clin Invest 2005;115:1082−91.

[96] Silvestri G, Fedanov A, Germon S, Kozyr N, Kaiser WJ, Garber DA, et al. Divergent host responses during primary simian immunodeficiency virus SIVsm infection of natural sooty mangabey and nonnatural rhesus macaque hosts. J Virol 2005;79:4043−54.

[97] Onanga R, Kornfeld C, Pandrea I, Estaquier J, Souquiere S, Rouquet P, et al. High levels of viral replication contrast with only transient changes in CD4+ and CD8+ cell numbers during the early phase of experimental infection with simian immunodeficiency virus SIVmnd-1 in *Mandrillus sphinx*. J Virol 2002;76:10256−63.

[98] Onanga R, Souquiere S, Makuwa M, Mouinga-Ondeme A, Simon F, Apetrei C, et al. Primary simian immunodeficiency virus SIVmnd-2 infection in mandrills (*Mandrillus sphinx*). J Virol 2006;80:3303−9.

[99] Souquière S, Onanga R, Makuwa M, Pandrea I, Ngari P, Rouquet P, et al. SIVmnd-1 and SIVmnd-2 have different pathogenic potentials in rhesus macaques upon experimental cross-species transmission. J Gen Virol 2009;90:488−99.

[100] Hendry RM, Wells MA, Phelan MA, Schneider AL, Epstein JS, Quinnan GV. Antibodies to simian immunodeficiency virus in African green monkeys in Africa in 1957−62. Lancet 1986;2:455.

[101] Mandell D, Gaufin T, Gautam R, Sandler N, Dufour J, Douek DC, et al. A single serial passage of SIVagm.sab in pigtailed macaques results in a dramatic increase in pathogenicity of infection. submitted 2011.

[102] Pandrea I, Gaufin T, Gautam R, Kristoff J, Mandell D, Montefiori DC, et al. Functional cure of SIVagm infection in rhesus macaques results in complete recovery of CD4+ T cells and is reverted by CD8+ cell depletion. Plos Pathogens 2011;7:e1002170.

[103] Beaumier CM, Harris LD, Goldstein S, Klatt NR, Whitted S, McGinty J, et al. CD4 downregulation by memory CD4+ T cells *in vivo* renders African green monkeys resistant to progressive SIVagm infection. Nat Med 2009;15:879−85.

[104] Favre D, Lederer S, Kanwar B, Ma ZM, Proll S, Kasakow Z, et al. Critical loss of the balance between Th17 and T regulatory cell populations in pathogenic SIV infection. Plos Pathogens 2009;5:e1000295.

[105] Milush JM, Mir KD, Sundaravaradan V, Gordon SN, Engram J, Cano CA, et al. Lack of clinical AIDS in SIV-infected sooty mangabeys with significant CD4+ T cell loss is associated with double-negative T cells. J Clin Invest 2011;121:1102−10.

[106] Moore JP, Kitchen SG, Pugach P, Zack JA. The CCR5 and CXCR4 coreceptors—central to understanding the transmission and pathogenesis of human immunodeficiency virus type 1 infection. AIDS Res Hum Retroviruses 2004;20:111−26.

[107] Chen Z, Gettie A, Ho DD, Marx PA. Primary SIVsm isolates use the CCR5 coreceptor from sooty mangabeys naturally infected in west Africa: A comparison of coreceptor usage of primary SIVsm, HIV-2, and SIVmac. Virology 1998;246:113−24.

[108] Zhang Y, Lou B, Lal RB, Gettie A, Marx PA, Moore JP. Use of inhibitors to evaluate coreceptor usage by simian and simian/human immunodeficiency viruses and human immunodeficiency virus type 2 in primary cells. J Virol 2000;74:6893−910.

[109] Gautam R, Carter AC, Katz N, Butler IF, Barnes M, Hasegawa A, et al. *In vitro* charac-terization of primary SIVsmm isolates belonging to different lineages. *In vitro* growth on

rhesus macaque cells is not predictive for *in vivo* replication in rhesus macaques. Virology 2007;362:257−70.

[110] Owen SM, Masciotra S, Novembre F, Yee J, Switzer WM, Ostyula M, et al. Simian immunodeficiency viruses of diverse origin can use CXCR4 as a coreceptor for entry into human cells. J Virol 2000;74:5702−8.

[111] Schols D, De Clercq E. The simian immunodeficiency virus mnd(GB-1) strain uses CXCR4, not CCR5, as coreceptor for entry in human cells. J Gen Virol 1998;79:2203−5.

[112] Chen Z, Kwon D, Jin Z, Monard S, Telfer P, Jones MS, et al. Natural infection of a homozygous delta24 CCR5 red-capped mangabey with an R2b-tropic simian immuno-deficiency virus. J Exp Med 1998;188:2057−65.

[113] Gautam R, Gaufin T, Butler I, Gautam A, Barnes M, Mandell D, et al. SIVrcm, a unique CCR2-tropic virus, selectively depletes memory CD4+ T cells in pigtailed macaques through rapid coreceptor expansion *in vivo*. J Virol 2009;83:7894−908.

[114] Pandrea I, Apetrei C, Gordon S, Barbercheck J, Dufour J, Bohm R, et al. Paucity of CD4+CCR5+ T cells is a typical feature of natural SIV hosts. Blood 2007;109: 1069−76.

[115] Pandrea I, Onanga R, Souquiere S, Mouinga-Ondéme A, Bourry O, Makuwa M, et al. Paucity of CD4+CCR5+ T-cells may prevent breastfeeding transmission of SIV in natural non-human primate hosts. J Virol 2008;82:5501−9.

[116] Pandrea I, Parrish N, Gaufin T, Gautam R, KMH, Kuhrt D, et al. Mucosal SIV transmission in natural hosts: Susceptibility to infection depends on the availability of target cells at the mucosal sites. J Virol 2011. submitted.

[117] Pandrea I, Silvestri G, Onanga R, Veazey RS, Marx PA, Hirsch V, et al. Simian immuno-deficiency viruses replication dynamics in African non-human primate hosts: Common patterns and species-specific differences. J Med Primatol 2006;35:194−201.

[118] Apetrei C, Gautam R, Sumpter B, Carter AC, Gaufin T, Staprans SI, et al. Virus subtype-specific features of natural simian immunodeficiency virus SIVsmm infection in sooty mangabeys. J Virol 2007;81:7913−23.

[119] Pandrea I, Onanga R, Kornfeld C, Rouquet P, Bourry O, Clifford S, et al. High levels of SIVmnd-1 replication in chronically infected *Mandrillus sphinx*. Virology 2003;317: 119−27.

[120] Mellors JW. Viral-load tests provide valuable answers. Sci Am 1998;279:90−3.

[121] Mellors JW, Rinaldo Jr CR, Gupta P, White RM, Todd JA, Kingsley LA. Prognosis in HIV-1 infection predicted by the quantity of virus in plasma. Science 1996;272:1167−70.

[122] Hirsch VM. What can natural infection of African monkeys with simian immunodeficiency virus tell us about the pathogenesis of AIDS? AIDS Rev 2004;6:40−53.

[123] Gaufin T, Pattison M, Gautam R, Stoulig C, Dufour J, MacFarland J, et al. Effect of B cell depletion on viral replication and clinical outcome of SIV infection in a natural host. J Virol 2009;83:10347−57.

[124] Gaufin T, Gautam R, Kasheta M, Ribeiro RM, Ribka E, Barnes M, et al. Limited ability of humoral immune responses in control of viremia during infection with SIVsmmD215 strain. Blood 2009;113:4250−61.

[125] Wang Z, Metcalf B, Ribeiro RM, McClure H, Kaur A. Th-I-type cytotoxic CD8+ T-lymphocyte responses to simian immunodeficiency virus (SIV) are a consistent feature of natural SIV infection in sooty mangabeys. J Virol 2006;80:2771−83.

[126] Dunham R, Pagliardini P, Gordon S, Sumpter B, Engram J, Moanna A, et al. The AIDS-resistance of naturally SIV-infected sooty mangabeys is independent of cellular immunity to the virus. Blood 2006;108:209−17.

[127] Barry AP, Silvestri G, Safrit JT, Sumpter B, Kozyr N, McClure HM, et al. Depletion of CD8+ cells in sooty mangabey monkeys naturally infected with simian immunodeficiency virus reveals limited role for immune control of virus replication in a natural host species. J Immunol 2007;178:8002–12.

[128] Zahn RC, Rett MD, Li M, Tang H, Korioth-Schmitz B, Balachandran H, et al. Suppression of adaptive immune responses during primary SIV infection of sabaeus African green monkeys delays partial containment of viremia but does not induce disease. Blood 115:3070–3078.

[129] Schmitz JE, Zahn RC, Brown CR, Rett MD, Li M, Tang H, et al. Inhibition of adaptive immune responses leads to a fatal clinical outcome in SIV-infected pigtailed macaques but not vervet African green monkeys. PLoS Pathog 2009;5:e1000691.

[130] Gaufin T, Ribeiro RM, Gautam R, Dufour J, Mandell D, Apetrei C, et al. Experimental depletion of CD8+ cells in acutely SIVagm-infected African green monkeys results in increased viral replication. Retrovirology 2010;7:42.

[131] Gordon SN, Klatt NR, Bosinger SE, Brenchley JM, Milush JM, Engram JC, et al. Severe depletion of mucosal CD4+ T cells in AIDS-free simian immunodeficiency virus-infected sooty mangabeys. J Immunol 2007;179:3026–34.

[132] Picker LJ, Hagen SI, Lum R, Reed-Inderbitzin EF, Daly LM, Sylwester AW, et al. Insufficient production and tissue delivery of CD4+ memory T cells in rapidly progressive simian immunodeficiency virus infection. J Exp Med 2004;200:1299–314.

[133] Bosinger SE, Li Q, Gordon SN, Klatt NR, Duan L, Xu L, et al. Global genomic analysis reveals rapid control of a robust innate response in SIV-infected sooty mangabeys. J Clin Invest 2009;119:3556–72.

[134] Pandrea I, Gaufin T, Brenchley JM, Gautam R, Monjure C, Gautam A, et al. Experimentally-induced immune activation in natural hosts of SIV induces significant increases in viral replication and CD4+ T cell depletion. J Immunol 2008;181:6687–91.

[135] Silvestri G, Sodora DL, Koup RA, Paiardini M, O'Neil SP, McClure HM, et al. Nonpathogenic SIV infection of sooty mangabeys is characterized by limited bystander immunopathology despite chronic high-level viremia. Immunity 2003;18:441–52.

[136] Estaquier J, Idziorek T, de Bels F, Barre-Sinoussi F, Hurtrel B, Aubertin AM, et al. Programmed cell death and AIDS: Significance of T-cell apoptosis in pathogenic and nonpathogenic primate lentiviral infections. Proc Natl Acad Sci USA 1994;91:9431–5.

[137] Zeng M, Smith AJ, Wietgrefe SW, Southern PJ, Schacker TW, Reilly CS, et al. Cumulative mechanisms of lymphoid tissue fibrosis and T cell depletion in HIV-1 and SIV infections. J Clin Invest 121:998–1008.

[138] Apetrei C, Gormus B, Pandrea I, Metzger M, ten Haaft P, Martin LN, et al. Direct inoculation of simian immunodeficiency virus from sooty mangabeys in black mangabeys (*Lophocebus aterrimus*): First evidence of AIDS in a heterologous African species and different pathologic outcomes of experimental infection. J Virol 2004;78: 11506–18.

[139] Grossman Z, Meier-Schellersheim M, Paul WE, Picker LJ. Pathogenesis of HIV infection: What the virus spares is as important as what it destroys. Nat Med 2006;12:289–95.

[140] Ploquin MJ, Desoutter JF, Santos PR, Pandrea I, Diop OM, Hosmalin A, et al. Distinct expression profiles of TGF-beta1 signaling mediators in pathogenic SIVmac and nonpathogenic SIVagm infections. Retrovirology 2006;3:37.

[141] Jacquelin B, Mayau V, Targat B, Liovat AS, Kunkel D, Petitjean G, et al. Nonpathogenic SIV infection of African green monkeys induces a strong but rapidly controlled type I IFN response. J Clin Invest 2009;119:3544–55.

[142] Coleman CA, Muller-Trutwin MC, Apetrei C, Pandrea I. T regulatory cells: Aid or hindrance in the clearance of disease? J Cell Mol Med 2007;11:1291−325.

[143] Harrington LE, Hatton RD, Mangan PR, Turner H, Murphy TL, Murphy KM, et al. Interleukin 17-producing CD4+ effector T cells develop via a lineage distinct from the T helper type 1 and 2 lineages. Nat Immunol 2005;6:1123−32.

[144] Korn T, Bettelli E, Oukka M, Kuchroo VK. IL-17 and Th17 cells. Annu Rev Immunol 2009;27:485−517.

[145] Brenchley JM, Paiardini M, Knox KS, Asher AI, Cervasi B, Asher TE, et al. Differential Th17 CD4 T-cell depletion in pathogenic and nonpathogenic lentiviral infections. Blood 2008;112:2826−35.

[146] Cecchinato V, Trindade CJ, Laurence A, Heraud JM, Brenchley JM, Ferrari MJ, et al. Altered balance between Th17 and Th1 cells at mucosal sites predicts AIDS progression in simian immunodeficiency virus-infected macaques. Mucosal Immunol 2008;1:279−88.

[147] Mandl JN, Barry AP, Vanderford TH, Kozyr N, Chavan R, Klucking S, et al. Divergent TLR7 and TLR9 signaling and type I interferon production distinguish pathogenic and nonpathogenic AIDS virus infections. Nat Med 2008;14:1077−87.

[148] Lederer S, Favre D, Walters KA, Proll S, Kanwar B, Kasakow Z, et al. Transcriptional profiling in pathogenic and non-pathogenic SIV infections reveals significant distinctions in kinetics and tissue compartmentalization. PLoS Pathog 2009;5:e1000296.

[149] Harris LD, Tabb B, Sodora DL, Paiardini M, Klatt NR, Douek DC, et al. Downregulation of robust acute type I interferon responses distinguishes nonpathogenic simian immunodeficiency virus (SIV) infection of natural hosts from pathogenic SIV infection of rhesus macaques. J Virol 2010;84:7886−91.

[150] Brenchley JM, Price DA, Schacker TW, Asher TE, Silvestri G, Rao S, et al. Microbial translocation is a cause of systemic immune activation in chronic HIV infection. Nat Med 2006;12:1365−71.

[151] Brenchley JM, Price DA, Douek DC. HIV disease: Fallout from a mucosal catastrophe? Nat Immunol 2006;7:235−9.

[152] d'Ettorre G, Paiardini M, Ceccarelli G, Silvestri G, Vullo V. HIV-associated immune activation: From bench to bedside. AIDS Res Hum Retroviruses 2011;27:355−64.

[153] Koopman G, Niphuis H, Newman W, Kishimoto TK, Maino VC, Heeney JL. Decreased expression of IL-2 in central and effector CD4 memory cells during progression to AIDS in rhesus macaques. AIDS 2001;15:2359−69.

[154] Paiardini M, Galati D, Cervasi B, Cannavo G, Galluzzi L, Montroni M, et al. Exogenous interleukin-2 administration corrects the cell cycle perturbation of lymphocytes from human immunodeficiency virus-infected individuals. J Virol 2001;75:10843−55.

[155] Nacsa J, Edghill-Smith Y, Tsai WP, Venzon D, Tryniszewska E, Hryniewicz A, et al. Contrasting effects of low-dose IL-2 on vaccine-boosted simian immunodeficiency virus (SIV)-specific CD4+ and CD8+ T cells in macaques chronically infected with SIVmac251. J Immunol 2005;174:1913−21.

[156] Sereti I, Anthony KB, Martinez-Wilson H, Lempicki R, Adelsberger J, Metcalf JA, et al. IL-2-induced CD4+ T-cell expansion in HIV-infected patients is associated with long-term decreases in T-cell proliferation. Blood 2004;104:775−80.

[157] Abrams D, Levy Y, Losso MH, Babiker A, Collins G, Cooper DA, et al. Interleukin-2 therapy in patients with HIV infection. N Engl J Med 2009;361:1548−59.

[158] Picker LJ, Reed-Inderbitzin EF, Hagen SI, Edgar JB, Hansen SG, Legasse A, et al. IL-15 induces CD4 effector memory T cell production and tissue emigration in nonhuman primates. J Clin Invest 2006;116:1514−24.

[159] Alpdogan O, van den Brink MR. IL-7 and IL-15: Therapeutic cytokines for immunodeficiency. Trends Immunol 2005;26:56—64.

[160] Ahmad A, Ahmad R, Iannello A, Toma E, Morisset R, Sindhu ST. IL-15 and HIV infection: Lessons for immunotherapy and vaccination. Curr HIV Res 2005;3:261—70.

[161] Mueller YM, Bojczuk PM, Halstead ES, Kim AH, Witek J, Altman JD, et al. IL-15 enhances survival and function of HIV-specific CD8+ T cells. Blood 2003;101:1024—9.

[162] Amicosante M, Poccia F, Gioia C, Montesano C, Topino S, Martini F, et al. Levels of interleukin-15 in plasma may predict a favorable outcome of structured treatment interruption in patients with chronic human immunodeficiency virus infection. J Infect Dis 2003;188:661—5.

[163] Lum JJ, Schnepple DJ, Nie Z, Sanchez-Dardon J, Mbisa GL, Mihowich J, et al. Differential effects of interleukin-7 and interleukin-15 on NK cell anti-human immunodeficiency virus activity. J Virol 2004;78:6033—42.

[164] Mueller YM, Petrovas C, Bojczuk PM, Dimitriou ID, Beer B, Silvera P, et al. Interleukin-15 increases effector memory CD8+ T cells and NK cells in simian immunodeficiency virus-infected macaques. J Virol 2005;79:4877—85.

[165] Mueller YM, Do DH, Altork SR, Artlett CM, Gracely EJ, Katsetos CD, et al. IL-15 treatment during acute simian immunodeficiency virus (SIV) infection increases viral set point and accelerates disease progression despite the induction of stronger SIV-specific CD8+ T cell responses. J Immunol 2008;180:350—60.

[166] Eberly MD, Kader M, Hassan W, Rogers KA, Zhou J, Mueller YM, et al. Increased IL-15 production is associated with higher susceptibility of memory CD4 T cells to simian immunodeficiency virus during acute infection. J Immunol 2009;182:1439—48.

[167] Hryniewicz A, Price DA, Moniuszko M, Boasso A, Edghill-Spano Y, West SM, et al. Interleukin-15 but not interleukin-7 abrogates vaccine-induced decrease in virus level in simian immunodeficiency virus mac251-infected macaques. J Immunol 2007;178:3492—504.

[168] Schluns KS, Lefrancois L. Cytokine control of memory T-cell development and survival. Nat Rev Immunol 2003;3:269—79.

[169] Seddon B, Tomlinson P, Zamoyska R. Interleukin 7 and T cell receptor signals regulate homeostasis of CD4 memory cells. Nat Immunol 2003;4:680—6.

[170] Moniuszko M, Fry T, Tsai WP, Morre M, Assouline B, Cortez P, et al. Recombinant interleukin-7 induces proliferation of naive macaque CD4+ and CD8+ T cells *in vivo*. J Virol 2004;78:9740—9.

[171] Bradley LM, Haynes L, Swain SL. IL-7: Maintaining T-cell memory and achieving homeostasis. Trends Immunol 2005;26:172—6.

[172] Napolitano LA, Grant RM, Deeks SG, Schmidt D, De Rosa SC, Herzenberg LA, et al. Increased production of IL-7 accompanies HIV-1-mediated T-cell depletion: Implications for T-cell homeostasis. Nat Med 2001;7:73—9.

[173] Fry TJ, Moniuszko M, Creekmore S, Donohue SJ, Douek DC, Giardina S, et al. IL-7 therapy dramatically alters peripheral T-cell homeostasis in normal and SIV-infected nonhuman primates. Blood 2003;101:2294—9.

[174] Beq S, Nugeyre MT, Ho Tsong Fang R, Gautier D, Legrand R, Schmitt N, et al. IL-7 induces immunological improvement in SIV-infected rhesus macaques under antiviral therapy. J Immunol 2006;176:914—22.

[175] Leone A, Rohankhedkar M, Okoye A, Legasse A, Axthelm MK, Villinger F, et al. Increased CD4+ T cell levels during IL-7 administration of antiretroviral therapy-treated simian immunodeficiency virus-positive macaques are not dependent on strong proliferative responses. J Immunol 2010;185:1650—9.

[176] Sereti I, Dunham RM, Spritzler J, Aga E, Proschan MA, Medvik K, et al. IL-7 administration drives T cell-cycle entry and expansion in HIV-1 infection. Blood 2009;113:6304−14.

[177] Levy Y, Lacabaratz C, Weiss L, Viard JP, Goujard C, Lelievre JD, et al. Enhanced T cell recovery in HIV-1-infected adults through IL-7 treatment. J Clin Invest 2009;119: 997−1007.

[178] Smithgall MD, Wong JG, Critchett KE, Haffar OK. IL-7 up-regulates HIV-1 replication in naturally infected peripheral blood mononuclear cells. J Immunol 1996;156:2324−30.

[179] Ducrey-Rundquist O, Guyader M, Trono D. Modalities of interleukin-7-induced human immunodeficiency virus permissiveness in quiescent T lymphocytes. J Virol 2002;76: 9103−11.

[180] Wang FX, Xu Y, Sullivan J, Souder E, Argyris EG, Acheampong EA, et al. IL-7 is a potent and proviral strain-specific inducer of latent HIV-1 cellular reservoirs of infected individuals on virally suppressive HAART. J Clin Invest 2005;115:128−37.

[181] Veazey RS, Ling B, Green LC, Ribka EP, Lifson JD, Piatak Jr M, et al. Topically applied recombinant chemokine analogues fully protect macaques from vaginal simian−human immunodeficiency virus challenge. J Infect Dis 2009;199:1525−7.

[182] Grant RM, Hamer D, Hope T, Johnston R, Lange J, Lederman MM, et al. Whither or wither microbicides? Science 2008;321:532−4.

[183] Lederman MM, Veazey RS, Offord R, Mosier DE, Dufour J, Mefford M, et al. Prevention of vaginal SHIV transmission in rhesus macaques through inhibition of CCR5. Science 2004;306:485−7.

[184] Gulick RM, Lalezari J, Goodrich J, Clumeck N, DeJesus E, Horban A, et al. Maraviroc for previously treated patients with R5 HIV-1 infection. N Engl J Med 2008;359:1429−41.

[185] Saag M, Goodrich J, Fatkenheuer G, Clotet B, Clumeck N, Sullivan J, et al. A double-blind, placebo-controlled trial of maraviroc in treatment-experienced patients infected with non-R5 HIV-1. J Infect Dis 2009;199:1638−47.

[186] Funderburg N, Kalinowska M, Eason J, Goodrich J, Heera J, Mayer H, et al. Effects of maraviroc and efavirenz on markers of immune activation and inflammation and associations with CD4+ cell rises in HIV-infected patients. PLoS One 5:e13188.

[187] Pett SL, Zaunders J, Bailey M, Murray J, MacRae K, Emery S, et al. A novel chemokine-receptor-5 (CCR5) blocker, SCH532706, has differential effects on CCR5+CD4+ and CCR5+CD8+ T cell numbers in chronic HIV infection. AIDS Res Hum Retroviruses 26:653−661.

[188] Hutter G, Nowak D, Mossner M, Ganepola S, Mussig A, Allers K, et al. Long-term control of HIV by CCR5 Delta32/Delta32 stem-cell transplantation. N Engl J Med 2009;360: 692−8.

[189] Allers K, Hutter G, Hofmann J, Loddenkemper C, Rieger K, Thiel E, et al. Evidence for the cure of HIV infection by CCR5Delta32/Delta32 stem cell transplantation. Blood 117:2791−2799.

[190] Zanin MK, Duvall MR. Back-burning to cure HIV: Temporary depletion of all CD4+ cells and elimination of the extracellular reservoir with HIV immunotoxin therapy. Med Hypotheses 2009;72:592−5.

[191] Pandrea I, Gaufin T, Brenchley JM, Gautam R, Monjure C, Gautam A, et al. Cutting edge: Experimentally induced immune activation in natural hosts of simian immunodeficiency virus induces significant increases in viral replication and CD4+ T cell depletion. J Immunol 2008;181:6687−91.

[192] Shafran I, Burgunder P. Rifaximin for the treatment of newly diagnosed Crohn's disease: A case series. Am J Gastroenterol 2008;103:2158−60.

[193] Bass NM, Mullen KD, Sanyal A, Poordad F, Neff G, Leevy CB, et al. Rifaximin treatment in hepatic encephalopathy. N Engl J Med 2010;362:1071−81.

[194] Sun PP, Perianayagam MC, Jaber BL. Endotoxin-binding affinity of sevelamer: A potential novel anti-inflammatory mechanism. Kidney Intl Suppl 2009:S20−25.

[195] Perez-Bosque A, Amat C, Polo J, Campbell JM, Crenshaw J, Russell L, et al. Spray-dried animal plasma prevents the effects of *Staphylococcus aureus* enterotoxin B on intestinal barrier function in weaned rats. J Nutr 2006;136:2838−43.

[196] Moreto M, Perez-Bosque A. Dietary plasma proteins, the intestinal immune system, and the barrier functions of the intestinal mucosa. J Anim Sci 2009;87:E92−100.

[197] Perez-Bosque A, Miro L, Polo J, Russell L, Campbell J, Weaver E, et al. Dietary plasma proteins modulate the immune response of diffuse gut-associated lymphoid tissue in rats challenged with *Staphylococcus aureus* enterotoxin B J Nutr 2008;138:533−7.

[198] Moreno-Fernandez ME, Rueda CM, Rusie LK, Chougnet CA. Regulatory T cells control HIV replication in activated T cells through a cAMP-dependent mechanism. Blood 2011;117:5372−80.

[199] Cecchinato V, Tryniszewska E, Ma ZM, Vaccari M, Boasso A, Tsai WP, et al. Immune activation driven by CTLA-4 blockade augments viral replication at mucosal sites in simian immunodeficiency virus infection. J Immunol 2008;180:5439−47.

[200] Ensoli B, Bellino S, Tripiciano A, Longo O, Francavilla V, Marcotullio S, et al. Therapeutic immunization with HIV-1 Tat reduces immune activation and loss of regulatory T-cells and improves immune function in subjects on HAART. PLoS One 2010;5:e13540.

[201] Qu Y, Zhang B, Liu S, Zhang A, Wu T, Zhao Y. 2-Gy whole-body irradiation significantly alters the balance of CD4+ CD25− T effector cells and CD4+ CD25+ Foxp3+ T regulatory cells in mice. Cell Mol Immunol 2010;7:419−27.

[202] Chang JH, Cha HR, Lee DS, Seo KY, Kweon MN. 1,25-Dihydroxyvitamin D3 inhibits the differentiation and migration of T(h)17 cells to protect against experimental autoimmune encephalomyelitis. PLoS One 5:e12925.

[203] Zold E, Szodoray P, Kappelmayer J, Gaal J, Csathy L, Barath S, et al. Impaired regulatory T-cell homeostasis due to vitamin D deficiency in undifferentiated connective tissue disease. Scand J Rheumatol 2010;39:490−7.

[204] Mus AM, Cornelissen F, Asmawidjaja PS, van Hamburg JP, Boon L, Hendriks RW, et al. Interleukin-23 promotes Th17 differentiation by inhibiting T-bet and FoxP3 and is required for elevation of interleukin-22, but not interleukin-21, in autoimmune experimental arthritis. Arthritis Rheum 2010;62:1043−50.

[205] Fontenot JD, Gavin MA, Rudensky AY. Foxp3 programs the development and function of CD4+CD25+ regulatory T cells. Nat Immunol 2003;4:330−6.

[206] Siegal F. Interferon-producing plasmacytoid dendritic cells and the pathogenesis of AIDS. Res Initiat Treat Action 2003;8:10−3.

[207] Marroni M, Gresele P, Landonio G, Lazzarin A, Coen M, Vezza R, et al. Interferon-alpha is effective in the treatment of HIV-1-related, severe, zidovudine-resistant thrombocytopenia. A prospective, placebo-controlled, double-blind trial. Ann Intern Med 1994;121:423−9.

[208] Skillman DR, Malone JL, Decker CF, Wagner KF, Mapou RL, Liao MJ, et al. Phase I trial of interferon alfa-n3 in early-stage human immunodeficiency virus type 1 disease: Evidence for drug safety, tolerance, and antiviral activity. J Infect Dis 1996;173:1107−14.

[209] Rivero J, Fraga M, Cancio I, Cuervo J, Lopez-Saura P. Long-term treatment with recombinant interferon alpha-2b prolongs survival of asymptomatic HIV-infected individuals. Biotherapy 1997;10:107−13.

[210] Mauss S, Klinker H, Ulmer A, Willers R, Weissbrich B, Albrecht H, et al. Response to treatment of chronic hepatitis C with interferon alpha in patients infected with HIV-1 is associated with higher CD4+ cell count. Infection 1998;26:16−9.

[211] Fauci AS, Rosenberg SA, Sherwin SA, Dinarello CA, Longo DL, Lane HC. NIH conference. Immunomodulators in clinical medicine. Ann Intern Med 1987;106:421−33.

[212] Laguno M, Murillas J, Blanco JL, Martinez E, Miquel R, Sanchez-Tapias JM, et al. Peginterferon alfa-2b plus ribavirin compared with interferon alfa-2b plus ribavirin for treatment of HIV/HCV co-infected patients. Aids 2004;18:F27−36.

[213] Asmuth DM, Murphy RL, Rosenkranz SL, Lertora JJ, Kottilil S, Cramer Y, et al. Safety, tolerability, and mechanisms of antiretroviral activity of pegylated interferon alfa-2a in HIV-1-monoinfected participants: A phase II clinical trial. J Infect Dis 2010;201:1686−96.

[214] Schlaepfer E, Speck RF. Anti-HIV activity mediated by natural killer and CD8+ cells after toll-like receptor 7/8 triggering. PLoS One 2008;3:e1999.

[215] Lu W, Andrieu JM. In vitro human immunodeficiency virus eradication by autologous CD8(+) T cells expanded with inactivated-virus-pulsed dendritic cells. J Virol 2001;75:8949−56.

[216] Lu W, Wu X, Lu Y, Guo W, Andrieu JM. Therapeutic dendritic-cell vaccine for simian AIDS. Nat Med 2003;9:27−32.

[217] Lu W, Arraes LC, Ferreira WT, Andrieu JM. Therapeutic dendritic-cell vaccine for chronic HIV-1 infection. Nat Med 2004;10:1359−65.

[218] Garcia F, Climent N, Assoumou L, Gil C, Gonzalez N, Alcami J, et al. A therapeutic dendritic cell-based vaccine for HIV-1 infection. J Infect Dis 2011;203:473−8.

[219] Kundu SK, Engleman E, Benike C, Shapero MH, Dupuis M, van Schooten WC, et al. A pilot clinical trial of HIV antigen-pulsed allogeneic and autologous dendritic cell therapy in HIV-infected patients. AIDS Res Hum Retroviruses 1998;14:551−60.

[220] Ide F, Nakamura T, Tomizawa M, Kawana-Tachikawa A, Odawara T, Hosoya N, et al. Peptide-loaded dendritic-cell vaccination followed by treatment interruption for chronic HIV-1 infection: A phase 1 trial. J Med Virol 2006;78:711−8.

[221] Connolly NC, Whiteside TL, Wilson C, Kondragunta V, Rinaldo CR, Riddler SA. Therapeutic immunization with human immunodeficiency virus type 1 (HIV-1) peptide-loaded dendritic cells is safe and induces immunogenicity in HIV-1-infected individuals. Clin Vaccine Immunol 2008;15:284−92.

[222] Gandhi RT, O'Neill D, Bosch RJ, Chan ES, Bucy RP, Shopis J, et al. A randomized therapeutic vaccine trial of canarypox-HIV-pulsed dendritic cells vs. canarypox-HIV alone in HIV-1-infected patients on antiretroviral therapy. Vaccine 2009;27:6088−94.

[223] Kloverpris H, Karlsson I, Bonde J, Thorn M, Vinner L, Pedersen AE, et al. Induction of novel CD8+ T-cell responses during chronic untreated HIV-1 infection by immunization with subdominant cytotoxic T-lymphocyte epitopes. Aids 2009;23:1329−40.

[224] Wang Y, Abel K, Lantz K, Krieg AM, McChesney MB, Miller CJ. The Toll-like receptor 7 (TLR7) agonist, imiquimod, and the TLR9 agonist, CpG ODN, induce antiviral cytokines and chemokines but do not prevent vaginal transmission of simian immunodeficiency virus when applied intravaginally to rhesus macaques. J Virol 2005;79:14355−70.

[225] Wang Y, Blozis SA, Lederman M, Krieg A, Landay A, Miller CJ. Enhanced antibody responses elicited by a CpG adjuvant do not improve the protective effect of an aldrithiol-2-inactivated simian immunodeficiency virus therapeutic AIDS vaccine. Clin Vaccine Immunol 2009;16:499−505.

[226] Martinson JA, Montoya CJ, Usuga X, Ronquillo R, Landay AL, Desai SN. Chloroquine modulates HIV-1-induced plasmacytoid dendritic cell alpha interferon: Implication for T-cell activation. Antimicrob Agents Chemother 2010;54:871−81.

[227] Murray SM, Down CM, Boulware DR, Stauffer WM, Cavert WP, Schacker TW, et al. Reduction of immune activation with chloroquine therapy during chronic HIV infection. J Virol 2010;84:12082−6.

[228] Piconi S, Parisotto S, Rizzardini G, Passerini S, Terzi R, Argenteri B, et al. Hydroxy-chloroquine drastically reduces immune activation in HIV-infected, ART-treated, immunological non-responders. Blood

[229] Aerts NE, De Knop KJ, Leysen J, Ebo DG, Bridts CH, Weyler JJ, et al. Increased IL-17 production by peripheral T helper cells after tumour necrosis factor blockade in rheumatoid arthritis is accompanied by inhibition of migration-associated chemokine receptor expression. Rheumatology (Oxford) 49:2264−2272.

[230] Klatt NR, Brenchley JM. Th17 cell dynamics in HIV infection. Curr Opin HIV AIDS 2010;5:135−40.

[231] Ribas A, Comin-Anduix B, Chmielowski B, Jalil J, de la Rocha P, McCannel TA, et al. Dendritic cell vaccination combined with CTLA4 blockade in patients with metastatic melanoma. Clin Cancer Res 2009;15:6267−76.

[232] Kader M, Bixler S, Piatak M, Lifson J, Mattapallil JJ. Anti-retroviral therapy fails to restore the severe Th-17: Tc-17 imbalance observed in peripheral blood during simian immunodeficiency virus infection. J Med Primatol 2009;38(Suppl 1):32−8.

[233] Kikly K, Liu L, Na S, Sedgwick JD. The IL-23/Th(17) axis: Therapeutic targets for autoimmune inflammation. Curr Opin Immunol 2006;18:670−5.

[234] Maek ANW, Buranapraditkun S, Klaewsongkram J, Ruxrungtham K. Increased interleukin-17 production both in helper T cell subset Th17 and CD4-negative T cells in human immunodeficiency virus infection. Viral Immunol 2007;20:66−75.

[235] Hou W, Kang HS, Kim BS. Th17 cells enhance viral persistence and inhibit T cell cytotoxicity in a model of chronic virus infection. J Exp Med 2009;206:313−28.

[236] Argyropoulos C, Mouzaki A. Immunosuppressive drugs in HIV disease. Curr Top Med Chem 2006;6:1769−89.

[237] Ciuffreda D, Pantaleo G, Pascual M. Effects of immunosuppressive drugs on HIV infection: Implications for solid-organ transplantation. Transpl Intl 2007;20:649−58.

[238] Starzl TE, Klintmalm GB, Porter KA, Iwatsuki S, Schroter GP. Liver transplantation with use of cyclosporin A and prednisone. N Engl J Med 1981;305:266−9.

[239] Italia JL, Bhardwaj V, Kumar MN. Disease, destination, dose and delivery aspects of cyclosporin: The state of the art. Drug Discov Today 2006;11:846−54.

[240] Bartz SR, Hohenwalter E, Hu MK, Rich DH, Malkovsky M. Inhibition of human immunodeficiency virus replication by nonimmunosuppressive analogs of cyclosporin A. Proc Natl Acad Sci USA 1995;92:5381−5.

[241] Franke EK, Luban J. Inhibition of HIV-1 replication by cyclosporine A or related compounds correlates with the ability to disrupt the Gag−cyclophilin A interaction. Virology 1996;222:279−82.

[242] Andrieu JM, Even P, Venet A, Tourani JM, Stern M, Lowenstein W, et al. Effects of cyclosporin on T-cell subsets in human immunodeficiency virus disease. Clin Immunol Immunopathol 1988;47:181−98.

[243] Levy R, Jais JP, Tourani JM, Even P, Andrieu JM. Long-term follow-up of HIV positive asymptomatic patients having received cyclosporin A. Adv Exp Med Biol 1995;374:229−34.

[244] Rizzardi GP, Harari A, Capiluppi B, Tambussi G, Ellefsen K, Ciuffreda D, et al. Treatment of primary HIV-1 infection with cyclosporin A coupled with highly active antiretroviral therapy. J Clin Invest 2002;109:681−8.

[245] Markowitz M, Vaida F, Hare CB, Boden D, Mohri H, Hecht FM, et al. The virologic and immunologic effects of cyclosporin as an adjunct to antiretroviral therapy in patients treated during acute and early HIV-1 infection. J Infect Dis 2010;201:1298—302.

[246] Calabrese LH, Lederman MM, Spritzler J, Coombs RW, Fox L, Schock B, et al. Placebo-controlled trial of cyclosporin-A in HIV-1 disease: Implications for solid organ transplantation. J Acquir Immune Defic Syndr 2002;29:356—62.

[247] Allison AC, Kowalski WJ, Muller CD, Eugui EM. Mechanisms of action of mycophenolic acid. Ann N Y Acad Sci 1993;696:63—87.

[248] Allison AC, Almquist SJ, Muller CD, Eugui EM. *In vitro* immunosuppressive effects of mycophenolic acid and an ester pro-drug, RS-61443. Transplant Proc 1991;23:10—4.

[249] Margolis D, Heredia A, Gaywee J, Oldach D, Drusano G, Redfield R. Abacavir and mycophenolic acid, an inhibitor of inosine monophosphate dehydrogenase, have profound and synergistic anti-HIV activity. J Acquir Immune Defic Syndr 1999;21:362—70.

[250] Heredia A, Margolis D, Oldach D, Hazen R, Le N, Redfield R. Abacavir in combination with the inosine monophosphate dehydrogenase (IMPDH)-inhibitor mycophenolic acid is active against multidrug-resistant HIV-1. J Acquir Immune Defic Syndr 1999;22:406—7.

[251] Hossain MM, Coull JJ, Drusano GL, Margolis DM. Dose proportional inhibition of HIV-1 replication by mycophenolic acid and synergistic inhibition in combination with abacavir, didanosine, and tenofovir. Antiviral Res 2002;55:41—52.

[252] Chapuis AG, Paolo Rizzardi G, D'Agostino C, Attinger A, Knabenhans C, Fleury S, et al. Effects of mycophenolic acid on human immunodeficiency virus infection *in vitro* and *in vivo*. Nat Med 2000;6:762—8.

[253] Sankatsing SU, Jurriaans S, van Swieten P, van Leth F, Cornelissen M, Miedema F, et al. Highly active antiretroviral therapy with or without mycophenolate mofetil in treatment-naive HIV-1 patients. Aids 2004;18:1925—31.

[254] Millan O, Brunet M, Martorell J, Garcia F, Vidal E, Rojo I, et al. Pharmacokinetics and pharmacodynamics of low dose mycophenolate mofetil in HIV-infected patients treated with abacavir, efavirenz and nelfinavir. Clin Pharmacokinet 2005;44:525—38.

[255] Barnes PJ. Anti-inflammatory actions of glucocorticoids: Molecular mechanisms. Clin Sci (Lond) 1998;94:557—72.

[256] Lu W, Salerno-Goncalves R, Yuan J, Sylvie D, Han DS, Andrieu JM. Glucocorticoids rescue CD4+ T lymphocytes from activation-induced apoptosis triggered by HIV-1: Implications for pathogenesis and therapy. Aids 1995;9:35—42.

[257] Andrieu JM, Lu W, Levy R. Sustained increases in CD4 cell counts in asymptomatic human immunodeficiency virus type 1-seropositive patients treated with prednisolone for 1 year. J Infect Dis 1995;171:523—30.

[258] McComsey GA, Whalen CC, Mawhorter SD, Asaad R, Valdez H, Patki AH, et al. Placebo-controlled trial of prednisone in advanced HIV-1 infection. Aids 2001;15:321—7.

[259] Andrieu JM, Lu W. Long-term clinical, immunologic and virologic impact of glucocorticoids on the chronic phase of HIV infection. BMC Med 2004;2:17.

[260] Ulmer A, Muller M, Bertisch-Mollenhoff B, Frietsch B. Low-dose prednisolone has a CD4-stabilizing effect in pre-treated HIV-patients during structured therapy interruptions (STI). Eur J Med Res 2005;10:227—32.

[261] Abraham RT, Wiederrecht GJ. Immunopharmacology of rapamycin. Annu Rev Immunol 1996;14:483—510.

[262] Molnar-Kimber KL. Mechanism of action of rapamycin (Sirolimus, Rapamune). Transplant Proc 1996;28:964—9.

[263] Sehgal SN. Rapamune (RAPA, rapamycin, sirolimus): Mechanism of action immunosuppressive effect results from blockade of signal transduction and inhibition of cell cycle progression. Clin Biochem 1998;31:335−40.

[264] Roy J, Paquette JS, Fortin JF, Tremblay MJ. The immunosuppressant rapamycin represses human immunodeficiency virus type 1 replication. Antimicrob Agents Chemother 2002;46:3447−55.

[265] Donia M, McCubrey JA, Bendtzen K, Nicoletti F. Potential use of rapamycin in HIV infection. Br J Clin Pharmacol 2010;70:784−93.

[266] Heredia A, Amoroso A, Davis C, Le N, Reardon E, Dominique JK, et al. Rapamycin causes downregulation of CCR5 and accumulation of anti-HIV beta-chemokines: An approach to suppress R5 strains of HIV-1. Proc Natl Acad Sci USA 2003;100:10411−6.

[267] Gao WY, Cara A, Gallo RC, Lori F. Low levels of deoxynucleotides in peripheral blood lymphocytes: A strategy to inhibit human immunodeficiency virus type 1 replication. Proc Natl Acad Sci USA 1993;90:8925−8.

[268] Lori F, Malykh A, Cara A, Sun D, Weinstein JN, Lisziewicz J, et al. Hydroxyurea as an inhibitor of human immunodeficiency virus-type 1 replication. Science 1994;266:801−5.

[269] Gao WY, Johns DG, Mitsuya H. Anti−human immunodeficiency virus type 1 activity of hydroxyurea in combination with 2′,3′-dideoxynucleosides. Mol Pharmacol 1994;46:767−72.

[270] Zachary KC, Davis B. Hydroxyurea for HIV infection. AIDS Clin Care 1998;10:25−6. 32.

[271] Lori F, Lisziewicz J. Hydroxyurea: Overview of clinical data and antiretroviral and immunomodulatory effects. Antivir Ther 1999;4(Suppl 3):101−8.

[272] Biron F, Lucht F, Peyramond D, Fresard A, Vallet T, Nugier F, et al. Anti-HIV activity of the combination of didanosine and hydroxyurea in HIV-1-infected individuals. J Acquir Immune Defic Syndr Hum Retrovirol 1995;10:36−40.

[273] Vila J, Biron F, Nugier F, Vallet T, Peyramond D. 1-year follow-up of the use of hydroxycarbamide and didanosine in HIV infection. Lancet 1996;348:203−4.

[274] Vila J, Nugier F, Bargues G, Vallet T, Peyramond D, Hamedi-Sangsari F, et al. Absence of viral rebound after treatment of HIV-infected patients with didanosine and hydroxycarbamide. Lancet 1997;350:635−6.

[275] Lisziewicz J, Jessen H, Finzi D, Siliciano RF, Lori F. HIV-1 suppression by early treatment with hydroxyurea, didanosine, and a protease inhibitor. Lancet 1998;352:199−200.

[276] Giacca M, Zanussi S, Comar M, Simonelli C, Vaccher E, de Paoli P, et al. Treatment of human immunodeficiency virus infection with hydroxyurea: virologic and clinical evaluation. J Infect Dis 1996;174:204−9.

[277] Simonelli C, Nasti G, Vaccher E, Tirelli U, Zanussi S, De Paoli P, et al. Hydroxyurea treatment in HIV-infected patients. J Acquir Immune Defic Syndr Hum Retrovirol 1996;13:462−4.

[278] Zala C, Rouleau D, Montaner JS. Role of hydroxyurea in treatment of disease due to human immunodeficiency virus infection. Clin Infect Dis 2000;30(Suppl 2):S143−150.

[279] Frank I, Bosch RJ, Fiscus S, Valentine F, Flexner C, Segal Y, et al. Activity, safety, and immunological effects of hydroxyurea added to didanosine in antiretroviral-naive and experienced HIV type 1-infected subjects: A randomized, placebo-controlled trial, ACTG 307. AIDS Res Hum Retroviruses 2004;20:916−26.

[280] Swindells S, Cohen CJ, Berger DS, Tashima KT, Liao Q, Pobiner BF, et al. Abacavir, efavirenz, didanosine, with or without hydroxyurea, in HIV-infected adults failing initial nucleoside/protease inhibitor-containing regimens. BMC Infect Dis 2005;5:23.

[281] Day CL, Kaufmann DE, Kiepiela P, Brown JA, Moodley ES, Reddy S, et al. PD-1 expression on HIV-specific T cells is associated with T-cell exhaustion and disease progression. Nature 2006;443:350−4.

[282] Macatangay BJ, Rinaldo CR. PD-1 blockade: A promising immunotherapy for HIV? Cellscience 2009;5:61–5.

[283] Velu V, Titanji K, Zhu B, Husain S, Pladevega A, Lai L, et al. Enhancing SIV-specific immunity *in vivo* by PD-1 blockade. Nature 2009;458:206–10.

[284] Finnefrock AC, Tang A, Li F, Freed DC, Feng M, Cox KS, et al. PD-1 blockade in rhesus macaques: Impact on chronic infection and prophylactic vaccination. J Immunol 2009;182:980–7.

HIV-1-Exposed Seronegative Individuals

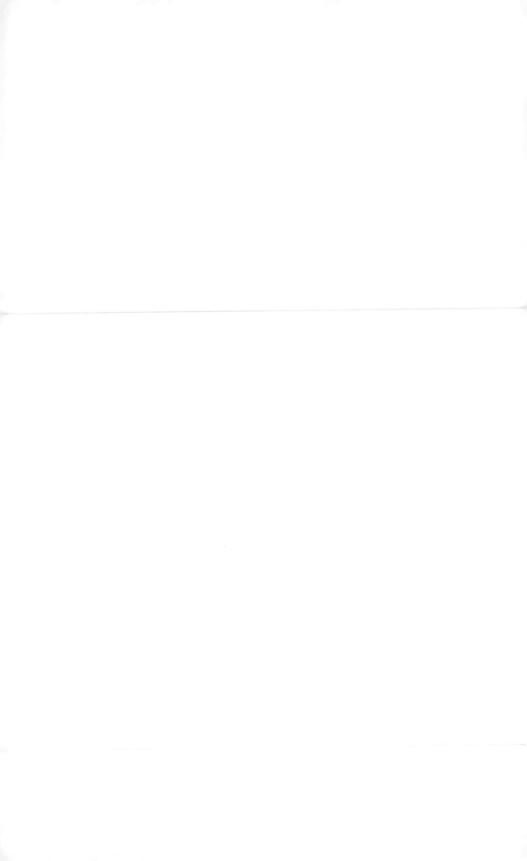

Chapter 4

Are Some People Protected Against HIV Infection?

Mario Clerici [1,2], Mara Biasin [1] and Gene M. Shearer [3]

[1] *Universita degli Studi di Milano, Milan, Italy,* [2] *Fondazione Don Gnocchi, ONLUS, Milan, Italy,*
[3] *Experimental Immunology Branch, Center for Cancer Research, NCI, NIH, Bethesda, Maryland, USA*

GENESIS OF THE FIELD

Differences in susceptibility to infection by members of distinct classes of infectious agents, such as bacteria, parasites and viruses, have been known for decades. This failure to observe infection upon repeated exposure to a particular infectious agent was often attributed to protection by host genetics and/or host immunity, and was typically observed in a minority of individuals in each exposed population. Despite these examples recorded in medical history, many researchers who attended the VIIth International Conference on AIDS (Florence, Italy, June 16—19, 1991) were surprised and skeptical of the data presented in a poster session by the late Janis Giorgi. Dr Giorgi and co-workers found that peripheral blood mononuclear cells (PBMCs) from HIV-uninfected homosexual men known to have repeated unprotected sexual interactions with HIV-infected men [1] generated strong *in vitro* CD4 T cell responses to multiple synthetic HIV envelope peptides [2]. Giorgi's poster was neither the first presentation of this seemingly resistant cohort of homosexual men from MACS [1], nor the first report of HIV-specific T helper cell responses in seronegative unprotected sexual partners of HIV-infected patients [3]. It was, however, the first presentation at a major scientific meeting to show an association between the absence of infection and development of HIV-specific cellular immunity.

Models of Protection Against HIV/SIV. DOI: 10.1016/B978-0-12-387715-4.00004-6

Negative data obtained from (i) unexposed healthy controls provided immunologic evidence that these at-risk individuals had been mucosally exposed to HIV; and from (ii) HIV chronically-infected patients suggested that HIV infection had prevented the development of potentially protective adaptive anti-HIV cellular immunity. Although the study did not establish a cause-and-effect relationship [4], it led to the Th1/Th2 hypothesis of HIV infection [5]. A small follow-up retrospective study in the SIV/macaque model suggested that low-dose exposure of this SIV pathogenic-susceptible non-human primate (NHP) species protected these animals against infection by a high-dose SIV infectious challenge 16 months after initial low-dose exposure [6].

Independently of the above-noted immunologic experiments, epidemiologic research was being conducted during the same time period by the laboratory of Dr Francis Plummer at the University of Manitoba in Winnipeg, Canada and their colleagues at the University of Nairobi in Kenya. Although their original objective had been to study sexually transmitted diseases in a cohort of female sex workers in Nairobi, these researchers found themselves in a hotbed of HIV infection. By carefully following this cohort longitudinally, the study identified a small subset (10—15 percent) of HIV frequently-exposed sex workers who remained seronegative throughout years of follow-up [7], and whose pattern of resistance and susceptibility fitted a statistical model that favored immunologic protection [8]. A more recent study of this cohort indicated that interruption of frequent unprotected sexual encounters resulted in increased susceptibility to HIV infection [9], raising the possibility that frequently repeated HIV exposure may be important for maintaining this protective phenotype.

The poster by Giorgi and co-workers [2] was followed by a series of cellular immunology papers demonstrating that PBMCs from HIV-exposed but uninfected individuals generated HIV-specific T helper cell [4,10,11] and CD8 cytotoxic T cell responses *in vitro* [12,13]. Both HIV-specific T cell subsets were detected in exposed seronegative adults [4,11,13] and in uninfected neonates born to HIV-infected mothers [10,12]. Later studies of HIV-exposed individuals indicated increased levels of anti-HIV soluble factors, including the CD8 anti-HIV factor (CAF) [14], as well as β-chemokines [15], α-defensins [16], APOBEC3G [17] and secretory IgA [18,19], as well as increased NK cell activity [20]. A recent comparative study of Toll-like receptor (TLR) activation between ESN and unexposed healthy controls indicated that TLR activation of leukocytes from ESN exhibit a more potent release of factors that induce stronger adaptive immune responses [21].

DIVERSITY OF COHORTS

Also noteworthy was the broad spectrum of distinct cohorts that were repeatedly exposed, in which only a small percentage of each remained uninfected. These included individuals who were involved in promiscuous sexual practices, stable unprotected sex with an HIV-infected partner, or intravenous drug abuse.

Also included were hemophiliacs who had received HIV-contaminated anti-clotting factors. A particularly interesting cohort was uninfected newborns of HIV-infected mothers. These neonates were unique in that most were uninfected at birth (65—75 percent), in contrast to the rare exposed uninfected adults. The infants were HIV seropositive, due to having passively received maternal anti-HIV antibodies *in utero*; and they were continuously exposed to an HIV+ environment during pregnancy, in contrast to frequent but interrupted exposures in the adults. Throughout the first two decades after the discovery of these cohorts, HIV-exposed uninfected individuals were frequently referred to as exposed seronegatives (ESN) or exposed uninfected (EU). It should be noted that the ESN designation does not fit the uninfected neonates, due to the presence of maternal anti-HIV antibodies.

All of the above cohorts were either repeatedly or continuously exposed to HIV, although a single sub-infectious dose exposure to infectious SIV appeared to have protected macaques against subsequent high-dose infectious challenge [6]. To investigate whether low or limited exposure to HIV would generate HIV-specific cellular immune responses, we tested PBMCs from a single exposure by accidental needle-stick HIV-exposed healthcare workers (HCWs) who did not seroconvert. We observed that that PBMCs from most of the HCWs tested repeatedly generated both HIV-specific T-helper [22] and CD8 cytotoxic T-effector [23] cell responses. Although these findings did not indicate whether these HCWs would have been protected against infectious challenge, the experiments did demonstrate that even a single percutaneous exposure to HIV could induce HIV-specific cellular immunity.

HOST GENETICS

Host genetic factors also play an important role in resistance to HIV infection shaping different steps in the viral cycle (penetration, attachment to target cells, integration and viral gene expression) as well as in immune responses to HIV antigens. The seminal discovery [24] that homozygosity for the allelic variant Δ32 of the chemokine receptor CCR5, the main coreceptor for the R5-HIV-1 viruses, is associated with a strong, although not complete, protection against sexually transmitted HIV-1 infection encouraged the search for other mutant genes possibly involved in resistance to HIV-1. The most significant genetic correlates of protection belong to two families: chemokine receptors/ligands and human leukocyte antigens (HLAs). Despite the established role exerted by the chemokine network in resistance to HIV infection, none of the analyzed factors has so far exhibited absolute protection against infection, and discrepant findings have been reported for: (i) polymorphisms in the regulatory region of the CCR5 gene [25]; (ii) a genetic variant of CCR2 (CCR2-64I) that is in strong linkage disequilibrium with a mutation in the CCR5 regulatory region [26]; (iii) an A-to-G substitution at position 801 within the 3′ untranslated region of the SDF-1 chemokine gene [27]; and (iv) promoter polymorphisms responsible for increased levels of CC-chemokine production (RANTES, MIP-1α, MIP-1β and MIP1αP) that can block R5-HIV-1 infection either by competition or by inducing receptor internalization [28]. More recently, analyses of the relationship between CCL3L1 copy number and susceptibility to HIV-1 infection have shown that CCL3L1 levels are inversely related to CCR5 expression on CD4+ T cells [29]. These findings might explain the mechanism by which chemokines exert their protective role: downregulation of CCR5 expression on the cell surface. Additional results performed in HTLV-2-infected individuals showed that the median copy number of the CCL3L1 and the CCL3L1/CCL3 mRNA ratios were increased in ESN individuals and in LTNP patients compared to those in healthy controls [30].

Immune responses to viral antigens are strictly dependent on host immune response genes. HLA genes are definitely the most prominent of such genes, due to their role in binding and presenting antigenic epitopes to T lymphocytes. Several publications describe associations of particular HLA alleles with different outcomes of HIV-1 infection; however, not all these reports have been confirmed. HLA alleles that have been definitively correlated with potent and possibly protective immune responses to HIV include (i) HLA-B*57, associated with particularly effective CTLs responses and lower viral load; (ii) B*27, involved in selective presentation of an immunodominant p24^{gag} epitope; and (iii) B*35, most consistently associated with an earlier AIDS progression among whites [31,32]. Additional studies performed in HIV-infected mothers showed that maternal/fetal HLA class I concordance was proportionally associated with a stepwise increased incidence of perinatal transmission, suggesting that discordant HLAs provide infants with a means of protection against HIV, possibly as a result of allogeneic infant antimaternal MHC immune responses [33]. More recently, the ESN phenotype has been associated with another gene involved in the antigen presentation pathway: the endoplasmic reticulum aminopeptidase 2 (ERAP2) [34]. This enzyme trims peptides to optimal size for loading onto HLA I molecules and shapes the antigenic repertoire presented to CD8+ T cells. The haplotype network of ERAP2 is highly structured, with two differentiated haplogroups: haplotype A and haplotype B. Haplotype A has a higher frequency in the ESN individuals and leads to the expression of a 960-amino-acid full-length protein. Conversely, haplotype B, because of an alternative splicing, generates a truncated protein of 534 amino acids [35]. The maintenance of the two haplogroups at similar frequencies, around 0.5 percent in all populations, suggests a functional difference between haplotype A and B that could modulate the susceptibility to HIV infection.

Among non-MHC genes involved in the regulation of host immune response, a novel and intriguing HIV-1 genetic resistant factor refers to new genotypes at chromosome 22q12-13 [36]. This region is homologous to the one on mouse chromosome 15 that harbors the Rfv3 locus, which is able to influence the production of virus-neutralizing antibodies against Friend virus infection [37]. A genotyping analysis of microsatellite markers at polymorphic loci spanning a region of human chromosome 22 pointed out that one or more genes within this region are strongly associated with resistance to HIV infection [36]. It is of particular interest that the APOBEC3 locus is present in the middle of the above chromosomal segment [36]. Notably, APOBEC3G levels are higher in ESN compared to unexposed-uninfected individuals [38]; polymorphisms in the APOBEC3 locus were also shown to affect the susceptibility to Friend virus infection in mice [39], and, finally, Rfv3 was recently shown to be encoded by APOBEC [40].

COALESCING THE FIELD

Although first discovered and studied in the early 1990s, the ESN/EU issue received little attention beyond the studies conducted by the investigators and laboratories that had made the original ESN/EU discoveries and observations. Thus, in November 2009 the First International Symposium on Natural Immunity to HIV was held in Winnipeg, Manitoba, Canada. This meeting was quickly followed by a second conference, HIV-Exposed and Resistant, in Rockville, Maryland, United States in June 2010. At the second meeting the decision was made to refer to HIV-resistant individuals as HESNs, an acronym for **H**IV-**E**xposed **S**ero**N**egatives or, alternatively, **H**ighly **E**xposed **S**ero**N**egatives. The fact that these meetings were held at all indicates some increased interest in the phenomenon, by both AIDS researchers and administrators. Evidence that other AIDS research groups are beginning to investigate the HESN phenomenon can now be seen in a recent multi-institute collaborative publication [41] that confirms and extends our original findings that T cells from HESNs generate HIV-specific immune responses [4].

CHALLENGES TO BE MET

Although several HESN cohorts have been identified and are currently being studied by different laboratories, the phenomenon suffers from certain limitations and a lack of better understanding—which is not surprising, considering the lack of financial support for HESN research during the past two decades. For example, not yet clarified are the relative contributions of genetics and immunity to HESN resistance. Also, the ability to study the early dynamics of HESN development is hindered by the definition of the resistance phenotype itself. Because a repeatedly exposed individual must remain seronegative for several years before being designated HESN, research to observe critically any early immunological and virological changes cannot be performed. Thus, researchers are left to observe and compare the consequences of potentially important changes that likely occurred years before HESN designation could be made. One possible approach to avoid this problem that could save time and resources would be to develop a SIV/macaque model similar to that we reported in 1994 [6]. In this model, macaques would be exposed to sub-infectious amounts of infectious SIV, and followed longitudinally by testing for innate and adaptive SIV immunologic changes in blood and tissue before and after systemic and mucosal challenge with infectious amounts of SIV.

THE WAY FORWARD

More than 15 years ago, we considered the possibility that the ESN (now HESN) phenotype might teach us some important lessons concerning the design and development of effective AIDS vaccines. Thus, we asked the question: Has nature done the experiment for us? [42]. Interestingly, Elite Controllers (ECs), who comprise a small percentage of HIV-infected patients but who maintain very low HIV viral loads and high CD4 T cell counts [43], are studied for the purpose of developing effective prophylactic AIDS vaccines. However, by definition, ECs have failed the first of test of an efficacious AIDS vaccine by having become infected. In contrast, HESNs do not permit infection to occur, and understanding the immunological aspects of HESN resistance could be informative for vaccine design. Arguments have been made that: (i) the HESN phenomenon involves the "study of a negative", which is difficult to understand; and (ii) little progress has been made in understanding the HESN phenomenon, despite having been discovered 20 years ago. The answer to (i) may reside in developing a low-dose exposure SIV/macaque model that (as noted above) could permit the generation of "positive" data collected during the critical days and weeks after the initial exposure. It may relevant that the challenge-protected macaques that received sub-infectious doses of SIV went through a period of transient SIV infection 2—4 weeks after low-dose exposure [6]. The answer to (ii) may reside in potential financial support by HIV/AIDS research granting agencies, and recent increased scientific interest by the HIV/AIDS research community [44].

REFERENCES

[1] Inagawa DT, Lee MH, Moon HL, Wolinski SM, Sano K, Morales F, et al. Human immunodeficiency virus type 1 infection in homosexual men who remain seronegative for prolonged periods. N Engl J Med 1989;320:1458—62.

[2] Giorgi JV, Clerici M, Berzofsky JA, Shearer GM. HIV-specific cellular immunity in high-risk HIV-1 seronegative homosexual men. Florence, Italy: VIIth International Conference on AIDS; June 1992. 1620. Abstract 1209.

[3] Ranki A, Mattinen S, Yarchoan R, Broder S, Ghrayeb J, Lahdevirta J, et al. T cell responses towards HIV in infected individuals with and without zidovudine therapy, and in HIV-exposed sexual partners. AIDS 1989;3:63—9.

[4] Clerici M, Giorgi JV, Chou CC, Gudeman VK, Zack JA, Gupta P, et al. Cell-mediated immune responses to human immunodeficiency virus (HIV) type 1 in seronegative homosexual men with recent sexual exposure to HIV-1. J Infect Dis 165:1012—1019.

[5] Clerici M, Shearer GM. A TH1/TH2 switch is a critical step in the etiology of HIV infection. Immunol Today 1993;14:107—11.

[6] Clerici M, Clark EA, Polacino P, Axberg I, Kuller L, Casey NI, et al. T-cell proliferation to subinfectious SIV correlates with lack of infection after challenge of macaques. AIDS 1994;8:1391—5.

[7] Plummer F, Fowke K, Nagelkerke NJ, Simonsen JN, Bwayo J, Ngugi E. Evidence for resistance to HIV among continuously exposed prostitutes in Nairobi, Kenya. Berlin, Germany: Presented at the 9th International AIDS Conference/4th STD World Congress; June 1993. Abstract WA-A07—3.

[8] Fowke KR, Nagelkerke NJ, Kimani J, Simonsen JN, Anzala AO, Bwayo JJ, et al. Resistance to HIV-1 infection among persistently seronegative prostitutes in Nairobi, Kenya. Lancet 1996;348:1347—51.

[9] Kaul R, Rowland-Jones SL, Kimani J, Dong T, Yang HB, Kiama P, et al. Late seroconversion in HIV-resistant Nairobi prostitutes despite pre-existing HIV-specific CD8+ responses. J Clin Invest 2001;107:341—9.

[10] Clerici M, Sison AV, Berzofsky JA, Rakusan TA, Brandt CD, Ellaurie M, et al. Cellular immune factors associated with mother-to-infant transmission of HIV. AIDS 1993;7:1427—33.

[11] Barcellini W, Rizzardi GP, Velati C, Borghi MO, Fain C, Lazzarin A, et al. *In vitro* production of type 1 and type 2 cytokines by peripheral blood mononuclear cells from high-risk-negative intravenous use drug users. AIDS 1995;9:691—4.

[12] Cheynier R, Langlade-Demoyen P, Marescot MR, Blanche S, Blondin G, Wain-Hobson S, et al. Cytotoxic T lymphocyte responses in the peripheral blood of children born to human immunodeficiency virus-1-infected mothers. Eur J Immunol 1992;22:2211—7.

[13] Langlade-Demoyen P, Ngo-Giang-Huong N, Ferchal F, Oksenhendler E. Human immunodeficiency virus (HIV) nef-specific cytotoxic T lymphocytes in noninfected heterosexual contact of HIV-infected patients. J Clin Invest 1994;93:1293—7.

[14] Mackewicz CE, Blackbourn DJ, Levy JA. CD8+ T cells suppress human immunodeficiency virus replication by inhibiting viral transcription. Proc Natl Acad Sci USA 1995;92:2308—12.

[15] Koning FA, Jansen CA, Dekker J, Kaslow RA, Dukers N, van Baarle D, et al. Correlates of resistance to HIV-1 infection in homosexual men with high-risk sexual behaviour. AIDS 2004;18:1117—26.

[16] Trabattoni D, Caputo SL, Maffeis G, Vichi F, Biasin M, Pierotti P, et al. Human alpha defensin in HIV-exposed but uninfected individuals. J Acquir Immune Defic Syndr 2004;35:455—63.

[17] Biasin M, Piacentini L, Lo Caputo S, Kanari Y, Magri G, Trabattoni D, et al. Apolipoprotein B mRNA-editing enzyme, catalytic polypeptide-like 3G: A possible role in the resistance to HIV of HIV-exposed seronegative individuals. J Infect Dis 2007;195:960—4.

[18] Mazzoli S, Trabattoni D, Lo Caputo S, Piconi S, Blé C, Meacci F, et al. HIV-specific mucosal and cellular immunity in HIV-seronegative partners of HIV-seropositive individuals. Nature Med 1997;3:1250—7.

[19] Devito C, Hinkula J, Kaul R, Lopalco L, Bwayo JJ, Plummer F, et al. Mucosal and plasma IgA from HIV-exposed seronegative individuals neutralize a primary HIV-1 isolate. AIDS 2000;14:1917—20.

[20] Scott-Algara D, Truong LX, Versmisse P, David A, Luong TT, Nguyen NV, et al. Cutting edge: Increased NK cell activity in HIV-1-exposed but uninfected Vietnamese intravascular drug users. J Immunol 2003;171:5663—7.

[21] Biasin M, Piacentini L, Lo Caputo S, Naddeo V, Pierotti P, Borelli M, et al. TLR activation pathways in HIV-1-exposed seronegative individuals. J Immunol 2010;184:2710—7.

[22] Clerici M, Levin JM, Kessler HA, Harris A, Berzofsky JA, Landay AL, et al. HIV-specific T-helper activity in seronegative health care workers exposed to contaminated blood. J Am Med Assoc 1994;271:42–6.

[23] Pinto LA, Sullivan J, Berzofsky JA, Clerici M, Kessler HA, Landay AL, et al. ENV-specific cytotoxic T lymphocyte responses in HIV seronegative health care workers occupationally exposed to HIV-contaminated body fluids. J Clin Invest 1995;96:867–76.

[24] Deng H, Liu R, Ellmeier W, Choe S, Unutmaz D, Burkhart M, et al. Identification of a major co-receptor for primary isolates of HIV-1. Nature 1996;381:661–6.

[25] Yang C, Li M, Limpakarnjanarat K, Young NL, Hodge T, Butera ST, et al. Polymorphisms in the CCR5 coding and non-coding regions among HIV type 1-exposed, persistently seronegative female sex-workers from Thailand. AIDS Res Hum Retrovir 2003;19:661–5.

[26] Louisirirotchanakul S, Liu H, Roongpisuthipong A, Nakayama EE, Takebe Y, Shioda T, et al. Genetic analysis of HIV-1 discordant couples in Thailand: Association of CCR2-64I homozygosity with HIV-1-negative status. J Acquir Immune Defic Syndr 2002;29:314–5.

[27] Soriano A, Martinez C, Garcia F, Plana M, Palou E, Lejeune M, et al. Plasma stromal cell-derived factor (SDF)-1 levels, SDF1–30A genotype, and expression of CXCR4 on T lymphocytes: Their impact on resistance to human immunodeficiency virus type 1 infection and its progression. J Infect Dis 2002;186:922–31.

[28] Wu L, LaRosa G, Kassam N, Gordon CJ, Heath H, Ruffing N, et al. Interaction of chemokine receptor CCR5 with its ligands: Multiple domains for HIV-1 gp120 binding and a single domain for chemokine binding. J Exp Med 1997;186:1373–81.

[29] Gonzalez E, Kulkarni H, Bolivar H, Mangano A, Sanchez R, Catano G, et al. The influence of CCL3L1 gene-containing segmental duplications on HIV-1/AIDS susceptibility. Science 2005;307:1434–40.

[30] Pilotti E, Elviri L, Vicenzi E, Bertazzoni U, Re MC, Allibardi S, et al. Postgenomic up-regulation of CCL3L1 expression in HTLV-2-infected persons curtails HIV-1 replication. Blood 2007;109:1850–6.

[31] Carrington M, O'Brien SJ. The influence of HLA genotype on AIDS. Annu Rev Med 2003;54:535–51.

[32] Carrington M, Bontrop RE. Effects of MHC class I on HIV/SIV disease in primates. AIDS 2002;16(Suppl. 4):S105–14.

[33] MacDonald KS, Embree J, Njenga S, Nagelkerke NJD, Ngatia I, Mohammed Z, et al. Mother–child class I HLA concordance increases perinatal human immunodeficiency virus type 1 transmission. J Infect Dis 1998;177:551–6.

[34] Cagliani R, Riva S, Biasin M, Fumagalli M, Pozzoli U, Lo Caputo S, et al. Genetic diversity at endoplasmic reticulum aminopeptidases is maintained by balancing selection and is associated with natural resistance to HIV-1 infection. Hum Mol Genet 2010; 19:4705–14.

[35] Andrés AM, Dennis MY, Kretzschmar WW, Cannons JL, Lee-Lin SQ, Hurle B, et al. Balancing selection maintains a form of ERAP2 that undergoes nonsense-mediated decay and affects antigen presentation. PLoS Genet 2010;6:e1001157.

[36] Kanari Y, Clerici M, Abe H, Kawabata H, Trabattoni D, Caputo S, et al. Genotypes at chromosome 22q12-13 are associated with HIV-1-exposed but uninfected status in Italians. AIDS 2005;19:1015–24.

[37] Kawabata H, Niwa A, Tsuji-Kawahara S, Uenishi H, Iwanami N, Matsukuma H, et al. Peptide-induced immune protection of CD8R T cell-deficient mice against Friend retrovirus-induced disease. Intl Immunol 2006;18:183–98.

[38] Biasin M, Piacentini L, Lo Caputo S, Kanari Y, Magri G, Trabattoni D, et al. APOBEC3G: A possible role in the resistance to HIV of HIV-exposed-seronegative individuals. J Infect Dis 2007;195:960−4.

[39] Takeda E, Tsuji-Kawahara S, Sakamoto M, Langlois MA, Neuberger MS, Rada C, et al. Mouse APOBEC3 restricts Friend leukemia virus infection and pathogenesis *in vivo*. J Virol 2008;82:10998−1008.

[40] Santiago ML, Montano M, Benitez R, Messer RJ, Yonemoto W, Chesebro B, et al. Apobec3 encodes Rfv3, A gene influencing neutralizing antibody control of retrovirus infection. Science 2008;321:1343−6.

[41] Ritchie AJ, Campion SL, Kopycinski J, Moodie Z, Wang ZM, Pandya K, et al. Differences in HIV specific T cell responses between HIV seronegative exposed and unexposed individuals. J Virol 2011;85:3507−16.

[42] Shearer GM, Clerici M. Protective immunity against HIV infection: Has nature done the experiment for us? Immunol Today 1996;17:21−4.

[43] Owen RE, Heitman JW, Hirschkorn DF, Lanteri MC, Biswas HH, Martin JN, et al. HIV+ elite controllers have low HIV-specific T-cell activation yet maintain strong, polyfunctional T-cell responses. AIDS 2010;24:1095−105.

[44] Young JM, et al. Summary of 06/2010 HESN mtg. AIDS Res Hum Retrovir, in press.

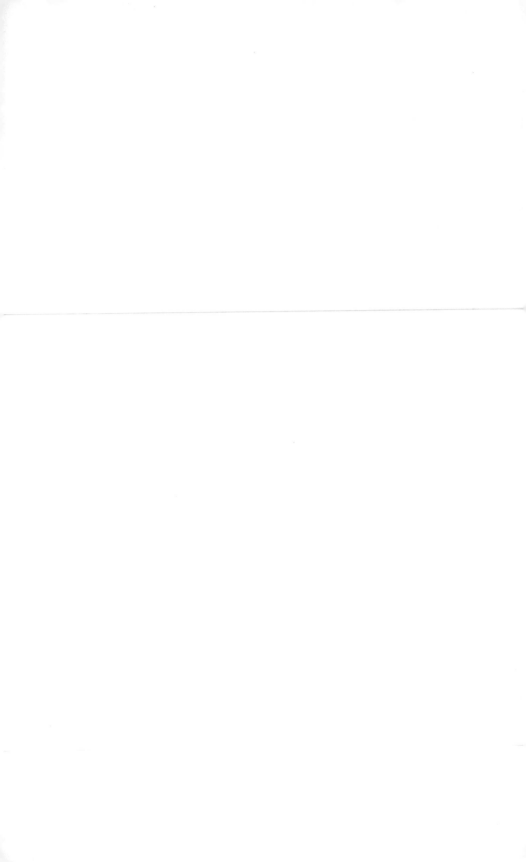

Chapter 5

The Genital Mucosa, the Front Lines in the Defense Against HIV

T. Blake Ball [1,2] and Kristina Broliden [3]

[1] *National Laboratory for HIV Immunology, National HIV & Retrovirology Laboratories, Public Health Agency of Canada, Winnipeg, Manitoba, Canada,* [2] *Department of Medical Microbiology, University of Manitoba, Winnipeg, Manitoba, Canada,* [3] *Karolinska Institutet, Department of Medicine Solna, Center for Molecular Medicine; Stockholm, Sweden*

Chapter Outline

Models of Protection Against HIV/SIV. DOI: 10.1016/B978-0-12-387715-4.00005-8

145

INTRODUCTION

In recent years, a focus has developed on trying to understand HIV transmission at the site of exposure: the genital mucosa. While much of the literature regarding HIV infection and mechanisms of protection against infection is based on studies performed within the systemic immune compartment, this does not reflect initial viral—host interactions. Initial exposure to HIV during sexual transmission, now accounts for the majority of transmission worldwide [1], and occurs at the genital tract. However, relative to what is known systemically, comparatively speaking, less is known about innate and adaptive immune responses capable of affecting HIV transmission at this site; in part due to difficulties in acquiring adequate samples for immunological studies of the genital tract, the lack of standardization in sample collection [2], differences in study design, and differences in the methodologies carried out to study mucosal immunology [3]. However, over the past several years considerable inroads have been made in understanding the early events in mucosal HIV transmission, and in greater understanding of the complexity of the immune environment at this site and the role it plays in HIV transmission. Some of the best data describing initial events during HIV transmission have come from studies of macaques inoculated intravaginally with the closely related simian immunodeficiency virus (SIV), representing the most relevant animal model for *in vivo* studies of HIV-1 infection [4,5]. In macaques, within the first 2—3 weeks of infection the virus is transmitted out of the mucosal compartment and becomes established in lymphatic tissue [6], the principle site of virus production, persistence and pathology [7,8]. It is only after this acute infection phase that cellular immune responses are generated in infected, susceptible hosts capable of containing viral replication [9,10,11]. By this time, the host's immune response is insufficient to clear infection. It is estimated that a vaccine of > 95 percent efficacy would be required to extinguish productive infection at the acute stage [10]. It therefore seems self-evident that the window of opportunity to eliminate HIV infection is during initial infection events. It is thus important not only to understand the early events in HIV infection and discover when and where the virus is most vulnerable, but also to comprehend how natural immunity limits these early events. A more complete understanding of innate and adaptive immune responses to HIV at the mucosal surface will inform the design of a mucosal-targeted vaccine, microbicide or other novel prevention technologies. In this chapter we will discuss issues surrounding sexual HIV transmission at mucosal surfaces, primarily at the female genital tract (FGT), and our current understanding of the putative role of the innate and adaptive responses in the genital mucosa in protecting highly HIV-exposed sero-negative (HESN) subjects from HIV infection.

SEXUAL EXPOSURE TO HIV INFECTIONS IN THE GENITAL MUCOSA

Several groups at risk of HIV infection have been defined as relatively resistant to virus infection, including the sexual partners of HIV-infected subjects [12]. In many cases, these subjects provide the most relevant model of protection against HIV infection. To understand specific correlates of protective immunity against sexual exposures to HIV, the specific anatomic site of viral penetration must be considered. Genetic, innate and adaptive immunologic defence mechanisms most likely need to act in synergy. The risks of exposure to HIV and, therefore, transmission vary substantially, from a single low-dose exposure of HIV-contaminated semen or genital secretions on an intact and non-inflamed mucosal surface to repeated, multiple exposures with high doses of infectious virus on damaged mucosal surfaces infiltrated by inflammatory cells. Different protective mechanisms are likely needed to compensate for these variations in dose of exposure and underlying inflammatory conditions. For example, secretory immune factors in genital fluid may be potentially sufficient for inhibiting low-dose exposure on intact mucosal surfaces, whereas submucosal cells and immune molecules must act in synergy to prevent systemic infection under high-dose and/or inflammatory conditions.

If mucosal innate or adaptive immune factors are responsible for protection in HESN subjects, they likely have several opportunities, and may need to act at multiple physiologic sites to inhibit HIV infection. Following sexual intercourse with an HIV-infected partner infectious virus could remain intact in the genital tract for some time, trapped in the genital fluid or in the stiff mucus layer covering some genital mucosal surfaces, or attached to epithelial cell structures, intra-epithelially or even in the submucosa, before it could be efficiently targeted by the immune system. It is important to understand whether self-limiting submucosal infections or long-standing compartmentalized viral foci can exist in sexually exposed HESN individuals, or whether the infection is ablated before passing the epithelial layer prior to transmission to the systemic compartment upon reaching the lymphatic system. Only a few studies have reported the detection of pro-viral DNA in the systemic compartment in HESN subjects, using ultrasensitive PCR [13,14]. These studies suggest that the virus obtained from PBMCs is the result of an archived, abortive infection, or that seronegative systemic viral replication in HESN subjects happens incredibly rarely. Together, these studies imply that viral infection in HESN subjects is likely aborted at the genital tract level, due to defective particles, or, as the wide array of data on the HESN subjects indicate, due to specific host factors, prior to widespread systemic dissemination. Nevertheless, the possibility of mucosal occult infections in HESN individuals cannot be ruled out following viral exposure.

In non-human primate studies, these questions are being resolved by examining the relevant tissue samples obtained via biopsies or necropsies [15].

Mucosal biopsies collected within a few days following sexual exposure to HIV cannot, for obvious reasons, be readily obtained in humans, and thus the question remains as to whether focal sites of viral replication exist in the absence of a systemic spread. While such questions cannot be answered in humans, they should continue to be explored and defined in studies of non-human primate models. The possibility of limited or abortive viral infections, either mucosally or systemically, does not exclude the likelihood that HESN individuals are indeed protected against HIV infection and define a "resistant phenotype" that can be informative towards understanding correlates of protection against HIV infection and disease. All individuals that can be classified as HESN by sexual transmission are by definition HIV-seronegative and show no evidence of systemic viral RNA replication even in rigorous, well-controlled studies [16], indicating that HESN subjects, even if subclinically infected, maintain control over active viral replication. However, the presence of an adaptive HIV-specific cellular and humoral immune response in the systemic circulation [17] and in the genital mucosa [18] of HESN individuals favors the hypothesis that at least one or a few rounds of viral replication may have occurred in the submucosa, as the stimulation of adaptive T cell responses, other than those arising by cross-presentation, normally requires antigen presentation by virus-infected cells in lymph nodes.

INFLUENCE OF IMMUNE FACTORS IN GENITAL SECRETIONS ON HIV TRANSMISSION

Semen is the main vector for HIV dissemination worldwide, and contains free HIV particles, virions associated to spermatozoa, and HIV-infected leukocytes [19,20]. HIV can thus be transmitted to mucosal target cells, including dendritic cells, macrophages and T cells [21]. It was recently shown that specific proteins in seminal fluid, such as semen derived enhancer of virus infection (SEVI), can induce fibril structures promoting the physical contact between the virus and epithelial surfaces, and thereby promote virus infection [22]. Semen also acts as a buffer of the low pH in the female genital tract, and thereby counteracts this natural antimicrobial defense. Furthermore, semen triggers induction of a local inflammatory response, induces dendritic cell projections to the luminal surface and promotes attraction of HIV target cells, including Langerhans cells, in the human FGT [23,24]. Additionally, HIV binds to C-type lectins and pattern recognition receptors (PRR) on both epithelial and antigen-presenting cells, and can result in activation of the immune system in a dose-dependent manner [25,26]. Thus, the route and dose of HIV exposure are issues that need to be considered when interpreting study results. Clearly, inflammatory immune signals likely influence the ability of HIV to target mucosal cells for replication, and/or transmission out of the mucosal compartment. Thus, innate or adaptive immune responses to semen and/or HIV in HESN subjects, especially in female genital secretions, may play a key role in altering HIV susceptibility at the FGT.

In Figure 5.1, both external and intrinsic factors that can affect the genital mucosal surface and thereby contribute to its susceptibility to virus infection are illustrated.

Female Genital Secretions Mediate both Antiviral and Inflammatory Activity

In the FGT, a layer of mucus is firmly attached to parts of the epithelial surface and functions as a barrier to HIV transmission [15]. The FGT is further protected from microbes by a cervical mucus plug that normally inhibits seminal fluid and microbes from entering the upper genital tract [27]. During ovulation the mucus plug is, however, more permissive to passage, and likely allows also free virus particles and HIV-infected leukocytes to passage to the upper genital tract regions. In the case of sexual exposure to HIV, there are numerous soluble factors and cells in genital and rectal secretions as well as in saliva that comprise the first line of defense against the virus. Here, a host of naturally occurring antimicrobial peptides, cytokines and chemokines may block the virus from attaching to target cells or epithelial surfaces, or may act by reducing cellular inflammation, the recruitment of susceptible target immune cells to this site. The altered expression of any of these factors may play a role in protecting against HIV.

A large number of innate proteins known (or suspected) to be able to inhibit HIV replication *in vitro* have been identified as being active in mucosal secretions, especially secretions from the FGT. These factors include anti-proteases such as secretory leukocyte protease inhibitor (SLPI) and elafin. Other cationic polypeptides with antiviral activity include α and β defensins, cathelicidins, calprotectin, lactoferrin and lysozyme, among others. These proteins act in a complex network including cytokines and chemokines such as IFN-α, MIP-1α, MIP-1β, Mip-3α and RANTES that can either promote or inhibit virus infection, depending on the time and location of their expression. Wira and colleagues recently reviewed and clarified the role of these mucosal factors in relation to HIV infection [25]. However, the ability of an innate factor to affect HIV replication *in vitro* does not necessarily correlate with the ability of these factors to do so in *vivo*. Several studies of HESN subjects have identified a number of FGT immune factors that correlate with protection from HIV infection and may shed light on whether any of these factors are indeed protective *in vivo*. These studies have identified the over-expression of certain β-chemokines, such as MIP-1α, MIP-1β and RANTES, in cells, secretions and cervical biopsies from HESN subjects [28–30]. Over-expression of proteins such as SLPI, elafin and lactoferrin has also been observed in cervical secretions in several HESN cohort studies [31–33], as has the over-expression of defensins and other small cationic antimicrobials [34,35]. Mucosal protection from infection may also be mediated by the absence or under-expression of inflammatory immune factors. Some studies have shown that HESN women had significantly lower levels of TNF-α and IFN-γ in their genital tract

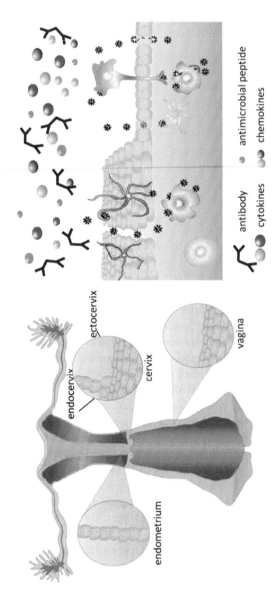

FIGURE 5.1   Model of factors that can protect from HIV infection in the female genital tract. The human female genital tract mucosa is covered by epithelial cells arranged in either a single layer (endocervix, endometrium) or multiple layers (ectocervix, vagina). A layer of mucus is firmly attached to the epithelial surface of the vagina and ectocervix, and constitutes a physical barrier to HIV transmission. In the case of sexual exposure to HIV, there are numerous soluble factors and cells in genital secretions that comprise the first line of defense against HIV. Here, a host of immune cells, antibodies, antimicrobial peptides, cytokines and chemokines may block the virus from attaching to epithelial surfaces and HIV target cells in the submucosa. The altered expression of any of these factors may influence the susceptibility to HIV infection. The balance between a pro- and an anti-inflammatory status of the mucosa may be one of the factors that determines the HESN status. Natural resistance to HIV infection and the inflammatory status are also critically influenced by physical and chemical external and intrinsic factors, including pH, presence of bacterial vaginosis, STIs, hormonal factors, seminal fluid and ruptions of the epithelial barrier.

compared with HIV-infected controls [36], while they had significantly higher levels of the HIV inhibitory factor MIP-1α. One caveat to these findings is that not all of these factors can be found at physiologic concentrations shown to inhibit HIV replication *in vitro*.

New approaches utilizing the tools of systems biology have identified several novel innate factors in genital secretions, providing a deeper appreciation of the complexity of mucosal fluids from this site. Using proteomic approaches, researchers have identified literally hundreds to thousands of specific proteins and isoforms in genital secretions [37]. Some of these approaches have been used to identify additional novel innate factors that associate with protection in HESN women. Using 2D-DIGE, a proteomics approach, over 15 new proteins were found to be differentially expressed between HIV-resistant women and controls, with the majority of over-expressed proteins being antiproteases, including serpins B1, B3, B4, and B13, A2ML1, and cystatin A [38]. In a larger confirmatory study, using multiple proteomic and standard immunologic approaches, these findings were expanded and confirmed the over-expression of antiproteases such as serpins and elafin in HESN subjects (A. Burgener and colleagues, personal communication). Serpins have a diverse set of functions, including regulation of the immune response and subduing general inflammatory responses in a variety of cell lines and tissues, including those at mucosal surfaces [39]. Additionally, some serpins exhibit potent antiviral activity against HIV infection of target cells present in the cervicovaginal compartment [40,41]. Interestingly, the majority of anti-proteases in genital secretions were found at physiologically concentrations shown to inhibit HIV and inflammation *in vitro*. As inflammation of the genital tract is known to increase susceptibility to HIV infection [42], anti-proteases such as elafin/trappin2 and serpins would have a plausible role in being protective.

One critical factor that must be addressed is that many of these factors (cytokines, chemokines, defensins, serpins, etc.) both act to inhibit HIV replication *in vitro* and are also potent in inflammatory processes and the recruitment of HIV target cells, critical for the establishment of HIV infection [43]. Many of these factors associate with conditions and infections that have been clearly demonstrated to increase susceptibility to HIV, such as bacterial vaginosis and genital tract inflammation. Consistent with this, higher genital levels of RANTES, able to block HIV infection *in vitro*, directly correlated with an increased number of mucosal CD4+ T cells in the cervix [44]. This means that the role of these immune factors must be carefully considered in the context of co-infection and immune activation at the FGT. Factors that correlate with protection may have pleiotropic effects, on the one hand recruiting susceptible target cells but on the other potentially inhibiting HIV infection at this site. The majority of these factors have been identified primarily through cross-sectional studies, in which causality of these factors is not established, and their association with confounding co-infections or inflammatory processes is unclear. In fact, one study demonstrated that lactoferrin, RANTES and SLPI (all capable of inhibiting HIV replication) were found to be associated with bacterial vaginosis and inflammation rather than exposure to HIV [33], while levels of α defensins and LL37 were shown to associate with genital infections and increased acquisition of HIV rather than protection in prospective studies [34]. Relatively few factors, such as elafin, have been shown to be causally associated with protection in prospective studies [31]. Thus, there are several lines of evidence to suggest that mucosal secretions from HESN subjects contain soluble factors capable of inhibiting HIV. Further well-controlled, prospective studies are critically needed to determine causality of these factors, where the effects of genital inflammation and infection can be well controlled and the impact of these events on expression of inhibitory factors in genital secretions can be accurately assessed.

ENDOGENOUS HOST MICROFLORA AFFECT INFLAMMATION AND SUSCEPTIBILITY TO HIV

In addition to the effects of concurrent STIs or genital tract infections, the endogenous host microflora in the FGT likely play a critical role in mediating the expression of specific factors in mucosal secretions. A biofilm of commensal bacteria usually covers the cervicovaginal epithelium, and is crucial for maintenance of natural immunity against invading microbes. Disruption of this balance causes changes in vaginal pH and influences the inflammatory status of the mucosa [45]. Due to the extremely complex nature of mucosal immune defenses, the composition of the normal microflora of the FGT varies in women from different continents as well as with allostimulation, the stage of the menstrual cycle and the use of hormonal contraceptives [46]. The epithelial cell—microflora interactions also regulate the control of the normal microbial flora through its constitutive as well as inducible antimicrobial peptide defense system [47]. With the advent of new technologies such as deep sequencing, and advances in microbial genotyping and quantification, a better understanding of the microbial ecology surrounding HIV susceptibility is now possible [48]. This was recently discussed in an excellent review by Mirmonset and colleagues [45]. Generally speaking, however, other than the role of bacterial vaginosis (BV), relatively few studies have examined the role of commensal bacteria in genital tract inflammation and HIV susceptibility. The role of BV in HIV susceptibility is relatively well understood, and can be defined as shift of vaginal microflora from *Lactobacillus*-dominated to overall non-*Lactobacillus* flora, including *Gardnerella* and *Prevotella*, among others [49]. BV is commonly associated with increased vulnerability to most STIs [50], including HIV [51]. Despite not inducing a classic inflammatory mucosal response, BV is strongly associated with increased levels of pro-inflammatory cytokines [52] and decreased mucosal innate factors such as elafin and others [53]. In contrast, lactobacilli are thought to produce lactic acid and reactive oxygen species such as hydrogen peroxide (H_2O_2), protecting the reproductive tract from exogenous pathogens [54]. The anti-inflammatory effects of "normal" vaginal flora dominated by lactobacillus in the vagina have not been well described, but the literature to date would suggest they are important in maintaining a relatively non-inflammatory state. To examine whether BV status and/or the composition of microbial flora was associated with the HESN phenotype, Schellenberg and colleagues utilized a deep sequencing analysis based on the chaperonin-60 universal target (*cpn*60 UT) [55]. They were thereby able to richly describe the composition of the microbial flora in HESN and uninfected controls, identifying over 54 species in 29 genera. However, few differences between HESN and HIV-uninfected, susceptible controls were observed; HESN subjects were just as likely to be diagnosed with BV in cross-sectional and longitudinal studies. No differences in overall bacterial richness, diversity or evenness were observed in HESN individuals [55]. Therefore, at least based upon this single study, there does not appear to be a determinative role for BV or microbial composition in the HESN phenotype, suggesting that differences in innate factor expression in the FGT are due to host factors rather than differences in microbial flora.

THE GENITAL EPITHELIUM PROTECTS AGAINST VIRAL INVASION BY MULTIPLE MECHANISMS

Epithelial cells in the genital tract are arranged either in a single layer (endo-cervix, endometrium) or in multiple layers (ectocervix, vagina, foreskin), and play an important role in protection from infectious agents [56]. In addition, there are also specialized cell-to-cell junctions that create a barrier between the surface and the adjacent connective tissue. The intercellular space between epithelial cells is minimal and devoid of any structure except where junctional attachments are present. Subclassifications of epithelium are usually based on the shape of the cells (squamous, cuboidal and columnar) and the number of cell layers (single or multiple) rather than on function [57]. The anatomy of human genital epithelial surfaces has not been studied with regard to the HESN phenotype as compared with HIV-susceptible individuals, but it stands to reason that these structures may be a critical component in mediating protection from infection.

The biologic properties of the various domains (apical, lateral, basal) of epithelial cells are determined by specific lipids and integral membrane proteins. These domains allow functional and morphologic polarity of the epithelial cells, and can determine the immunologic function of the various cell types. For example, the epithelial cell polymeric Ig receptor (pIgR) can traverse the epithelial cell from the basolateral side to the apical side to release IgA into the lumen. Some have argued that this is mechanism by which HIV may be prevented from transversing the epithelial layers ([58], but this has yet to be examined *in vivo* in HESN subjects. Certainly, as is discussed later, IgA responses against HIV have been detected in HESN subjects, and this might be one mechanism by which they may act. Together with other genetic factors [59] these epithelial mechanisms may contribute to the HESN status. Furthermore, tight junction barriers permit epithelial cells to polarize functionally to respond to different stimuli and serve as a directional conduit for a number of secreted factors. Uterine epithelial cells have been shown to secrete cytokines such as TGF-β preferentially at the basolateral surface, and TNF-α at the apical surface [60]. In regard to sexual exposure from HIV-infected genital secretions, the various types of epithelial cells form different anatomic barriers for the passage of viral particles to the underlying stroma. These cells are also under the influence of sex hormones, and must maintain a role in balancing reproductive potential with protection against sexually transmitted pathogens [61]. Since it is not clear where HIV enters the human genital tract and establishes the first local round of replication, it is important to study all sites that could be exposed to infected secretions. These sites must be individually evaluated for HIV susceptibility in order to understand and direct the development of prophylactic vaccine or microbicide compounds. The composition and densities of HIV target cells, receptors and antiviral immune responses are fundamentally different throughout the genital tract, and therefore a multitude of strategies are required to combat HIV infection. In non-human primate models experimentally challenged with high-dose viral particles, the endocervical region was the only site of initial HIV replication [62]. Based on this observation, and from a purely anatomical viewpoint, the endocervix and especially the cervical transformation zone, seems to be the most likely site for human HIV transmission.

Obviously, breaches or inflammation in any of these epithelial types allow increased access for pathogens to the submucosa, with subsequent viral dissemination to regional lymph nodes and the systemic circulation. Disruption of the epithelium due to these entities is unfortunately a common status in many HESN individuals as a result of frequent sexual intercourse and repeated subclinical and clinical mucosal infections. We do not know whether HESN individuals have any structural or functional advantages regarding the role of epithelial cells in protection against invasive HIV particles. Human genital epithelial cells express a variety of pattern recognition receptors, including Toll-like receptors (TLRs), and are therefore prepared to respond to a range of pathogens, including HIV, by triggering the innate immune response. The role of epithelial cells directly responding to HIV has only recently been a major focus of research, and it has been shown that genital epithelial cells are active in mounting host responses to HIV and likely play a critical role in HIV transmission [26]. As discussed above, a number of innate immune factors, many capable of being induced by TLR-mediated stimulation of epithelial cells, have been shown to be differentially expressed in genital secretions from HESN subjects. The regulation and site-specificity of the expression of these factors, if they are indeed protective against HIV infection, should be a priority. Levels of serpins, for example, shown to be primarily secreted by epithelial cells, may play a more direct role against HIV as HIV passes through epithelial surfaces. Importantly, secretion of many of these factors is also regulated by sex hormones, and studies on human subjects must take this effect into account when interpreting results on their role in HIV susceptibility. Regardless, the virus can, under certain conditions, enter the submucosal space by overcoming the protective secretions on the luminal side of the epithelium, penetrating the mucus layer and entering through breaches in the epithelial layer or attaching to projections of dendritic cells reaching out to the luminal surface. Virus particles also seem to actively diffuse through the outer layers of genital multistratified epithelium, where they can attach to intraepithelial lymphocytes and dendritic cells, including Langerhans cells [63]. A better understanding of how these processes may be altered in HESN individuals due to innate or adaptive immune responses to HIV, or the secretion of antiviral innate factors at these specific sites, should shed light on the natural mechanisms by which HIV passes through these sites in the vast majority of successful HIV transmission events.

THE ROLE OF CONNECTIVE TISSUE IN MUCOSAL IMMUNE DEFENSE

Connective tissue cells are conspicuously separated from one another, and the extracellular matrix (ECM) occupies the intervening spaces. Subclassification of connective tissue takes into account not only the resident cells but also the composition and organization of the ECM. Most epithelia rest on loose connective tissue, and the ECM in the FGT contains loosely arranged collagen fibers and numerous cells. The cells include fibroblasts, which form and maintain the ECM; however, most cells in this space are migrants from the vascular system and mediate important immune functions against invading pathogens [64]. While the interactions between migratory immune cells and components of the ECM have been well described in pathogenesis of various diseases such as cancer, renal disease, allergy and arthritis, and have been studied in the context of neuronal HIV pathogenesis and degeneration [65], little is known about the role of these types of interactions in HIV transmission and susceptibility, and no studies have been carried out in HESN individuals. However, as elements that comprise the ECM have been shown to play a role in such critical immune responses as antigen presentation [66] and T cell migration [67] and epithelial integrity, it stands to reason that interactions between HIV, transitory immune cells and the ECM are likely important in HIV susceptibility. Additional studies in this area are critically needed.

Expression of HIV-Binding Receptors in the Genital Mucosa

Clearly, the distribution of immune cells and HIV-binding receptors in the upper FGT is critical in the sexual transmission of HIV. To the best of our knowledge, these studies have yet to be performed in HESN subjects. In healthy controls the HIV receptors CD4 and galactosyl ceramide, as well as CCR5 and CXCR4, are expressed on uterine endometrial epithelial cells, and the expression changes as a function of menstrual cycle [68]. Furthermore, CD1a+Langerin+ Langerhans cells and CD11c+DC-SIGN+ dendritic cells are expressed just beneath the epithelial cells [69]. Together with abundant expression of T cells at this site and the permissiveness of the endocervical mucus plug to allow passage of HIV attached to spermatozoa, the uterus cannot be excluded as a site for HIV transmission. The endocervical epithelium contains numerous CD4+ cells including both T cells and antigen-presenting cells as well as Langerhans cells expressing CCR5 and CXCR4 [70]. Under certain hormonal conditions the single-cell layer epithelium can also reach out to the cervicovaginal lumen (cervical ectopy), thus affecting the risk of HIV transmission. The presence of the thin epithelium in direct contact with intact seminal fluid is likely to increase susceptibility to HIV infection. Another sexually transmitted pathogen, the human papilloma virus, is known to infect target cells in the vulnerable junction between the ectocervical multilayer epithelium and the endocervical single-cell layer [71]. This junction is called the transformation zone and is located in the lower part of the endocervical canal, and could also be a highly likely site for HIV penetration. SIV-exposed monkeys, human explant models and epidemiologic studies indicate that sexual transmission of the virus can occur across vaginal and cervical epithelial linings [72−74]. Although both the vaginal and ectocervical mucosal sites are likely first sites of contact with HIV following heterosexual transmission, the ectocervical mucosa contains higher concentrations of CD4+ intraepithelial lymphocytes and CD1a+ Langerhans cells than the vaginal mucosa [69]. Detailed phenotypic characterization of HIV target cells and receptors has not been performed in human vaginal tissue, whereas several studies have characterized the ectocervical tissue obtained from HESN women [75,76,77]. CD1a+Langerin+ Langerhans cells were found to be localized in the epithelium whereas CD11c+DC-SIGN+ dendritic cells and CD68+MR+ macrophages were restricted to the ectocervical lamina propria. Interestingly, the density of CLR expression was significantly higher in the high-risk as compared with the low-risk women. Detailed investigations discriminating epithelial from submucosal distribution of the CLRs revealed upregulated expression of Langerin in the epithelium, whereas DC-SIGN and MR were selectively upregulated in the submucosa [75]. Although limited in study numbers, there was no obvious difference between low-risk women of European *versus* African origin. The overall increased expression of CLRs in high-risk women as compared with low-risk control subjects was not a result of a higher influx of DCs in general, or a general inflammatory status, since the numbers of HLA-DR, CD11c, CD4 and CD8 did not differ between the groups in either ectocervical epithelium or the submucosa. Thus, the ectocervix remains a potential target for HIV transmission, yet transmission through the vaginal epithelium and upper FGT cannot be excluded.

The male foreskin epithelium is multi-stratified, and covered by a keratinized luminal surface. Intraepithelial as well as submucosal target cells are abundant, and express several HIV receptors. As in the ectocervix, the foreskin contains intraepithelial CD4+ T lymphocytes as well as CD1a+Langerin+ Langerhans cells. Abundant CD11c+DC-SIGN+MR+ dendritic cells as well as CD68+MR+ macrophages are located in the submucosa, and may also serve as initial target cells for HIV infection following contact with HIV-infected secretions. In addition, submucosal lymphoid aggregates are present in foreskin tissue from healthy men, and contain HLA-DR+, CD4+ and CD3+ cells. These aggregates, which are located close to the epithelium, could thus likely serve as replicative sites for incoming virus particles.

More studies are definitely needed on the status of the female and male genital submucosa in HESN individuals, since these are highly immunologically active sites. An altered distribution of HIV target cells and receptors in relation to antiviral immune mechanisms may be differently regulated in HESN individuals, and thus contribute to their resistant status.

THE IMMUNE RESPONSE IN HESN INDIVIDUALS

Mucosal Humoral Immune Responses in HESN Individuals

Antibody responses remain the focus for the generation of sterilizing protection against viral infection, and are the main correlate of protection in the majority of successful vaccines developed against viral pathogens [78]. Mucosal antibodies can be naturally occurring as well as induced by pathogen exposure, and they exert their antiviral effect at multiple sites, including genital secretions, the epithelium and the submucosa. In addition, systemic antibodies derived from the circulation are also secreted through mucosal surfaces; however, the mucosal and systemic activities are not coordinated, and the function is not always directly correlated between different mucosal sites (oral, genital and rectal). IgG is the main immunoglobin found in genital secretions, but its concentration varies at different anatomic sites [79]. Regarding mucosal immune responses, secretory IgA antibodies are also important, and their antiviral role is attractive since they: (i) function at lower concentrations than IgG at mucosal surfaces: (ii) are more resistant to degrading proteases; (iii) eliminate pathogens before they bind to epithelial cells; (iv) neutralize pathogens intraepithelially and in the submucosa; and (v) activate complement and opsonize pathogens to a very limited extent. Together these functional properties can be considered as "non-inflammatory", and this mucosal status is likely a desired property with regard to HIV risk exposures [80]. Studies on functional anti-HIV antibody responses in the genital mucosa of HESN individuals could possibly contribute to a better understanding of the nature of such a response.

The identification of IgA responses (with both HIV specific and non-specific biologic activities) in HESN subjects has been controversial, and hotly debated in the literature. The first identification of HIV-specific IgA was described in the genital tract of uninfected partners of seropositive individuals in 1997 [30], and subsequently HIV-specific IgA was found to be elevated in HIV-resistant sex workers compared to low-risk control women [81]. However, these results have not been replicated in other cohorts [82,83]. The presence of HIV specific IgA appears to be dependent on the frequency of HIV exposure (number of HIV-infected sexual partners, type of sexual activity and viral load in semen) [84]. Part of the controversy around this field is due to the difficulty in reliably and reproducibly detecting the specificity of IgA from cervicovaginal secretions. In fact, a recent study demonstrated that while HIV-specific IgG responses to HIV could be reliably detected in mucosal secretions, there was little concordance among six different laboratories in measuring IgA responses or viral neutralizing capacity [2]. Additionally, it has been shown that the IgA fraction including multiple specificities, rather than HIV-specific IgA *per se*, has been shown to neutralize HIV, and it is obvious that the measurement of antibody functionality is a more relevant assessment. Studies have previously detected two types of functional and/or biologic activity: HIV-1-neutralizing IgA antibodies in a peripheral blood mononuclear cell-based neutralization assay, and IgA-mediated inhibition of HIV-1 transcytosis across epithelial cells in HESN individuals [85,86]. Regarding specificity, the neutralizing IgA derived from HESN commercial sex worker cohorts have a reportedly broad cross-clade activity (i.e., is able to neutralize several HIV-1 clades). In contrast, IgA derived from exposed uninfected discordant partner cohorts seems to lack this characteristic [87,88].

Previous studies defining the presence of HIV-neutralizing IgA responses in exposed uninfected individuals were mainly based on cross-sectional studies including a limited number of study subjects. More recent studies have provided new data from prospective studies, as well as longitudinally followed HESNs regarding the possible biological relevance of these antibodies. In a blinded, carefully controlled prospective analysis of HIV transmission, HIV-neutralizing IgA was associated to protection against HIV infection [89]. Further, salivary and systemic IgA neutralizing responses can be maintained in HESN subjects over time during continuous exposure to the virus [90]. Interestingly, genetic and functional analysis of HIV gp41-specific monoclonal mucosal IgAs derived from HESN individuals showed that these antibodies could indeed block HIV epithelial transcytosis and mediate neutralization of CD4(+) cell infection [91]. In a subsequent study, immunization with HIV gp41 subunit virosomes induced mucosal IgA and IgG antibodies protecting non-human primates against vaginal SHIV challenges [92]. Although these recent studies have correlated HIV-neutralizing IgA to protection against infection, this function is just one of many other correlates of protection in HESN individuals. Furthermore, it remains to be determined whether the presence of these responses is a footprint of exposure or a true correlate of protection.

ADAPTIVE CELLULAR IMMUNE RESPONSES IN HESN INDIVIDUALS

While systemic HIV-specific cellular immune responses have been shown to play an important role in control of HIV replication in infected individuals [93], the role of these responses in HESN individuals has been debated. Compared to studies done on gut and gastrointestinal tract mucosal surfaces, there has been a paucity of studies examining the role of T cell responses to HIV in the genital mucosa either in HIV-infected subjects or in HESN individuals. This is due to difficulties in obtaining adequate samples via biopsy, or other invasive methods, from the FGT for traditional T cell assays. Several studies in HIV-infected subjects have utilized the relatively few cells obtained by cervical cytobrushes to show T cell responses are present in the FGT, and are similar clonally to those found systemically [94,95]. Methods have been developed to polyclonally expand cells from the genital tract; however, care must be taken, when assessing these cells post-expansion, that they retain their *in vivo* functional phenotype prior to expansion [96,97]. The functional relevance of cytotoxic T cell (CTL) responses in the FGT for reduction of HIV shedding, or control of viral replication, are just now being evaluated. Some have shown that while increased genital inflammatory cytokine expression correlated with cervical viral shedding [98], this was in contrast to what is observed systemically. Systemically, elevated viral loads generally correlate with increased CTL activity, assumed to be playing a role in viral suppression. This suggests that as genital shedding did not associate with levels of mucosal CTL, CTL responses in the FGT may be playing different roles and their functions may not reflect those found systemically [99]. Kaul and colleagues were able to demonstrate mucosal CTL responses in some HESN individuals [18], and the magnitude and frequency of responses to particular epitopes were increased compared to matched samples from those same individuals examined in blood [100]. This suggests that mucosal cellular responses again differ compared to systemic responses, and that mucosal CTL responses may play a role in protection from infection in HESN subjects. There have been few other studies examining cell-mediated responses to HIV in the FGT—an obvious shortcoming in the field. Difficulties remain in collecting enough cells from the FGT to accurately assess mucosal immune responses, and in that many current assays, even sensitive molecular assays, while capable of measuring systemic responses, fail to find these responses in FGT samples, even in HIV-infected subjects with robust systemic responses [101]. Again, it seems that further studies are critically needed to address the role of cell-mediated immunity at the genital tract. Studies of other cellular immune mechanisms that have been suggested to play a role in protection in

HESN subjects, such as NK responses or altered monocyte function [102], need to be replicated in studies at mucosal sites.

SYNTHESIS OF A MODEL OF PROTECTION IN HESN INDIVIDUALS: THE IQ HYPOTHESIS

In addition to the mucosal correlates of protection identified so far in HESN subjects and discussed above, other chapters in this book discuss the role of systemic cellular immune responses and of host genetics in mediating protection from infection in these unique experiments of nature. Some have tried to synthesize these findings into an overall view of the HESN phenotype. We have developed an overarching hypothesis that combines the majority of these findings into a unifying testable theory; that is, that HESN individuals seemingly naturally resistant to HIV infection are immunologically in a state of low baseline immune activation, but can respond appropriately to antigenic challenge. Data from our chapter, and discussed elsewhere, suggest that women described as resistant to HIV infection are *immunologically quiescent*. This generalized phenotype is characterized by: (i) reduced mRNA expression in pathways critical for HIV replication such as T cell signalling, host restriction factors, and immune activation pathways [103] (E. M. Songok and colleagues, personal communication); (ii) reduced systemic cellular immune activation and increased levels of regulatory T cells [104]; (iii) reduced mucosal inflammatory cytokine and elevated anti-inflammatory cytokine expression [36]; (iv) elevated expression of immunosuppressive anti-proteases at the genital mucosa [31,38]; (v) genetic polymorphisms in immunoregulatory genes controlling immune activation [59,105]; and (vi) a normal ability to generate *de novo* immune responses and a normal ability to respond to recall antigens [103]. This hypothesis does not solely rely on any of the above individual contributions, but rather reflects the sum of their parts. We propose a two-step mechanism for HIV resistance operational at the initial stages of exposure to HIV. Initially the IQ phenotype, likely driven by multiple factors, including regulatory T cells, a number of different innate immunomodulatory and HIV inhibitory factors and the right combination of host genetics, leads to a reduction in the numbers of activated lymphocytes utilized by HIV for replication in the genital mucosa. This would provide an advantage to HIV-resistant women due to reduced cellular susceptibility to HIV during vaginal exposure. This may permit the evolution of HIV-specific adaptive responses that would ultimately eliminate an initial mucosally-limited HIV infection and prevent the establishment of systemic infection. It is likely that as HIV only targets activated lymphocytes for productive infection, rather than epithelial cells and other cell types utilized by the majority of other sexually transmitted pathogens, that this protective phenotype is specific to HIV. This would tip the critical balance towards protection from HIV infection rather than replication and eventual transmission of HIV out of the mucosal compartment. This would also explain these women's equivalent susceptibility to classic STIs, which has been observed in our HESN cohort as well as others. As emphasized in recent studies, Haase notes that for an HIV vaccine to be developed, limiting mucosal target cells is required [15], and Virgin and Walker comment that appropriate pre-existing immunity has the potential to prevent infection [106]. Our proposed two-step model of protection incorporates both of these points.

CONCLUDING REMARKS

In a theoretical model of acquired HIV resistance, protection in high-risk individuals could be gained by repeated contact with low doses of infectious HIV, or even with non-infectious viral particles or viral debris, by exposure from an HIV-infected partner. The low-dose exposure could then be initially controlled by the innate immune response, and subsequently a local and systemic adaptive immune response would respond to the sub-infectious dose of viral particles. Indeed, altered innate as well as humoral and cellular HIV-specific adaptive immune responses have repeatedly been detected in both blood and mucosal samples of HESN individuals. These immune responses are normally not present in healthy control subjects from non-endemic areas of HIV-infection. However, occasionally HIV-specific immune responses are also detected in these latter control subjects, most likely representing exposures to HIV or cross-reactivity to other cellular or microbial antigens. This assumption is based on the fact that even in well-controlled clinical study settings the "low-risk" controls have some risk of HIV and STI exposure, and often acquire other STDs. Thus, carefully controlled epidemiologic analysis is critical to determine what constitutes a HESN phenotype.

Regardless, it is clear that the immune defences of the FGT already do a remarkable job of protecting against HIV infection, with an estimated risk of sexual transmission of 3–50 per 10,000 sexual exposures [107], such that the risk of transmission per act can range from 0.1 to 1 percent [108], indicating a protective efficacy of almost 99 percent—much greater than any biomedical intervention described to date. We have discussed the factors associated with sexual transmission, such as the need to consider the immunomodulatory effects of semen and the dose and type of exposure to infectious virus. The various physical barriers of the FGT, mucous genital secretions, endogenous microbial flora and the epithelial barrier, and the way HIV may target these sites, should also considered. The underlying ability of HIV to bind or target cells within the uterus, endocervix, ectocervix and vaginal vault as well as the underlying submucosa is also a critical component in HIV transmission. It seems self-evident that alterations in the expression any of the innate resident regulatory factors at these sites may affect HIV transmission. For example, upregulation of innate anti-HIV factors or downregulation of HIV-susceptible target cells at a specific tissue site would obviously affect HIV replication at these sites. Thus, "protective" alterations in the genital mucosa may comprise at least part of the mechanism protecting HESN subjects against infection. These factors alone, or the induction of adaptive immune responses to HIV at these sites, should be the focus of future studies in HESNs and other models of protection against HIV. The identification of innate factors truly demonstrated to have some causal effects in protection from infection—serpins or elafin, for example—can then be considered for development for novel intervention strategies against HIV. The induction of HIV-neutralizing cellular or IgA responses should clearly be the focus of vaccination strategies. As far as possible, future studies need to replicate conditions that most closely reflect the complex *in vivo* conditions of mucosal surfaces. Challenge studies should include semen or sperm, as it has the potential to affect mucosal responses, which in turn will affect HIV transmission. The complex nature of the FGT needs to be considered, along with interactions with endogenous microflora, genital tract sexually transmitted or other infections, or inflammatory processes at all tissue sites. The regulation of these factors by sex hormones, the menstrual cycle and other confounding factors also needs to be considered. Carefully controlled, prospective studies need to be a focus for future studies and, as far as possible, a control for these factors.

REFERENCES

[1] UNAIDS. UNAIDS Global Report, 2008−2009. Geneva: UNAIDS; 2009.

[2] Mestecky J, Alexander RC, Wei Q, Moldoveanu Z. Methods for evaluation of humoral immune responses in human genital tract secretions. Am J Reprod Immunol 2011;65: 361−7.

[3] Kaul R, Ball TB, Hirbod T. Defining the genital immune correlates of protection against HIV acquisition: Co-infections and other potential confounders. Sex Transm Infect 2011;87:125−30.

[4] Barouch DH. Challenges in the development of an HIV-1 vaccine. Nature 2008;455:613−9.

[5] Pope M, Haase AT. Transmission, acute HIV-1 infection and the quest for strategies to prevent infection. Nat Med 2003;9:847−52.

[6] Haase AT. Population biology of HIV-1 infection: viral and CD4+ T cell demographics and dynamics in lymphatic tissues. Annu Rev Immunol 1999;17:625−56.

[7] Tenner-Racz K, Racz P, Bofill M, Schulz-Meyer A, Dietrich M, Kern P, et al. HTLV-III/LAV viral antigens in lymph nodes of homosexual men with persistent generalized lymphadenopathy and AIDS. Am J Pathol 1986;123:9−15.

[8] Pantaleo G, Butini J, Graziosi C. Human immunodeficiency virus (HIV) infection in CD4+ T lymphocytes genetically deficient in LFA-1: LFA-1 is required for HIV-mediated cell fusion but not for viral transmission. J Exp Med 1991;173:511−4.

[9] Zhang L, Lewin SR, Markowitz M, Lin HH, Skulsky E, Karanicolas R, et al. Measuring recent thymic emigrants in blood of normal and HIV-1-infected individuals before and after effective therapy. J Exp Med 1999;190:725−32.

[10] Little SJ, McLean AR, Spina CA, Richman DD, Havlir DV. Viral dynamics of acute HIV-1 infection. J Exp Med 1999;190:841−50.

[11] Koup RA, Hesselton RM, Safrit JT, Somasundaran M, Sullivan JL. Quantitative assessment of human immunodeficiency virus type 1 replication in human xenografts of acutely infected Hu-PBL-SCID mice. AIDS Res Hum Retrovir 1994;10:279−84.

[12] Horton RE, McLaren PJ, Fowke K, Kimani J, Ball TB. Cohorts for the study of HIV-1-exposed but uninfected individuals: benefits and limitations. J Infect Dis 2010; 202(Suppl. 3):S377−81.

[13] Zhu T, Corey L, Hwangbo Y, Lee JM, Learn GH, Mullins JI, et al. Persistence of extraordinarily low levels of genetically homogeneous human immunodeficiency virus type 1 in exposed seronegative individuals. J Virol 2003;77:6108−16.

[14] Koning FA, van der Vorst TJ, Schuitemaker H. Low levels of human immunodeficiency virus type 1 DNA in high-risk seronegative men. J Virol 2005;79:6551−3.

[15] Haase AT. Targeting early infection to prevent HIV-1 mucosal transmission. Nature 2010;464:217−23.

[16] Delwart E, Bernardin F, Lee TH, Winkelman V, Liu C, Sheppard H, et al. Absence of reproducibly detectable low-level HIV viremia in highly exposed seronegative men and women. AIDS 2011;25:619−23.

[17] Fowke KR, Kaul R, Rosenthal KL, Oyugi J, Kimani J, Rutherford WJ, et al. HIV-1-specific cellular immune responses among HIV-1-resistant sex workers. Immunol Cell Biol 2000;78:586−95.

[18] Kaul R, Plummer FA, Kimani J, Dong T, Kiama P, Rostron T, et al. HIV-1-specific mucosal CD8+ lymphocyte responses in the cervix of HIV-1-resistant prostitutes in Nairobi. J Immunol 2000;164:1602−11.

[19] Klasse PJ, Shattock RJ, Moore JP. Which topical microbicides for blocking HIV-1 transmission will work in the real world? PLoS Med 2006;3:e351.

[20] Hladik F, Dezzutti CS. Can a topical microbicide prevent rectal HIV transmission? PLoS Med 2008;5:e167.

[21] Ceballos A, Remes Lenicov F, Sabatte J, Rodriguez Rodrigues C, Cabrini M, Jancic C, et al. Spermatozoa capture HIV-1 through heparan sulfate and efficiently transmit the virus to dendritic cells. J Exp Med 2009;206:2717−33.

[22] Munch J, Rucker E, Standker L, Adermann K, Goffinet C, Schindler M, et al. Semen-derived amyloid fibrils drastically enhance HIV infection. Cell 2007;131:1059−71.

[23] Robertson SA, Sharkey DJ. The role of semen in induction of maternal immune tolerance to pregnancy. Semin Immunol 2001;13:243−54.

[24] Berlier W, Cremel M, Hamzeh H, Levy R, Lucht F, Bourlet T, et al. Seminal plasma promotes the attraction of Langerhans cells via the secretion of CCL20 by vaginal epithelial cells: Involvement in the sexual transmission of HIV. Hum Reprod 2006;21: 1135−42.

[25] Wira CR, Patel MV, Ghosh M, Mukura L, Fahey JV. Innate immunity in the human female reproductive tract: Endocrine regulation of endogenous antimicrobial protection against HIV and other sexually transmitted infections. Am J Reprod Immunol 2011;65: 196−211.

[26] Kaushic C. HIV-1 infection in the female reproductive tract: Role of interactions between HIV-1 and genital epithelial cells. Am J Reprod Immunol 2011;65:253−60.

[27] Becher N, Waldorf KA, Hein M, Uldbjerg N. The cervical mucus plug: Structured review of the literature. Acta Obstet Gynecol Scand 2009;88:502−13.

[28] Hirbod T, Nilsson J, Andersson S, Uberti-Foppa C, Ferrari D, Manghi M, et al. Upregulation of interferon-alpha and RANTES in the cervix of HIV-1-seronegative women with high-risk behavior. J Acquir Immune Defic Syndr 2006;43:137−43.

[29] Iqbal SM, Ball TB, Kimani J, Kiama P, Thottingal P, Embree JE, et al. Elevated T cell counts and RANTES expression in the genital mucosa of HIV-1-resistant Kenyan commercial sex workers. J Infect Dis 2005;192:728−38.

[30] Mazzoli S, Trabattoni D, Lo Caputo S, Piconi S, Ble C, Meacci F, et al. HIV-specific mucosal and cellular immunity in HIV-seronegative partners of HIV-seropositive individuals. Nat Med 1997;3:1250−7.

[31] Iqbal SM, Ball TB, Levinson P, Maranan L, Jaoko W, Wachihi C, et al. Elevated elafin/trappin-2 in the female genital tract is associated with protection against HIV acquisition. AIDS 2009;23:1669−77.

[32.] Farquhar C, VanCott TC, Mbori-Ngacha DA, Horani L, Bosire RK, Kreiss JK, et al. Salivary secretory leukocyte protease inhibitor is associated with reduced transmission of human immunodeficiency virus type 1 through breast milk. J Infect Dis 2002;186:1173−6.

[33] Novak RM, Donoval BA, Graham PJ, Boksa LA, Spear G, Hershow RC, et al. Cervicovaginal levels of lactoferrin, secretory leukocyte protease inhibitor, and RANTES and the effects of coexisting vaginoses in human immunodeficiency virus (HIV)-seronegative women with a high risk of heterosexual acquisition of HIV infection. Clin Vaccine Immunol 2007;14:1102−7.

[34] Levinson P, Kaul R, Kimani J, Ngugi E, Moses S, MacDonald KS, et al. Levels of innate immune factors in genital fluids: Association of alpha defensins and LL-37 with genital infections and increased HIV acquisition. AIDS 2009;23:309−17.

[35] Trabattoni D, Caputo SL, Maffeis G, Vichi F, Biasin M, Pierotti P, et al. Human alpha defensin in HIV-exposed but uninfected individuals. J Acquir Immune Defic Syndr 2004;35:455−63.

[36] Lajoie J, Poudrier J, Massinga-Loembe M, Guedou F, Agossa-Gbenafa C, Labbe AC, et al. Differences in immunoregulatory cytokine expression patterns in the systemic and genital tract compartments of HIV-1-infected commercial sex workers in Benin. Mucosal Immunol 2008;1:309−16.

[37] Zegels G, Van Raemdonck GA, Tjalma WA, Van Ostade XW. Use of cervicovaginal fluid for the identification of biomarkers for pathologies of the female genital tract. Proteome Sci 2010;8:63.

[38] Burgener A, Boutilier J, Wachihi C, Kimani J, Carpenter M, Westmacott G, et al. Identification of differentially expressed proteins in the cervical mucosa of HIV-1-resistant sex workers. J Proteome Res 2008;7:4446−54.

[39] Mangan MS, Kaiserman D, Bird PI. The role of serpins in vertebrate immunity. Tissue Antigens 2008;72:1−10.

[40] Elmaleh DR, Brown NV, Geiben-Lynn R. Anti-viral activity of human antithrombin III. Intl J Mol Med 2005;16:191−200.

[41] Congote LF. The C-terminal 26-residue peptide of serpin A1 is an inhibitor of HIV-1. Biochem Biophys Res Commun 2006;343:617−22.

[42] Shattock RJ, Moore JP. Inhibiting sexual transmission of HIV-1 infection. Nat Rev Microbiol 2003;1:25−34.

[43] Zhou Z, Barry de Longchamps N, Schmitt A, Zerbib M, Vacher-Lavenu MC, Bomsel M, et al. HIV-1 Efficient entry in inner foreskin is mediated by elevated CCL5/RANTES that recruits T cells and fuels conjugate formation with Langerhans cells. PLoS Pathog 2011;7:e1002100.

[44] Kaul R, Rebbapragada A, Hirbod T, Wachihi C, Ball TB, Plummer FA, et al. Genital levels of soluble immune factors with anti-HIV activity may correlate with increased HIV susceptibility. AIDS 2008;22:2049−51.

[45] Mirmonsef P, Gilbert D, Zariffard MR, Hamaker BR, Kaur A, Landay AL, et al. The effects of commensal bacteria on innate immune responses in the female genital tract. Am J Reprod Immunol 2011;65:190–5.

[46] Spear GT, Sikaroodi M, Zariffard MR, Landay AL, French AL, Gillevet PM. Comparison of the diversity of the vaginal microbiota in HIV-infected and HIV-uninfected women with or without bacterial vaginosis. J Infect Dis 2008;198:1131–40.

[47] Ling Z, Liu X, Chen X, Zhu H, Nelson KE, Xia Y, et al. Diversity of cervicovaginal microbiota associated with female lower genital tract infections. Microb Ecol 2011;61:704–14.

[48] Lamont RF, Sobel JD, Akins RA, Hassan SS, Chaiworapongsa T, Kusanovic JP, et al. The vaginal microbiome: New information about genital tract flora using molecular based techniques. Br J Obst Gynaecol 2011;118:533–49.

[49] Livengood CH. Bacterial vaginosis: An overview for 2009. Rev Obstet Gynecol 2009;2:28–37.

[50] Larsson PG, Bergstrom M, Forsum U, Jacobsson B, Strand A, Wolner-Hanssen P. Bacterial vaginosis. Transmission, role in genital tract infection and pregnancy outcome: An enigma. Acta Pathol Microbol Immunol Scand 2005;113:233–45.

[51] Atashili J, Poole C, Ndumbe PM, Adimora AA, Smith JS. Bacterial vaginosis and HIV acquisition: A meta-analysis of published studies. AIDS 2008;22:1493–501.

[52] Mitchell CM, Balkus J, Agnew KJ, Cohn S, Luque A, Lawler R, et al. Bacterial vaginosis, not HIV, is primarily responsible for increased vaginal concentrations of proinflammatory cytokines. AIDS Res Hum Retrovir 2008;24:667–71.

[53] Stock SJ, Duthie L, Tremaine T, Calder AA, Kelly RW, Riley SC. Elafin (SKALP/Trappin-2/proteinase inhibitor-3) is produced by the cervix in pregnancy and cervicovaginal levels are diminished in bacterial vaginosis. Reprod Sci 2009;16:1125–34.

[54] Hillier SL. The vaginal microbial ecosystem and resistance to HIV. AIDS Res Hum Retrovir 1998;14(Suppl. 1):S17–21.

[55] Schellenberg JJ, Links MG, Hill JE, Dumonceaux TJ, Kimani J, Jaoko W, et al. Molecular definition of vaginal microbiota in East African commercial sex workers. Appl Environ Microbiol 2011;77:4066–74.

[56] Iwasaki A. Antiviral immune responses in the genital tract: Clues for vaccines. Nat Rev Immunol 2010;10:699–711.

[57] Coombs RW, Reichelderfer PS, Landay AL. Recent observations on HIV type-1 infection in the genital tract of men and women. AIDS 2003;17:455–80.

[58] Wright A, Lamm ME, Huang YT. Excretion of human immunodeficiency virus type 1 through polarized epithelium by immunoglobulin A. J Virol 2008;82:11526–35.

[59] Ball TB, Ji H, Kimani J, McLaren P, Marlin C, Hill AV, et al. Polymorphisms in IRF-1 associated with resistance to HIV-1 infection in highly exposed uninfected Kenyan sex workers. AIDS 2007;21:1091–101.

[60] Grant KS, Wira CR. Effect of mouse uterine stromal cells on epithelial cell transepithelial resistance (TER) and TNFalpha and TGFbeta release in culture. Biol Reprod 2003;69:1091–8.

[61] Wira CR, Fahey JV, Ghosh M, Patel MV, Hickey DK, Ochiel DO. Sex hormone regulation of innate immunity in the female reproductive tract: The role of epithelial cells in balancing reproductive potential with protection against sexually transmitted pathogens. Am J Reprod Immunol 2010;63:544–65.

[62] Haase AT. Early events in sexual transmission of HIV and SIV and opportunities for interventions. Annu Rev Med 2011;62:127–39.

[63] Hladik F, Hope TJ. HIV infection of the genital mucosa in women. Curr HIV/AIDS Rep 2009;6:20–8.

[64] Zaidel-Bar R, Cohen M, Addadi L, Geiger B. Hierarchical assembly of cell-matrix adhesion complexes. Biochem Soc Trans 2004;32:416–20.

[65] Chao C, Ghorpade A. Production and roles of glial tissue inhibitor of metalloproteinases-1 in human immunodeficiency virus-1-associated dementia neuroinflammation: A review. Am J Infect Dis 2009;5:314–20.

[66] Leonetti M, Gadzinski A, Moine G. Cell surface heparan sulfate proteoglycans influence MHC class II-restricted antigen presentation. J Immunol 2010;185:3847–56.

[67] Bi S, Hong PW, Lee B, Baum LG. Galectin-9 binding to cell surface protein disulfide isomerase regulates the redox environment to enhance T-cell migration and HIV entry. Proc Natl Acad Sci USA 2011;108:10650–5.

[68] Yeaman GR, Howell AL, Weldon S, Demian DJ, Collins JE, O'Connell DM, et al. Human immunodeficiency virus receptor and coreceptor expression on human uterine epithelial cells: Regulation of expression during the menstrual cycle and implications for human immunodeficiency virus infection. Immunology 2003;109:137–46.

[69] Pudney J, Quayle AJ, Anderson DJ. Immunological microenvironments in the human vagina and cervix: Mediators of cellular immunity are concentrated in the cervical transformation zone. Biol Reprod 2005;73:1253–63.

[70] Prakash M, Kapembwa MS, Gotch F, Patterson S. Chemokine receptor expression on mucosal dendritic cells from the endocervix of healthy women. J Infect Dis 2004;190:246–50.

[71] Veldhuijzen NJ, Snijders PJ, Reiss P, Meijer CJ, van de Wijgert JH. Factors affecting transmission of mucosal human papillomavirus. Lancet Infect Dis 2010;10:862–74.

[72] Spira AI, Marx PA, Patterson BK, Mahoney J, Koup RA, Wolinsky SM, et al. Cellular targets of infection and route of viral dissemination after an intravaginal inoculation of simian immunodeficiency virus into rhesus macaques. J Exp Med 1996;183:215–25.

[73] Hladik F, Sakchalathorn P, Ballweber L, Lentz G, Fialkow M, Eschenbach D, et al. Initial events in establishing vaginal entry and infection by human immunodeficiency virus type-1. Immunity 2007;26:257–70.

[74] Padian NS, van der Straten A, Ramjee G, Chipato T, de Bruyn G, Blanchard K, et al. Diaphragm and lubricant gel for prevention of HIV acquisition in southern African women: a randomised controlled trial. Lancet 2007;370:251–61.

[75] Hirbod T, Kaldensjo T, Lopalco L, Klareskog E, Andersson S, Uberti-Foppa C, et al. Abundant and superficial expression of C-type lectin receptors in ectocervix of women at risk of HIV infection. J Acquir Immune Defic Syndr 2009;51:239–47.

[76] Yeaman GR, Asin S, Weldon S, Demian DJ, Collins JE, Gonzalez JL, et al. Chemokine receptor expression in the human ectocervix: Implications for infection by the human immunodeficiency virus-type I. Immunology 2004;113:524–33.

[77] Patterson BK, Landay A, Andersson J, Brown C, Behbahani H, Jiyamapa D, et al. Repertoire of chemokine receptor expression in the female genital tract: Implications for human immunodeficiency virus transmission. Am J Pathol 1998;153:481–90.

[78] Hoxie JA. Toward an antibody-based HIV-1 vaccine. Annu Rev Med 2010;61:135–52.

[79] Mestecky J, Moldoveanu Z, Smith PD, Hel Z, Alexander RC. Mucosal immunology of the genital and gastrointestinal tracts and HIV-1 infection. J Reprod Immunol 2009;83:196–200.

[80] Cerutti A, Chen K, Chorny A. Immunoglobulin responses at the mucosal interface. Annu Rev Immunol 2011;29:273–93.

[81] Kaul R, Trabattoni D, Bwayo JJ, Arienti D, Zagliani A, Mwangi FM, et al. HIV-1-specific mucosal IgA in a cohort of HIV-1-resistant Kenyan sex workers. AIDS 1999;13:23−9.

[82] Dorrell L, Hessell AJ, Wang M, Whittle H, Sabally S, Rowland-Jones S, et al. Absence of specific mucosal antibody responses in HIV-exposed uninfected sex workers from the Gambia. AIDS 2000;14:1117−22.

[83] Mestecky J, Wright PF, Lopalco L, Staats HF, Kozlowski PA, Moldoveanu Z, et al. Scarcity or absence of humoral immune responses in the plasma and cervicovaginal lavage fluids of heavily HIV-1-exposed but persistently seronegative women. AIDS Res Hum Retroviruses 2011;27:469−86.

[84] Horton RE, Ball TB, Wachichi C, Jaoko W, Rutherford WJ, McKinnon L, et al. Cervical HIV-specific IgA in a population of commercial sex workers correlates with repeated exposure but not resistance to HIV. AIDS Res Hum Retroviruses 2009;25:83−92.

[85] Devito C, Broliden K, Kaul R, Svensson L, Johansen K, Kiama P, et al. Mucosal and plasma IgA from HIV-1-exposed uninfected individuals inhibit HIV-1 transcytosis across human epithelial cells. J Immunol 2000;165:5170−6.

[86] Devito C, Hinkula J, Kaul R, Lopalco L, Bwayo JJ, Plummer F, et al. Mucosal and plasma IgA from HIV-exposed seronegative individuals neutralize a primary HIV-1 isolate. AIDS 2000;14:1917−20.

[87] Devito C, Hinkula J, Kaul R, Kimani J, Kiama P, Lopalco L, et al. Cross-clade HIV-1-specific neutralizing IgA in mucosal and systemic compartments of HIV-1-exposed, persistently seronegative subjects. J Acquir Immune Defic Syndr 2002;30:413−20.

[88] Clerici M, Barassi C, Devito C, Pastori C, Piconi S, Trabattoni D, et al. Serum IgA of HIV-exposed uninfected individuals inhibit HIV through recognition of a region within the alpha-helix of gp41. AIDS 2002;16:1731−41.

[89] Hirbod T, Kaul R, Reichard C, Kimani J, Ngugi E, Bwayo JJ, et al. HIV-neutralizing immunoglobulin A and HIV-specific proliferation are independently associated with reduced HIV acquisition in Kenyan sex workers. AIDS 2008;22:727−35.

[90] Hasselrot K, Saberg P, Hirbod T, Soderlund J, Ehnlund M, Bratt G, et al. Oral HIV-exposure elicits mucosal HIV-neutralizing antibodies in uninfected men who have sex with men. AIDS 2009;23:329−33.

[91] Tudor D, Derrien M, Diomede L, Drillet AS, Houimel M, Moog C, et al. HIV-1 gp41-specific monoclonal mucosal IgAs derived from highly exposed but IgG-seronegative individuals block HIV-1 epithelial transcytosis and neutralize CD4(+) cell infection: An IgA gene and functional analysis. Mucosal Immunol 2009;2:412−26.

[92] Bomsel M, Tudor D, Drillet AS, Alfsen A, Ganor Y, Roger MG, et al. Immunization with HIV-1 gp41 subunit virosomes induces mucosal antibodies protecting nonhuman primates against vaginal SHIV challenges. Immunity 2011;34:269−80.

[93] Streeck H, Jolin JS, Qi Y, Yassine-Diab B, Johnson RC, Kwon DS, et al. Human immunodeficiency virus type 1-specific CD8+ T-cell responses during primary infection are major determinants of the viral set point and loss of CD4+ T cells. J Virol 2009;83:7641−8.

[94] Musey L, Hu Y, Eckert L, Christensen M, Karchmer T, McElrath MJ. HIV-1 induces cytotoxic T lymphocytes in the cervix of infected women. J Exp Med 1997;185:293−303.

[95] Musey L, Ding Y, Cao J, Lee J, Galloway C, Yuen A, et al. Ontogeny and specificities of mucosal and blood human immunodeficiency virus type 1-specific CD8(+) cytotoxic T lymphocytes. J Virol 2003;77:291−300.

[96] Bere A, Denny L, Burgers WA, Passmore JA. Polyclonal expansion of cervical cytobrush-derived T cells to investigate HIV-specific responses in the female genital tract. Immunology 2010;130:23−33.

[97] Bere A, Denny L, Hanekom W, Burgers WA, Passmore JA. Comparison of polyclonal expansion methods to improve the recovery of cervical cytobrush-derived T cells from the female genital tract of HIV-infected women. J Immunol Methods 2010;354:68−79.

[98] Bebell LM, Passmore JA, Williamson C, Mlisana K, Iriogbe I, van Loggerenberg F, et al. Relationship between levels of inflammatory cytokines in the genital tract and CD4+ cell counts in women with acute HIV-1 infection. J Infect Dis 2008;198:710−4.

[99] Nkwanyana NN, Gumbi PP, Roberts L, Denny L, Hanekom W, Soares A, et al. Impact of human immunodeficiency virus 1 infection and inflammation on the composition and yield of cervical mononuclear cells in the female genital tract. Immunology 2009;128:e746−57.

[100] Kaul R, Thottingal P, Kimani J, Kiama P, Waigwa CW, Bwayo JJ, et al. Quantitative *ex vivo* analysis of functional virus-specific CD8 T lymphocytes in the blood and genital tract of HIV-infected women. AIDS 2003;17:1139−44.

[101] Chege D, Chai Y, Huibner S, McKinnon L, Wachihi C, Kimani M, et al. Evaluation of a quantitative real-time PCR assay to measure HIV-specific mucosal CD8+ T cell responses in the cervix. PLoS One 2010;5:e13077.

[102] Tomescu C, Abdulhaqq S, Montaner LJ. Evidence for the innate immune response as a correlate of protection in human immunodeficiency virus (HIV)-1 highly exposed sero-negative subjects (HESN). Clin Exp Immunol 2011;164:158−69.

[103] McLaren PJ, Ball TB, Wachihi C, Jaoko W, Kelvin DJ, Danesh A, et al. HIV-exposed seronegative commercial sex workers show a quiescent phenotype in the CD4+ T cell compartment and reduced expression of HIV-dependent host factors. J Infect Dis 2010;202(Suppl. 3):S339−44.

[104] Card CM, McLaren PJ, Wachihi C, Kimani J, Plummer FA, Fowke KR. Decreased immune activation in resistance to HIV-1 infection is associated with an elevated frequency of CD4(+)CD25(+)FOXP3(+) regulatory T cells. J Infect Dis 2009;199:1318−22.

[105] Su RC, Sivro A, Kimani J, Jaoko W, Plummer FA, Ball TB. Epigenetic control of IRF1 responses in HIV-exposed seronegative *versus* HIV-susceptible individuals. Blood 2011;117:2649−57.

[106] Virgin HW, Walker BD. Immunology and the elusive AIDS vaccine. Nature 2010;464:224−31.

[107] Galvin SR, Cohen MS. The role of sexually transmitted diseases in HIV transmission. Nat Rev Microbiol 2004;2:33−42.

[108] Gray RH, Wawer MJ, Brookmeyer R, Sewankambo NK, Serwadda D, Wabwire-Mangen F, et al. Probability of HIV-1 transmission per coital act in monogamous, heterosexual, HIV-1-discordant couples in Rakai, Uganda. Lancet 2001;357:1149−53.

Host Genetics and Resistance to HIV-1 Infection

Ma Luo [1,2], Paul J. McLaren [3] and Francis A. Plummer [1,2]

[1] *Department of Medical Microbiology, University of Manitoba, Winnipeg, Manitoba, Canada,*
[2] *National Microbiology Laboratory, Public Health Agency of Canada, Winnipeg, Manitoba, Canada,* [3] *Department of Medicine, Division of Genetics, Brigham & Women's Hospital, Harvard Medical School, Boston, Massachusetts, USA*

Models of Protection Against HIV/SIV. DOI: 10.1016/B978-0-12-387715-4.00006-X
169

INTRODUCTION

The outcome of infections by infectious pathogens depends on the interactions between pathogen and host. In addition to the genetic variations of the pathogens, host genetic background plays an important role in determination of the outcome of infection. Variability in susceptibility to infectious disease has long been observed in human history, either within a population or among different populations. When exposed to an infectious pathogen, some individuals do not appear to become infected, or respond with mild symptoms and recover very quickly after being infected, while others succumb to the infection. Similarly, heterogeneity in susceptibility to HIV-1 has been observed in several cohort studies [1–6]. Most individuals are susceptible to HIV-1 infection through sexual transmission, blood transfusion, or other high-risk exposure. Some rare individuals, about 5 percent of the population, appear to be resistant to HIV-1 infection despite repeated exposure through high-risk sexual exposure or blood transfusion. Through two decades of research it has become clear that multiple factors are involved in the heterogeneous responses to HIV-1 infection, and the genetic factors underlying the phenomenon are complex and diverse [5–22]. Polymorphisms of host genetic factors involved in host immune responses and biological processes of HIV-1 infection, establishment and spread appear to play an important role in the heterogeneity in susceptibility to HIV-1 infection [17,23–52]. Several genetic factors, such as CCR5-Δ32 mutation [11,53–64], Trim5alpha polymorphisms [32,52,65–67], IRF-1 polymorphisms [10,68] and specific HLA class I and class II alleles [69–72], have been reported to influence a person's response to HIV-1 infection. Most of these genetic factors were identified through studying the rare individuals who are resistant to HIV-1 infection despite repeated high-risk exposure. However, identification of such individuals requires not only keen scientific observations, but also long-term follow-up of populations with high-risk exposure to HIV-1 infection. The Pumwani Sex Worker cohort is one of a few such populations in the world, and the only well-followed study population, established at the beginning of the HIV-1 epidemic in sub-Saharan Africa [73–86], where HIV/AIDS infection accounts for two-thirds of the world's HIV-infected population [87]. Thus, in this chapter, in addition to providing an evaluation of currently reported genetic factors contributing to the resistance or susceptibility to HIV-1 infection we have devoted a special section to the Pumwani Sex Worker cohort and the genetic factors identified in a subgroup of women who have been epidemiologically defined as resistant to HIV-1 infection [1].

GENETIC FACTORS ASSOCIATED WITH PROTECTION IN HIV-EXPOSED SERONEGATIVE INDIVIDUALS

Along with the description, by many groups, of individuals who are multiply exposed to HIV yet remain uninfected have come several investigations into the possible virologic, immunologic and genetic mechanisms underlying this resistance. The search for genetic factors associating with exposed uninfected status has led to major discoveries, such as the CCR5-Δ32 polymorphism, which has spawned several novel therapies and even discussion of a cure for infected patients. However, many other polymorphisms have been reported and remain unreplicated or controversial. Additionally, genetic studies in multiple ethnic groups with small sample sizes and varying levels of exposure make direct comparison of studies, even on the same gene, difficult. In this chapter, we will review the literature on genetic polymorphisms associated with HIV-exposed uninfected status and discuss the evidence supporting them.

CCR5

Within a few years of discovery and classification of HIV as the causative agent of AIDS, the CD4 molecule on T cells was determined to be the primary receptor required for viral entry into host cells. However, after a series of experiments determining that CD4 was necessary but not sufficient for HIV entry [88,89], a large number of groups began searching for potential coreceptors. The observation that the chemokines MIP-1α (CCL2), MIP-1β (CCL4) and RANTES (CCL5) could inhibit *in vitro* infection of highly susceptible CD4+ T cell clones, an effect that was blocked by adding neutralizing antibodies specific for those molecules, implicated the receptors for these molecules [90]. Shortly after these experiments, a series of reports in the journals *Science* and *Nature* described the identification of CCR5 and CXCR4 as critical coreceptors for the infection process [55,91–96].

Following this discovery, several groups described high rates of homozygosity for a 32 base-pair deletion mutation in *CCR5* (*CCR5-Δ32*) in multiply exposed but HIV-uninfected individuals of European ancestry [7,97,98]. It was further shown that the Δ32 heterozygous state results in reduced (but not eliminated) expression of CCR5 on the cell surface, and dramatically slows disease progression in infected individuals.

The *CCR5-Δ32* deletion results in a frame shift and early stop codon that, when present in a homozygous state, results in no functional CCR5 protein being expressed on the cell surface. This provides an obvious mechanistic link between the polymorphism and HIV resistance, as the coreceptor is required for infection. However, homozygosity for *CCR5-Δ32* is not totally protective, as rare examples of HIV infection, presumably by CXCR4-tropic viral isolates, have been observed [15,99,100].

The *CCR5-Δ32* polymorphism is present at the highest frequency in individuals of Northern European ancestry (~16 percent), at a lower frequency in Southern Europeans (~4 percent), and has not been detected in African or Asian populations [42,101]. Because of this population distribution, it was hypothesized that the Δ32 allele rose to high frequency due to dramatic positive selection pressure, possibly exerted by another infectious disease requiring CCR5 for infection, such as smallpox or bubonic plague [102]. However, later studies using more complete genetic maps of closely linked markers, larger sample pools and data showing high frequencies of this mutation in Bronze Age individuals have refuted this theory [62,103].

The observation that the CCR5 null state can occur in individuals without cost to general health has inspired a new class of anti-HIV drugs called CCR5 inhibitors (e.g., Maraviroc) that may be used in individuals with CCR5-tropic virus who show resistance to other drug classes. Additionally, an HIV-positive patient with relapsed acute myeloid leukemia was treated with transplanted stem cells from a *CCR5-Δ32* homozygous individual, and has since shown no further signs of HIV infection [104]. Although it is unclear whether the virus still resides in reservoirs and is undetectable by standard assays, several groups are now pursuing methods to delete the *CCR5* gene from autologous pluripotent stem cells as a potential HIV treatment or even cure.

The protection associated with the *CCR5* deletion mutation has led to targeted sequencing studies looking for other polymorphisms in the *CCR5* gene that may result in protection. A single base substitution at amino acid position 101, called m303 (rs1800560), has been reported to offer protection against infection when present with *CCR5-Δ32* [105,106]. However, this has only been observed in a small number of individuals, and the low frequency of this polymorphism makes replication difficult. Moreover, a set of SNPs in the promoter region of CCR5 forming a haplotype denoted as human haplogroup E (also called haplotype P1) has been associated with increased acquisition of HIV when found in the homozygous state, possibly through inducing over-expression of CCR5 [21,60,107]. Other CCR5 variants have also been identified in some Asian populations [108,109], and a heterozygous mutation has been shown to associate with a reduced CCR5 expression and a resistance to

HIV-1 R5 infection of CD4+ T cells in several Vietnamese HESN individuals [110].

HLA and KIR

Several studies of exposed uninfected individuals have shown evidence of HIV-specific immunity, discussed in detail in Chapter 7. Following these descriptions there has been association testing of genes involved in adaptive immunity, in particular human leukocyte antigen (HLA) genes, alleles which are known to play a strong role in determining disease outcome.

HLA concordance at class I loci has been convincingly associated with enhanced transmission from mother to child [111−114]. An analogous effect has been investigated in discordant couples, with some studies showing that HLA concordance increases speed of transmission, with *HLA-B* possibly having the largest effect [115,116]. However, another (although much smaller) study did not observe this effect [14]. Although the mechanism for enhanced susceptibility is not known, direct immune pressure selecting for viruses capable of escape in the uninfected recipient or muted allogenic responses to host cells or viral particles containing host protein are both plausible.

Due to the unequivocal impact that particular HLA alleles (such as HLA-B*57:01 and B*27:05) have on outcome after infection, multiple studies have searched for similar effects on acquisition. Interestingly, despite their large effect on lowering viral loads and slowing disease progression, neither B*57:01 nor B*27:05 has been shown to impact HIV transmission [115,117,118]. Association with a set of HLA-A alleles forming the A2/6802 supertype was originally reported in highly exposed yet uninfected Kenyan sex workers [72]. This was further substantiated by a similar trend of reduced mother-to-child transmission in the same Kenyan population [119] and association with protection against infection in high-risk men who have sex with men in North America [117]. In the latter study, the association was attributed to the A*02:05 subgroup of alleles within the supertype. Interestingly, this same study also implicated a polymorphism in *TAP2*, a gene involved in transporting antigens from the cytoplasm to the endoplasmic reticulum, and in MHC class I peptide loading. However, this association has not been replicated.

Multiple other studies have implicated particular HLA alleles in both increased and reduced susceptibility [112,118−124]. However, there is little to no consistency in the particular alleles shown to associate in each study. This may be due to a multitude of factors, such as differing allele frequencies in different ethnic groups, differing modes of transmission, differences in circulating viral strains, and false positive association. To clarify this area, efforts to replicate associations in samples matched over those factors would be required.

In addition to their role in adaptive immunity, HLA class I molecules also interact with killer immunoglobulin-like receptors (KIR) on the surface of natural killer (NK) cells. KIR molecules are a complex system of activating and inhibitory receptors encoded by 15 polymorphic genes on chromosome 19 that mediate the effector function of NK cells. As with HLA alleles, certain KIR molecules have been associated with varying rates of disease progression [125–127]. A study of HLA and KIR genotypes in a small number of highly exposed uninfected sex workers from Côte d'Ivoire showed they had an increased frequency of the inhibitory *KIR2DL2* and *KIR2DL5* and tended to possess *KIR2DL2* and *KIR2DL3* in the absence of their cognate HLA alleles [128]. The impact of KIR type on susceptibility was also investigated in exposed-uninfected individuals from Montreal, which showed that homozygosity for KIR3DS1 and possessing both HLA-B*57 and KIRDL*h/*y were protective against infection [129,130]. Both the studies in the African and North American population remain as the result of single association studies.

Controversies in the Field

In recent years, candidate gene studies of HIV susceptibility and disease progression in large cohorts have described several novel associations in genes with plausible biologic effects that have ultimately led to controversy. The *CCL3L1* (*MIP-1αP*) gene encodes a protein that is a potent ligand for CCR5 and exists in a complex area of the genome with good evidence for structural polymorphism (i.e., gene duplication). A report looking at the impact of the number of copies of this gene on HIV acquisition in a large, multiethnic sample showed that having fewer than the population mean number of copies of *CCL3L1* was associated with susceptibility to both mother-to-child and adult-to-adult infection [35]. It was hypothesized that an increased expression of *CCL3L1* that accompanied a higher gene dose may act by blocking CCR5 and preventing fusion. However, two studies attempting to replicate this effect in high-risk men who have sex with men showed no association [13,131]. A third study attempting to unravel the complexity of this locus identified technical issues that may have led to the original false positive association [132].

A similar controversy surrounded the description of resistance to HIV associated with a polymorphism in the Duffy Antigen Receptor for Chemokine gene (*DARC*). DARC is a glycosylated membrane protein primarily expressed on red blood cells that is known to bind a variety of pro-inflammatory cytokines and has been shown to bind HIV *in vitro* [133,134]. Polymorphism in this gene has been shown to impact infectious disease susceptibility as the *DARC-46C/C* variant, which results in a DARC null state, has been driven to fixation in many African populations due to it conferring resistance to malaria caused by *Plasmodium vivax* [135]. Its ability to bind HIV-suppressive chemokines such as CCL5 (RANTES) and to directly bind the virus has led to investigation of its role in mediating susceptibility in African Americans. The same group that originally described the association with *CCL3L1* (see above) also demonstrated a greatly increased susceptibility to infection in individuals homozygous for the *DARC-46C/C* variant [136]. The authors further speculated that the effect size of this variant, if extrapolated to African populations, could explain up to 11 percent of the HIV burden in that region. However, as with *CCL3L1*, multiple studies tested this claim in independent cohorts of exposed uninfected individuals, none of which could replicate the effect [137–139]. It was suggested by multiple authors of the contradictory studies that failure to account for admixture (combination of ancestral backgrounds) in the African Americans in the original study sample led to the false positive association—a claim the original authors dispute.

It is also of note that for both *DARC* and *CCL3L1* the original claims of reduced susceptibility to infection included investigations of disease progression. As with the susceptibility associations, these could not be replicated by multiple groups. This aspect of the controversy is discussed in Chapter 12 in this volume.

Dendritic-cell-specific ICAM-3-grabbing non-integrin (*DC-SIGN*, also known as *CD209*) and its homologue *DC-SIGNR* (also *CD209L*) encode for C-type lectin transmembrane receptors present on the surface of dendritic cells/ macrophages and hepatic/lymph node endothelial cells, respectively. Both proteins have been shown to bind HIV gp120 and promote *trans* infection of susceptible CD4+ cells [140,141]. Both proteins share similar structures, with a C-type lectin carbohydrate recognition domain, an N-terminal transmembrane domain and a tandem-repeat neck region. The neck region, encoded by exon 4, contains a 69-bp repeat segment that is variable in the population and may impact the interaction with gp120 [141,142]. The effect of the number of repeats in this region on HIV acquisition has been investigated for both genes. In a study of high-risk sexually exposed individuals from a multiethnic Seattle cohort, heterozygosity for repeats in *DC-SIGN* was associated with exposed-seronegative status, although these genotypes were found at a very low frequency [9]. Additionally, a study in an Asian population of discordant couples reported an association with reduced susceptibility and having fewer than five repeats in the *DC-SIGN* neck region [143]. Although different study populations, transmission risk and analytical strategies reported similar findings, the role of these repeats in limiting HIV acquisition should be tested and confirmed in functional studies. Additionally, a single study investigating promoter polymorphisms in *DC-SIGN* reported an increase in susceptibility to parenterally transmitted infection associated with the C allele at position −336 [45]. However, no association was seen with mucosal transmission, and no other published report has investigated this effect. An initial study of variation in the length of the neck region polymorphism in *DC-SIGNR* comparing HIV+ individuals to HIV− healthy volunteers reported no impact on susceptibility [144]. However, investigation in individuals with multiple sexual exposure to HIV in a Seattle cohort and the Multicenter AIDS Cohort Study (MACS) reported homozygosity for seven repeats in the neck region, and heterozygosity for seven and five repeats in *DC-SIGNR*, to be associated with increased susceptibility and resistance to infection, respectively [145]. These effects were also investigated in a Thai population of discordant couples [146] and an Indian population of high-risk uninfected individuals [147], with the former study showing agreement with the previously reported effect and the latter showing no effect. Thus, the impact of these polymorphisms is still unclear.

Mannose-binding lectin 2 (MBL2) is a component of the innate immune system present in the serum that activates complement and has been shown to inhibit HIV infection *in vitro*. Polymorphism in the *MBL2* coding and promoter regions has been described, with the wild-type allele being referred to as the "A allele" while variant alleles, coded B, C and D, are often collectively referred to as the "O allele". Early studies of the impact of these variants demonstrated that the O allele results in an unstable protein product and lowered serum concentration of the protein, which has clinical consequences. Several studies have investigated the role of these variants in impacting HIV transmission. In adult populations, several comparisons of HIV-infected to high-risk uninfected and/or healthy HIV− individuals have suggested that homozygosity for the O genotype results in increased susceptibility to infection [148−150]. A similar result has been seen in exposed-uninfected children born to HIV+ mothers [151,152]. However, in the largest published adult study comparing more than 1,000 HIV+ individuals to more than 2,000 HIV− controls with unreported risk characteristics, no effect of the promoter polymorphism on HIV acquisition was detected [153]. Similar to the *DC-SIGN/DC-SIGNR* polymorphisms, the differences in study populations, transmission routes and levels of HIV exposure make any conclusion regarding the effect of *MBL2* polymorphism on HIV acquisition an area of controversy.

Cytokines, Chemokines, Chemokine Receptors and Innate Antiviral Molecules

As knowledge of host factors that impact HIV replication, including but not limited to cytokines, chemokines and their receptors, has matured during the course of the HIV pandemic. Polymorphisms in genes encoding these factors have been investigated for their impact on susceptibility. Although many of these polymorphisms are either controversial or remain unconfirmed by independent replication (Table 6.1), there are a few of particular note.

With the knowledge that HIV preferentially targets cells of the immune system and utilizes chemokine receptors for entry comes the hypothesis that variation in genes that interact with CCR5 and/or CXCR4 may impact susceptibility. Stromal-derived factor 1 (*SDF1*, also known as *CXCL12*) is the principal ligand for CXCR4, and has been investigated by multiple studies for an influence on HIV transmission and disease progression. An early study of this gene in the MACS identified a variant allele called *SDF1-3′A* that was associated with protection in high-risk exposed-uninfected individuals, but not when extended to non-high-risk individuals [154]. Following this report, other groups studying high-risk uninfected individuals

TABLE 6.1 Reported polymorphisms in host genes impacting HIV life cycle with limited replication or discrepant effects

Class	Gene	Polymorphism	Proposed function	Effect	Reference
Cytokine/chemokine receptor	CX3CR1	T280	Reduced binding	Increased susceptibility	101
				No effect	102
	CD45	C77G	Altered T cell responses	Increased susceptibility	103
	IL-4RA	U haplotype	Hyperresponsiveness to IL-4	Increased susceptibility (parenteral); decreased susceptibility (mucosal)	104
Cytokine/chemokine	CCL2/CCL7/CCL11	H7 haplotype	Increased immune activation	Resistance	105
		MCP-1 −2578G (CCL2)			106
	CCL4	L2	Impaired CD8 function	Increased susceptibility	107
	CCL5	AC haplotype (−403A/−28C)	Increased immune activation	Increased susceptibility	111 112
				No effect	113 65
	IL-10	−403,In1.1C, 3'222C	Lower CCL5 expression	Increased susceptibility	114
	IL-18	5'A	Lowered IL-10 production	Increased susceptibility	115
	MIP1A	C-607A	Increased IL-18	Increased susceptibility	116
		TT haplotype ss46566437, ss46566438, s46566439	None	Resistance	111
			Higher expression	Resistance	117
Innate antiviral	DEFB1	−44CC	None	Increased susceptibility	118
Other	SLC11A1	5' [GT]n, 274C, 469+14G, 823C, 5' [GT]n g.43G > C	None	Increased susceptibility	119
				No effect No effect	120

A complete catalogue of natural history modifiers of HIV infection is available at http://www.hiv-pharmacogenomics.org

found the same association in Hispanics [155] and a Thai population [156]. However, several other studies investigating populations with various modes of transmission and exposure rates have failed to replicate the initial result [9,157—160], with still other studies reporting an effect in the opposite direction [51,161].

Both *APOBEC3G* and *TRIM5α* have been identified in recent years as genes that interact with HIV-1 and can inhibit infection [162,163]. The *APOBEC* family of genes binds directly to the reverse transcriptase machinery in the viral capsid interfering with replication capacity, a function that is counteracted by the viral protein Vif. Polymorphisms in both *APOBEC3G* and the related *APOBEC3B* have been investigated in cohorts of exposed-seronegative individuals for impact on HIV acquisition, with an intronic single base change in *APOBEC3G* and a homozygous deletion in *APOBEC3B* being associated with increased acquisition [164,165]. *TRIM5α* is another innate antiretroviral element found in primates that can exert an early block on retroviral infection. Species-specific variants of *TRIM5α* have been shown to differentially impact HIV-1 susceptibility, with the *TRIM5α* found in rhesus macaques exerting an inhibitory effect while the human variant is inactive against the virus [162]. A study of population frequencies of *TRIM5α* variants reported an increased frequency of the 136Q variant in HIV-uninfected individuals compared to HIV+ patients. *In vitro* studies of this variant also showed slightly higher ability to restrict HIV-1 infection compared to other variant proteins [166]. The host protein Cyclophilin A (encoded by the gene *PPIA*) has long been known to be incorporated into the HIV-1 virion and enhance infection [167,168]. Investigations into the impact of polymorphism in this gene on susceptibility have shown an increased frequency of a variant, so-called SNP5, in HIV+ individuals, suggesting that it acts to enhance infection [169].

Prospects for Future Studies of Host Genetic Factors Restricting HIV Infection

To date, only homozygosity for *CCR5-Δ32* stands out as a confirmed causal genetic influence on HIV-1 susceptibility [7,8]. However, this polymorphism is only present in people of European ancestry, and explains just a small proportion of exposed-uninfected individuals. There are several promising new candidate loci and several associations that need to be further confirmed either in different populations or by functional studies.

In many cases, discovery and replication samples have varied with respect to ancestry, risk factors and level of exposure, making direct comparison difficult. In order to separate which of these are true associations and which are false positives, future studies of large samples, well matched for the above criteria, will be essential. Available genomic approaches, such as genome-wide SNP chips and next-generation sequencing of whole genomes/exomes, have been tremendously successful in identifying common and rare genetic influences on common traits. However, to date there has been only one published genome-wide association study (GWAS) focusing on HIV-1 susceptibility. This study compared HIV+ to HIV− Malawian individuals determined through attendance at sexually transmitted infection clinics. Although this study found no significant hits, with reported power to detect common variants (> 12 percent) with an odds ratio > 2.0 at the genome-wide significance level, it did find nominal replication for a variant in *IL-18* (although the meta-analysis *P*-value of this variant was still well below genome-wide significance). Although this initial lack of discovery may seem disappointing, it lays important groundwork for future GWASs and meta-analysis of this phenotype. Currently, both whole-genome sequencing projects [170] and a community-wide meta-analysis comparing all available genotyped HIV infected individuals to general population controls are ongoing. These studies will be important steps forward for the HIV community, although much work needs to be done to fully elucidate the genetic mediators of HIV-1 susceptibility.

GENETIC FACTORS ASSOCIATED WITH RESISTANCE OR SUSCEPTIBILITY TO HIV-1 INFECTION IN THE PUMWANI SEX WORKER COHORT

The Pumwani Sex Worker Cohort

The Pumwani Sex Worker cohort was established in 1985 in Nairobi, Kenya, as an observational cohort study of the immunobiology and epidemiology of sexually transmitted infections (STI) [75,79,84−86,171−181]. It is an open prospective cohort located in the heart of the Pumwani slum. The patients enrolled in the cohort have been followed biannually since the cohort was established. In addition to research, it provides services related to STI and HIV prevention and care, including consultation, provision of free condoms, and treatment of other infections. Despite effective intervention programmes, the annual incidence of HIV-1 infection among initially seronegative women is currently 4 per 100 person years (PY)—a dramatic decrease from the initial annual incidence of 45 percent. Due to the introduction of the PEPFAR program (US President's Emergency Plan for AIDS Relief), after 2003 antiretroviral drug treatment was made available for HIV+ women whose CD4 counts dropped below $200/mm^3$. There was no program for antiretroviral drug treatment from 1985 to 2003.

The majority of women enrolled in the Pumwani Sex Worker cohort are from small towns in Tanzania and Uganda around Lake Victoria, and small towns of rural Kenya (see Figure 6.1). More than 90 percent of these women are Bantu speakers, and less than 10 percent are Nilos. Between 1985 and 2010, more than 3,000 sex workers were enrolled in the cohort. Through more than 20 years of biannual biological and clinical follow-ups, a sub-group of women who are resistant to HIV-1 infection have been identified. These women have remained seronegative and PCR-negative for HIV-1 for prolonged periods

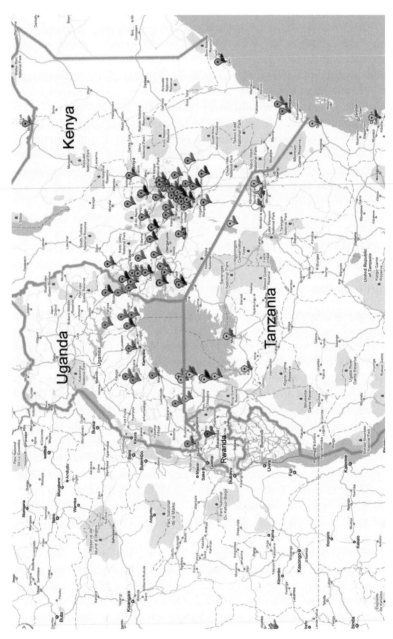

FIGURE 6.1   **Map of birth place of women enrolled in the Pumwani Sex Worker cohort.** Blue marker, Kenya locations; light blue marker, Tanzania locations; green marker, Uganda locations; purple marker, Rwanda locations.

despite heavy exposure to the virus through active sex work [1]. By contrast, many individuals from the same regions seroconverted shortly after enrolment [87].

The HIV prevalence in Urban Kenya and Tanzania from the late 1980s to 1990s—the period when the majority of HESN individuals in this cohort were enrolled—ranges from 23 to 30 percent among antenatal clinic attendees and around 70 percent in the Pumwani Sex Worker cohort [1,2,4,69−71,182−185]. The detailed long-term biological and clinical observations in the midst of the HIV-1 epidemic allow us not only to clearly define the biological phenotypes of these women for case−control analysis, but also to conduct longitudinal analysis to examine the effect of identified alleles on seroconversion. The genetic factors associated with resistance or susceptibility to HIV-1 infection discussed below were identified by studying women with the best-defined HESN phenotype. These HIV-1-resistant women have been followed for an average of 9.6 ± 4.3 years, and remain uninfected at the time of the study. Although many potential genetic factors may contribute to the resistance phenotype, in this section we will focus on those that have already been published or are in the more advanced stages of the review process.

HLA Class I and Class II Antigens and Resistance/Susceptibility to HIV-1 Infection

HLA class I and class II genes are centrally involved in the host adaptive immune responses to infectious pathogens. Together with NK cell receptor genes, HLA class I genes are also involved in the host innate immune response. HLA class I and class II genes are very polymorphic, and account for varied host immune responses to many infectious pathogens. HLA class I proteins present antigenic peptides to CD8+ T cells, which destroy the infected cells [186−189]. HLA class II antigens present antigenic epitopes to CD4+ T cells to initiate CD4+ T cell responses. The polymorphisms in exons 2 and 3 of class I antigens and exon 2 of class II antigens contribute to the variable binding abilities to different peptides and the spectrum of antigen presentation. Specific HLA class I and class II alleles have been associated with differential outcomes for various diseases [190,191]. HLA alleles, allele groups and supertypes have also been associated with different rates of disease progression among HIV-infected individuals [4,183−185,192−194]. However, few associations of HLA class I alleles with resistance or susceptibility to HIV-1 infection have been reported [4,69−72,121,195,196] for reasons discussed above. Through analysis of HLA class I and class II antigens of more than 700 enrollees of the Pumwani cohort, we identified a number of novel associations with resistance or susceptibility to HIV-1 infection. Since associations of HLA alleles with different outcomes of HIV-1 infection and disease progression are most likely due to the differences in the HIV epitopes being presented and the induced immune responses following antigen recognition, HLA alleles associated with different outcomes of HIV-1 infection and disease might be vital clues for developing an HIV-1 vaccine.

Associations of HLA-A, -B, and -C Alleles, Allele Groups with Resistance and Susceptibility to HIV-1 Infection in the Pumwani Sex Worker Cohort

Among many identified genetic factors influencing HIV-1 infection and the rate of progression towards AIDS, HLA class I alleles play the most important role [188,192,194,197–205]. Studies have shown convincingly that the adaptive immune response initiated by HLA class I genes is critical in controlling viral load in HIV-1-infected elite controllers [185,199,200] and in maintaining high CD4+ T cell counts in HIV-1-infected long-term non-progressors [185,199,200].

Analysis of HLA class I allele frequencies of more than 100 HIV-1-resistant women and more than 700 HIV-infected controls has identified a number of HLA class I alleles and allele groups that are enriched in HIV-1-resistant women or in the HIV-1 infected. The frequency of alleles and/or phenotypes of A*23:01, A*66:01, B*07:02, C*02:10 and C*07:02 is higher in the HIV-infected women, while that of A*01:01, B*18:01, B*47:01, B*57:02, B*41:01, C*07:01 and C*07:04 shows association with HESN status. These associations are allele-specific, as grouping by predicted peptide-binding properties [111,112] showed no association. Importantly, this observation was not influenced by time of enrolment as observed by an Hurvitz-Thompson analysis.

The cross-sectional results were used to examine whether women who entered the cohort HIV-1 negative were more or less likely to seroconvert if they had the alleles associated with increased or decreased susceptibility. Kaplan-Meier survival analysis of time to seroconversion for women who were HIV-1 negative at enrolment showed that patients with HLA-A*01, B*15:17, C*06:02 and C*07:01 were significantly less likely to seroconvert than those who did not have any of these alleles (Figure 6.2). Conversely, HIV-1-negative women with A*23:01, B*07:02, B*42:01, B7 supertype, C*02:10 and C*07:02 seroconverted significantly faster than those patients who did not have any of these alleles/supertype (Figure 6.3). Several alleles enriched in the HIV-1-resistant women showed a consistent but non-significant trend towards slower seroconversion, including B*18:01, B*41:01, B*47:01, B*57:02 and C*07:04 (data not shown), while A*66:01, enriched in the HIV-1-infected women, trended towards faster seroconversion (data not shown). In general, women with alleles enriched in the resistant group seroconverted more slowly, while those with alleles enriched in the HIV infected group seroconverted more quickly. The only exception was C*06:02, an allele at only slightly higher frequency in the resistant group that associated strongly with longer time to seroconversion (Figure 6.2). Women homozygous at any of the class I loci were more likely to seroconvert than those who were heterozygous at all class I loci,

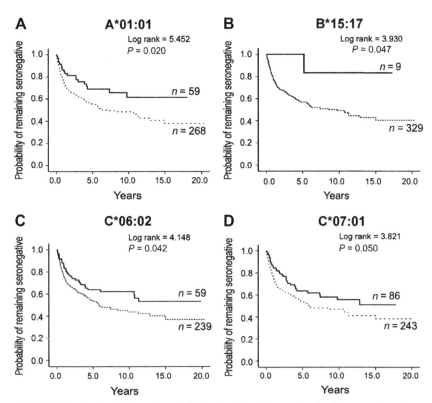

FIGURE 6.2 Kaplan-Meier plot of alleles significantly associated with protection from seroconversion. (A) A*01:01; (B) B*15:17; (C) C*06:02; (D) C*07:01. Solid line, women with the specified HLA allele; dashed line, women without the specified HLA allele.

although the difference was not significant even after excluding alleles associated with resistance to HIV-1 infection.

Since HLA class I genes are closely located on chromosome 6, the associations may be attributed to linkage disequilibrium between different class I alleles. Multivariate analysis and linkage disequilibrium analysis showed that the observed associations are largely independent of each other. Binary logistic regression analysis showed that A*23:01, A*66:01, B*42:01 and C*02:10 were independently associated with susceptibility to infection, with a potential overlap between B*07:02 and C*07:02. A*01, B*15:17, B*18:01, B*41:01, B*57:02, C*07:01 and C*07:04 were independently associated with resistance to infection. Cox regression analysis also showed that A*01, B*15:17, C*06:02 and C*07:01 were independently associated with a decreased rate of seroconversion. A*23:01, B*42:01 and C*02:10 were independently associated with an increased rate of seroconversion, with a potential overlap between B*07:02 and C*07:02. Overall, these results suggest a potential role for several HLA alleles from all three classical class I

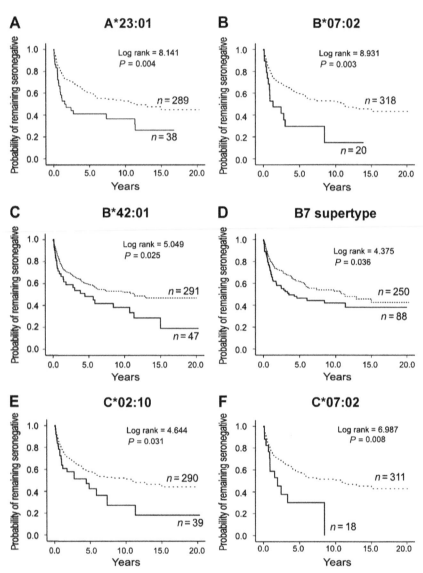

FIGURE 6.3   Kaplan-Meier plot of alleles/supertypes significantly associated with increased risk to HIV-1 seroconversion. (A) A*23:01; (B) B*07:02; (C) B*42:01; (D) B7 supertype; (E) C*02:10; (F) C*07:02. Solid line, women with the specified HLA allele; dashed line, women without the specified HLA allele.

genes acting in an additive manner (Figure 6.4) contributing to HIV resistance in this cohort.

Some of these findings confirmed previously reported associations. For example, B*18 was previously reported to be associated with resistance to

HIV-1 infection in a sex worker cohort in Thailand [100,101], and protection in a mother—child HIV-1 transmission cohort in Nairobi, Kenya [104]. However, B*18 was associated with susceptibility to HIV-1 infection in a study in Argentina [205]. In this case ethnicity may not explain the difference, since Thai and Kenyan populations yielded similar findings. Different HIV-1 subtypes predominantly found in different regions may account for these dissimilar associations. In Kenya, subtype A accounted for ~70 percent of infection and subtype 01_AE was responsible for > 90 percent of the infected population in Thailand (http://www.hiv.lanl.gov/), whereas in Argentina subtype B and recombinant subtype B predominate. The HIV subtype-dependent HLA associations with resistance to infection need to be studied further. A*23:01 was associated with increased risk of seroconversion in the Pumwani Sex Worker cohort in an earlier study of a subgroup of enrollees [72], and the association was confirmed in a large population study 10 years later with better defined phenotype. The allele has also been associated with an increased risk in mother—child HIV-1 transmission [122] in another Kenyan cohort.

Associations of HLA Class II Antigens: DRB, DQA1, DQB1, DPA1 and DPB1 Alleles and Haplotypes with Resistance and Susceptibility to HIV-1 Infection in the Pumwani Sex Worker Cohort

HLA class II molecules are expressed on professional antigen presenting cells (APCs) and present exogenously derived epitopes to CD4+ helper T cells. These cells are important to many aspects of the immune response, including antibody and cytokine production, and CD8+ T cell help. CD4+ T helper cells play an integral role in HIV-1 infection and immunity, and the CD4+ T cell responses of HIV-1-resistant sex workers are lower in magnitude and narrower in spectrum [114]. Studies showed that the frequency distributions of several HLA DRB, DQA1, DQB1, DPA1 and DPB1 alleles, phenotypes and haplotypes are different in the HIV-1-resistant women when compared with the HIV-1-infected controls [57—59]. The DRB1*01, DRB1*11:02, DRB1*11:02—DRB3*02:02:01 haplotype, DQB1*06:03, DQB1*06:09, DQA1*01:02:01—DQB1*06:03 haplotype, DPA1*01:03:01, DPA1*01:03:01—DPB1*30:01 and DPA1*03:01—DPB1*55:01 haplotypes are significantly enriched in HIV-1-resistant women [69—71]. Moreover, HIV-1-negative women who carry these alleles and haplotypes were significantly less likely to seroconvert than those who do not. Conversely, the DRB1*15—DRB5 haplotype, DRB1*07:01:01—DRB4*01:01:01 haplotype, DQA1*01:02:01—DQB1*06:02 haplotype, DPA1*03:02, DPB1*04:02 homozygotes, DPA1*03:02—DPB1*04:02 haplotype, DPB1*01:01:01—DPB1*18:01 genotype, and DPA1*02:01:01 homozygotes are enriched in the HIV-1-infected individuals [57—59]. HIV-1-negative women who have these alleles, haplotypes and genotypes seroconvert significantly faster than women without these alleles.

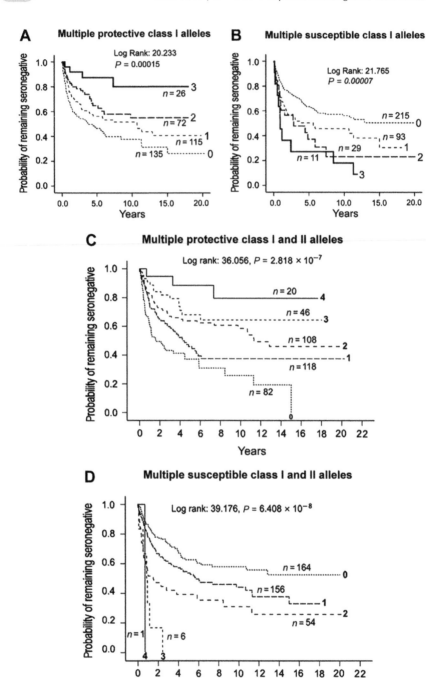

Some of these associations have also been reported in other studies. DRB1*01, associated with resistance in the Pumwani cohort, was also associated with the HIV-negative group in a study from Botswana [206]; DRB1*15:03, which conferred susceptibility in the Pumwani cohort, was also associated with increased HIV-1 seroconversion in Zambian discordant couples [207]. A 2006 study also showed that DR2 (DRB1*1516—DRB5 haplotype) was associated with susceptibility to HIV-1 infection in a South Indian cohort [208]; therefore, the findings from the Pumwani cohort might also be applicable to other populations such as the European or south-east Asian populations, which have different allele compositions and frequency distributions.

The advantage of possessing a rare HLA class I supertype in HIV-1 disease progression has been previously reported [200]. HIV is more likely to adapt to the most common HLA types in a given population. Individuals carrying rare HLA class I alleles would have an advantage [204]. This phenomenon, however, has not been observed for class II antigens in the Pumwani cohort. HLA—DRB alleles that were associated with resistance in the Pumwani cohort are quite common in the population. Similarly, DPA1*01:03:01, a very common allele in the Pumwani Sex Worker cohort and in different ethnic populations in the world, is associated with resistance to HIV-1 infection. The rare allele advantages in class I *versus* the associations of common DRB and DPA1 alleles with resistance may reflect different roles for CD8+ and CD4+ T cells in anti-HIV immune responses. HLA class II is directly involved in the initiation of the CD4+ T cell immune response. This response is mainly cytokine based, and is implicated in the proliferation of activated CD8+ T cells as well as the enhancement of the overall CD8+ T cell response [209—214].

FIGURE 6.4 **Kaplan-Meier plot showing the additive effect of multiple protective or susceptible HLA class I alleles on rates of HIV-1 seroconversion and progression to AIDS.** (A) Multiple protective class I alleles and rates of seroconversion. Thin dotted line (0), individuals without any identified resistant alleles; thin dashed line (1), individuals with one of the identified resistant alleles; thick dashed line (2), individuals with two of the identified resistant alleles; thick solid line (3), women with three or more of the identified resistant alleles. (B) Multiple susceptible class I alleles and rates of seroconversion. Thin dotted line (0), individuals without any identified susceptible alleles; thin dashed line (1), individuals with one of the identified susceptible alleles; thick dashed line (2), individuals with two of the identified susceptible alleles; thick solid line (3), women with three or more of the identified susceptible alleles. (C) Multiple protective class I and class II alleles and rates of seroconversion. Dotted line (0), individuals without any identified resistant alleles; long dashed line (1), individuals with one of the identified resistant alleles; mid-dashed line (2), individuals with two of the identified resistant alleles; short dashed line (3), individuals with three of the identified resistant alleles; thick solid line (4), women with four of the identified resistant alleles. (D) Multiple susceptible class I and class II alleles and rates of seroconversion. Dotted line (0), individuals without any identified susceptible alleles; long dashed line (1), individuals with one of the identified susceptible alleles; mid-dashed line (2), individuals with two of the identified susceptible alleles; short dashed line (3), individuals with three of the identified susceptible alleles; thick solid line (4), women with four of the identified susceptible alleles.

The CD4+ T cell immune response is also directly involved in the activation of antigen presenting cells, dendritic cells and B cells. The CD8+ T cell response is mainly responsible for controlling viral spread during the acute and chronic phases of infection [215–218].

The importance of these alleles in the immune response is highlighted by previous reports that have identified these alleles as being associated with allergies, and infectious and autoimmune diseases. DRB1*15 has been associated with susceptibility to a variety of autoimmune diseases, such as aplastic anemia [219], multiple sclerosis [220] and rheumatoid arthritis [221–223]. The DQA1*01:02–DQB1*06:02 haplotype was associated with increased susceptibility to narcolepsy [224] and multiple sclerosis [225], and decreased susceptibility to Type 1 diabetes [226,227]. DQB1*05:03:01 was associated with increased risk of vitiligo [228] and pemphigus vulgaris in a Chinese population [229], but had a protective effect against Type 1 diabetes in Czechs [230]. This suggests that individuals with this HLA genotype tend to have a higher level of immune activation. Higher immune activation could lead to higher rates of HIV-1 transmission due to an increased number of activated CD4+ T cells. The prevalence of autoimmune diseases in the Pumwani cohort has not been examined. Follow-up studies are necessary to determine the relationship between autoimmunity, DRB1*15:03 and susceptibility to HIV-1 infection. Although DRB1*01 and DRB1*15:03 have been associated with different outcomes of HIV-1 infection, both alleles were correlated with susceptibility to autoimmune diseases in non-African populations [170]. Factors such as immune stimulus, different ethnic backgrounds and environment may account for differences seen in allele associations between these populations. The complexity of anti-HIV-1 immunity further emphasizes the importance of comprehensive studies of large, well-characterized populations.

Additive Effect of HLA Associations with Resistance or Susceptibility to HIV-1 Infection

We identified multiple HLA class I and class II alleles associated with resistance or susceptibility to HIV-1 infection [69–71], and binary logistic regression and Cox regression analysis showed that the effects of these class I and class II alleles are largely independent of each other. There is an additive effect of having several of these class I and class II alleles (manuscript under review). Having more of the beneficial alleles significantly protected the women from seroconversion, whereas having more alleles associated with susceptibility to seroconversion is extremely detrimental. The majority of the women who are resistant to HIV-1 infection can be explained by having at least one (90 percent), two (71.7 percent), three (39.2 percent) or four (20 percent) of all the identified class I and class II alleles that are associated with resistance to HIV-1 infection in this population (Figure 6.4); conversely, the majority of

HIV-1-infected women can be explained by having at least one (79.4 percent) or two (44.2 percent) of all the identified class I and class II alleles that are associated with susceptibility to HIV-1 infection. HIV-1-negative women who have more of these alleles seroconvert rapidly after cohort enrolment (Figure 6.4).

The additive effects of multiple beneficial or detrimental HLA class I and/or class II alleles suggest that antigen presentation by different HLA alleles and the immune responses induced are not equal. Although the specific mechanisms of these additive effects need to be investigated, it suggests that the target of prophylactic vaccines should be selective. These vaccines should include multiple beneficial epitopes that can induce protective immune responses to HIV-1 and avoid the epitopes of susceptible alleles. It is possible that multiple susceptible alleles could result in excessive immune activation, thus generating easier targets for HIV-1, or prevent beneficial immune responses to HIV-1 from being induced. A thorough investigation of the epitopes of beneficial and detrimental HLA class I and class II alleles and immune responses induced by these epitopes could lead to a better approach for both preventive and therapeutic HIV-1 vaccines.

Genetic Polymorphism of Trim5alpha and Resistance or Susceptibility to HIV-1 Infection

It has become clear that in addition to the role of adaptive immunity in HIV-1 infection, intrinsic immune responses play an important role in such infection and may hold the key to an effective and accessible prophylactic to HIV-1 infection [231]. *TRIM5* is one such candidate, as TRIM5α, a splice variant of TRIM5, has the ability to provide innate protection against retroviruses [65,162,232−235]. While human TRIM5α (huTRIM5α) does not completely inhibit HIV-1 infection, it has shown slight anti-HIV activity and is known to restrict other retroviruses, such as the N-tropic murine-leukemia virus [65,232,233]. Several studies have suggested that certain polymorphisms in human *TRIM5* may enhance or impair the protein's affinity for HIV-1. This has also been examined in resistance or susceptibility to HIV-1 infection in the Pumwani Sex Worker cohort.

As described previously in this chapter, studies have shown, with conflicting results, that certain polymorphisms may alter the potency of huTRIM5α against HIV-1 [65,166,236,237]. Two SNPs in particular have been at the center of many investigations: a G to A change in rs10838525 (R136Q in exon 2), and a C to T change in rs3740996 (H43Y in exon 2). Genetic variation of TRIM5α exon 2 has also been investigated in the Pumwani cohort. In a study of 1,032 women, the SNP and haplotype frequencies in the cohort were investigated and correlations with resistance or susceptibility to HIV-1 infection were determined. Thirteen single nucleotide polymorphisms within the 1-kb genomic fragment containing exon 2 of *TRIM5* were identified, with seven being non-synonymous, two synonymous, three intronic, and one in the 5' UTR. Of the coding SNPs identified, three are located in the RING, three in the B-box and two in the coiled-coil domains [52]. Although many SNPs were at too low a frequency to be sufficiently tested for association, two SNPs identified were at frequencies above 3 percent (rs3740996/T (43Y) at 4.84 percent and rs10838525/A (136Q) at 10.8 percent]. rs3740996/T (43Y), which was enriched in HIV-1-negative individuals in previous studies [18], was evenly distributed between HIV-1-positive and -resistant women in the Pumwani cohort. Similarly, the amino acid change H43Y, shown to be associated with protection against HIV-1 by others [18], showed no such association in the Pumwani cohort. The SNP-induced amino acid change R136Q had been associated with both protection [18] and susceptibility [3] to HIV-1 in previous studies. This SNP is strongly correlated with resistance to HIV-1 infection in the Pumwani cohort, with an adjusted P value of 4.5×10^{-7} and odds ratio of 3.65.

TRIM5 haplotypes were also analyzed for any associations with HIV-1 resistance or susceptibility. Haplotype new2 was enriched in resistant women (37.1 percent) when compared to HIV-1-positive women (13.9 percent), with an adjusted P value of 5.7×10^{-7} and odds ratio of 3.65. Most observed haplotypes were exceedingly rare, which made it difficult to determine whether any significant distribution differences existed between the two groups of women. Alternatively, the effect of haplotypes as a whole was investigated by combining all individuals with polymorphic TRIM5α as compared to individuals with wild-type TRIM5α. Wild-type TRIM5α was more common in HIV-1-positive individuals (97.8 percent) than in resistant individuals (91.4 percent), suggesting that any polymorphism may be advantageous. These results were largely supported by analysis of time to seroconversion, with R136Q and carrying variant TRIM5 delaying time to seroconversion.

Codon 136 is located within the coiled-coil domain of TRIM5α, which is required for effective recognition and binding of HIV-1 [238,239]. It has also been suggested that the coiled-coil is needed for multimerization of TRIM5α particles, allowing for effective viral binding [239—242]. It is possible that variations in the amino acid sequence of the coiled-coil may alter multimerization and, in turn, the affinity of viral binding to the protein surface. Of note, most non-human primate TRIM5α (excluding chimpanzees) encodes a glutamine at codon 136 [166,243]. Many of these non-human forms of TRIM5α have been proven to effectively restrict HIV-1 [65,162,232,243]. Thus, a switch from arginine to glutamine at codon 136 in huTRIM5α could indicate a shift towards a protein that is more active against HIV-1. The SNP encoding R136Q varies greatly in population frequency, being 34.2 percent in Caucasian populations and only 4.4 percent and 2.3 percent in Chinese and Japanese populations, respectively. If R136Q exhibits a protective effect in all populations, the frequency of the SNP could have huge implications in the ease of HIV-1 transmission and spread of the epidemic.

Polymorphisms of Genes that Regulate Immune Response and Influence HIV-1 Infection Play an Important Role in the Resistance or Susceptibility to HIV-1 Infection in the Pumwani Sex Worker Cohort

Study of the *IL4* gene cluster identified associations of three polymorphisms in *IRF1* with resistance to HIV-1 infection [39] which correlated with reduced IRF1 protein expression and responsiveness to exogenous IFN-γ stimulation [10,39]. *IRF1* belongs to the Interferon Regulatory Factor family of trans-criptional activators and repressors [244], and is responsible for the expression of factors important in innate responses and the development and function of adaptive immunity [245,246]. *In vitro* evidence also suggests a role for *IRF1* expression in HIV-1 replication, as upregulation of *IRF1* has been shown in Jurkat T cell lines to be essential in transactivating the HIV-1 LTR [247,248]. Moreover, lymphocytes from HIV-uninfected individuals with protective *IRF1* genotypes exhibited a markedly reduced level of HIV-1 LTR transactivation and viral replication [249]. Thus, the protective *IRF1* genotype is associated with lower levels of induced *IRF1* protein expression, increased protein turnover, and reduced HIV replicative capacity. Interestingly, it appears that *IRF1* may also be regulated at the epigenetic level. Epigenetic downregulation of *IRF1* is critical in regulating these altered *IRF1* responses in HIV-resistant women [68]. Levels of histone acetylation at the *IRF1* promoter correlated with *IRF1* transcript levels during IFN-γ stimulation. Moreover, histone deacetylase-2 recruitment (an epigenetic repressor) corresponded to silencing of IRF1 responses, suggesting epigenetic-mediated silencing of these responses [68]. Together, these studies suggest that tight regulation of IRF1 levels may be critical to immune activation, and may play a role in resistance to HIV infection.

The presence of a common non-synonymous SNP (C868T) in *CD4* was identified because of the observation that some people of African descent had CD4 molecules that were unable to bind an IgG monoclonal antibody directed at an epitope in the third domain of CD4 called OKT4 [250–252]. The change of cytosine to thymidine at nucleotide position 868 results in an amino acid change from arginine to tryptophan at the amino acid location 240 within the third domain (D3) of CD4 [253]. Therefore, the C868T polymorphism results in a protein called CD4-Trp240 [252]. Replacement of the basic Arginine residue with the more hydrophobic Tryptophan in the centre of a β-sheet has been predicted to have a significant effect on the tertiary structure of CD4 [253]. Evidence from CD4 structure and mutagenesis studies has shown that the redox state of a disulfide bond in D2 of CD4 and the alteration in the D3 of CD4 can affect the binding of HIV gp120 to D1 of CD4 [254,255]. The C868T allele frequency is higher (20 percent) among African Americans and much lower (< 1 percent) among Caucasians

[256]. The *CD4* C868T polymorphism was significantly associated with HIV prevalence and incidence in the Pumwani Sex Worker cohort [257], and a cell line expressing CD4-Trp240 was more susceptible to infection with HIV-1$_{IIIB}$ virus and Kenyan primary viral isolate than were cells with wild-type CD4. This was confirmed in *ex vivo* cultures of PBMCs from subjects with different *CD4* genotypes. Together, these data suggest that a polymorphism in the CD4 gene that is expressed at a high frequency in populations of African descent is a significant risk factor for HIV infection.

Identification of Genetic Factors of Resistance to HIV-1 Infection by a Systems Biology Approach

Systems biology is a holistic approach to understanding biology that aims at system-level understanding, rather than the characteristics of isolated parts of a cell or organism [258]. Many properties of life arise at the systems level, and the behavior of the system cannot be explained by its constituents. The systems biology approach is to obtain, integrate and analyze complex data from multiple experimental sources using interdisciplinary tools [259]. This approach consists of five steps: (1) generating a set of candidate genes using gene−gene interaction data sets; (2) reconstructing a genetic network with the set of candidate genes from gene expression data; (3) identifying differentially regulated genes between normal and abnormal samples in the network; (4) validating regulatory relationship between the genes in the network by perturbing the network using RNAi and monitoring the response using RT-PCR; and (5) genotyping the differentially regulated genes and testing their association with the diseases by direct association studies.

The systems biology approach is an unbiased and comprehensive approach to studying genes involved in resistance to HIV-1 infection. Microarray analysis of gene expression of splicing variant expression and genome-wide SNPs analysis can generate a large amount of data. By synthesizing information obtained from different datasets, it can help to identify key biological pathways or a set of key candidate genes that may play an important role in the resistance to HIV-1 infection. For example, gene enrichment and pathway analysis can be conducted separately for the gene expression data obtained from Affymetrix GeneChip® U133 Microarray, the gene expression and splicing variant expression data obtained using the Affymetrix GeneChip® Exon 1.0 Microarray, the genes contained in or near the SNPs (Affymetrix GeneChip® 5.0) that are significantly associated with the resistant phenotype, and the genes with significant copy number variations. Overlap of the top hits from different datasets (such as genome-wide SNP/CNV data and gene expression data) can help to prioritize the functional tests to confirm the most significant signal transduction pathways and the genes involved. Identification of DPP4 [259] and Serpins [260] as two of the factors contributing to some of the resistant phenotypes to HIV-1 is such an example.

Dipeptidyl peptidase-4 (DPP4), also named CD26, was identified as playing a role in the resistance to HIV-1 infection in the Pumwani Sex Worker cohort through a systems biology approach [259]. Affymetrix® microarray analysis of mRNA expression of whole blood of 43 HIV-1-resistant women and 43 HIV-1-negative controls showed that mRNA expression of DPP4 is highly elevated in the HIV-1-resistant women (fold change 2.3, $P = 2.4 \times 10^{-7}$). Similarly, DPP4 plasma concentration was significantly elevated among the HIV-R group (mean 1315 ng/ml) than among the HIV-negative (910 ng/ml) and HIV-infected volunteers (870 ng/ml, $P < 0.001$). FACs analysis of peripheral mononuclear cells derived from the HIV-R, HIV-negative and HIV-positive women revealed higher CD26 expression on CD4+ T cells from the HIV-resistant group compared to both the HIV+ and HIV− low-risk controls (90.30 percent *versus* 82.30 and 80.90 percent, respectively; $P < 0.001$ for HIV− low risk, $P = 0.002$ for HIV+). Mean fluorescent intensity (MFI) analysis showed a higher DPP4 MFI on CD4+ T cells of HIV-1-resistant women compared to HIV− low-risk controls (median 118 *versus* 91, $P = 0.0003$; Figure 6.4B), suggesting that more DPP4 molecules are expressed per CD4+T cell in HIV-R subjects. No difference in DPP4 expression was observed on CD8+ T cells between the groups.

DPP4 is a multifunctional protein ubiquitously expressed in both soluble and cell surface forms in various endothelial and epithelial cells, including T cells, and exerts different functions depending on the cell type and conditions under which it is expressed [261]. It acts as a proteolytic enzyme, receptor and co-stimulatory protein, and its substrates have been reported to be involved in various physiological processes, including immunomodulation and homeostasis. Dysregulation of DPP4 has been suggested to play a role in rheumatoid arthritis, melanoma, Crohn's disease and Type 2 diabetes, among other diseases [261,262]. Studies have shown that susceptibility of cells to HIV infection is correlated with DPP4 expression, and HIV transactivator Tat and envelope protein gp120 are reported to interact with DPP4 and implicate it in HIV cell entry [263,264]. DPP4 has been shown to control the anti-HIV and chemotactic activities of RANTES (Regulated on Activation, Normal T cell Expressed and Secreted) and stromal cell-derived factor-1 (SDF-1) [263−267]. Whether genetic polymorphisms of DPP4 exist in HIV-1-resistant women and the mechanisms of high expression of DPP4 contribute to the resistance to HIV-1 infection needs to be further investigated.

CONCLUSION

Identification of genetic factors in resistance to HIV-1 infection requires clearly defined biological phenotype and functional studies to confirm the role of identified candidate genes in HIV-1 infection. *CCR5-Δ32* was identified originally in only 2 of 25 exposed uninfected individuals [7,8]; it was the solid functional study that convincingly showed the deletion mutation preventing

HIV-1 infection [7,8], not the *P* value of the original association. Thus, functional study is essential for the candidate genes identified through genetic association studies, either by a candidate gene approach or by genome-wide association studies, especially for the genes that we have no prior knowledge of their function in HIV-1 infection.

REFERENCES

[1] Fowke KR, Nagelkerke NJ, Kimani J, Simonsen JN, Anzala AO, Bwayo JJ, et al. Resistance to HIV-1 infection among persistently seronegative prostitutes in Nairobi, Kenya. Lancet 1996;348:1347—51.

[2] Plummer FA, Ball TB, Kimani J, Fowke KR. Resistance to HIV-1 infection among highly exposed sex workers in Nairobi: what mediates protection and why does it develop? Immunol Lett 1999;66:27—34.

[3] Rowland-Jones S, Sutton J, Ariyoshi K, Dong T, Gotch F, McAdam S, et al. HIV-specific cytotoxic T-cells in HIV-exposed but uninfected Gambian women. Nat Med 1995;1:59—64.

[4] Trachtenberg EA, Erlich HA. A review of the role of the human leukocyte antigen (HLA) system as a host immunogenetic factor influencing HIV transmission and progression to AIDS. In: Korber BT, Brander C, Haynes BF, Koup R, Kuiken C, Moore JP, et al. editors. HIV Molecular Immunology. Los Alamos, NM: Theoretical Biology and Biophysics Group, Los Alamos National Laboratory; 2001.

[5] Pereyra F, Addo MM, Kaufmann DE, Liu Y, Miura T, Rathod A, et al. Genetic and immunologic heterogeneity among persons who control HIV infection in the absence of therapy. J Infect Dis 2008;197:563—71.

[6] Koning FA, Jansen CA, Dekker J, Kaslow RA, Dukers N, Van Baarle D, et al. Correlates of resistance to HIV-1 infection in homosexual men with high-risk sexual behaviour. AIDS 2004;18:1117—26.

[7] Liu R, Paxton WA, Choe S, Ceradini D, Martin SR, Horuk R, et al. Homozygous defect in HIV-1 coreceptor accounts for resistance of some multiply-exposed individuals to HIV-1 infection. Cell 1996;86:366—77.

[8] Paxton WA, Martin SR, Tse D, O'Brien TR, Skurnick J, VanDevanter NL, et al. Relative resistance to HIV-1 infection of CD4 lymphocytes from persons who remain uninfected despite multiple high-risk sexual exposure. Nat Med 1996;2:412—7.

[9] Liu H, Hwangbo Y, Holte S, Lee J, Wang C, Kaupp N, et al. Analysis of genetic polymorphisms in CCR5, CCR2, stromal cell-derived factor-1, RANTES, and dendritic cell-specific intercellular adhesion molecule-3-grabbing nonintegrin in seronegative individuals repeatedly exposed to HIV-1. J Infect Dis 2004;190:1055—8.

[10] Ball TB, Ji H, Kimani J, McLaren P, Marlin C, Hill AV, et al. Polymorphisms in IRF-1 associated with resistance to HIV-1 infection in highly exposed uninfected Kenyan sex workers. AIDS 2007;21:1091—101.

[11] Balotta C, Bagnarelli P, Violin M, Ridolfo AL, Zhou D, Berlusconi A, et al. Homozygous delta 32 deletion of the CCR-5 chemokine receptor gene in an HIV-1-infected patient. AIDS 1997;11:F67—71.

[12] Becker Y. The molecular mechanism of human resistance to HIV-1 infection in persistently infected individuals—a review, hypothesis and implications. Virus Genes 2005;31:113—9.

[13] Bhattacharya T, Stanton J, Kim EY, Kunstman KJ, Phair JP, Jacobson LP, et al. CCL3L1 and HIV/AIDS susceptibility. Nat Med 2009;15:1110—2.

[14] Bienzle D, MacDonald KS, Smaill FM, Kovacs C, Baqi M, Courssaris B, et al. Factors contributing to the lack of human immunodeficiency virus type 1 (HIV-1) transmission in HIV-1-discordant partners. J Infect Dis 2000;182:123−32.

[15] Biti R, Ffrench R, Young J, Bennetts B, Stewart G, Liang T. HIV-1 infection in an individual homozygous for the CCR5 deletion allele. Nat Med 1997;3:1240−3.

[16] Broliden K, Hinkula J, Devito C, Kiama P, Kimani J, Trabbatoni D, et al. Functional HIV-1 specific IgA antibodies in HIV-1 exposed, persistently IgG seronegative female sex workers. Immunol Lett 2001;79:29−36.

[17] Carrington M, Dean M, Martin MP, O'Brien SJ. Genetics of HIV-1 infection: Chemokine receptor CCR5 polymorphism and its consequences. Hum Mol Genet 1999;8: 1939−45.

[18] Devito C, Broliden K, Kaul R, Svensson L, Johansen K, Kiama P, et al. Mucosal and plasma IgA from HIV-1-exposed uninfected individuals inhibit HIV-1 transcytosis across human epithelial cells. J Immunol 2000;165:5170−6.

[19] Kulkarni PS, Butera ST, Duerr AC. Resistance to HIV-1 infection: Lessons learned from studies of highly exposed persistently seronegative (HEPS) individuals. AIDS Rev 2003;5:87−103.

[20] Rowland-Jones SL, Pinheiro S, Kaul R, Hansasuta P, Gillespie G, Dong T, et al. How important is the "quality" of the cytotoxic T lymphocyte (CTL) response in protection against HIV infection? Immunol Lett 2001;79:15−20.

[21] Tang J, Shelton B, Makhatadze NJ, Zhang Y, Schaen M, Louie LG, et al. Distribution of chemokine receptor CCR2 and CCR5 genotypes and their relative contribution to human immunodeficiency virus type 1 (HIV-1) seroconversion, early HIV-1 RNA concentration in plasma, and later disease progression. J Virol 2002;76:662−72.

[22] Yang C, Li M, Limpakarnjanarat K, Young NL, Hodge T, Butera ST, et al. Polymorphisms in the CCR5 coding and noncoding regions among HIV type 1-exposed, persistently seronegative female sex-workers from Thailand. AIDS Res Hum Retroviruses 2003;19:661−5.

[23] Castelli EC, Mendes-Junior CT, Donadi EA. HLA-G alleles and HLA-G 14 bp polymorphisms in a Brazilian population. Tissue Antigens 2007;70:62−8.

[24] Castelli EC, Mendes-Junior CT, Deghaide NH, de Albuquerque RS, Muniz YC, Simoes RT, et al. The genetic structure of 3'untranslated region of the HLA-G gene: Polymorphisms and haplotypes. Genes Immun 11:134−41.

[25] Chen XY, Yan WH, Lin A, Xu HH, Zhang JG, Wang XX. The 14 bp deletion polymorphisms in HLA-G gene play an important role in the expression of soluble HLA-G in plasma. Tissue Antigens 2008;72:335−41.

[26] Colobran R, Adreani P, Ashhab Y, Llano A, Este JA, Dominguez O, et al. Multiple products derived from two CCL4 loci: High incidence of a new polymorphism in HIV+ patients. J Immunol 2005;174:5664−5.

[27] Duggal P, An P, Beaty TH, Strathdee SA, Farzadegan H, Markham RB, et al. Genetic influence of CXCR6 chemokine receptor alleles on PCP-mediated AIDS progression among African Americans. Genes Immun 2003;4:245−50.

[28] Fabris A, Catamo E, Segat L, Morgutti M, Arraes LC, de Lima−Filho JL, et al. Association between HLA-G 3'UTR 14-bp polymorphism and HIV vertical transmission in Brazilian children. AIDS 2009;23:177−82.

[29] Fellay J, Ge D, Shianna KV, Colombo S, Ledergerber B, Cirulli ET, et al. Common genetic variation and the control of HIV-1 in humans. PLoS Genet 2009;5:e1000791.

[30] Fellay J, Shianna KV, Ge D, Colombo S, Ledergerber B, Weale M, et al. A whole-genome association study of major determinants for host control of HIV-1. Science 2007;317:944−7.

[31] Geczy AF, Kuipers H, Coolen M, Ashton LJ, Kennedy C, Ng G, et al. HLA and other host factors in transfusion-acquired HIV-1 infection. Hum Immunol 2000;61:172−6.

[32] Goldschmidt V, Bleiber G, May M, Martinez R, Ortiz M, Telenti A. Role of common human TRIM5alpha variants in HIV-1 disease progression. Retrovirology 2006;3:54.

[33] Gonzalez E, Dhanda R, Bamshad M, Mummidi S, Geevarghese R, Catano G, et al. Global survey of genetic variation in CCR5, RANTES, and MIP-1alpha: impact on the epidemiology of the HIV-1 pandemic. Proc Natl Acad Sci USA 2001;98:5199−204.

[34] Gonzalez E, Rovin BH, Sen L, Cooke G, Dhanda R, Mummidi S, et al. HIV-1 infection and AIDS dementia are influenced by a mutant MCP-1 allele linked to increased monocyte infiltration of tissues and MCP-1 levels. Proc Natl Acad Sci USA 2002;99:13795−800.

[35] Gonzalez E, Kulkarni H, Bolivar H, Mangano A, Sanchez R, Catano G, et al. The influence of CCL3L1 gene-containing segmental duplications on HIV-1/AIDS susceptibility. Science 2005;307:1434−40.

[36] Gonzalez S, Tirado G, Revuelta G, Yamamura Y, Lu Y, Nerurkar VR, et al. CCR5 chemokine receptor genotype frequencies among Puerto Rican HIV-1-seropositive individuals. Bol Asoc Med P R 1998;90:12−5.

[37] Haddad R, Ciliao Alves DC, Rocha-Junior MC, Azevedo R, do Socorro Pombo-de-Oliveira M, Takayanagui OM, et al. HLA-G 14-bp insertion/deletion polymorphism is a risk factor for HTLV-1 infection. AIDS Res Hum Retroviruses 2011;23:283−8.

[38] Harrison GA, Humphrey KE, Jakobsen IB, Cooper DW. A 14 bp deletion polymorphism in the HLA-G gene. Hum Mol Genet 1993;2:2200.

[39] Ji H, Ball TB, Kimani J, Plummer FA. Novel interferon regulatory factor-1 polymorphisms in a Kenyan population revealed by complete gene sequencing. J Hum Genet 2004;49:528−35.

[40] Ji H, Ball TB, Liang BB, Kimani J, Plummer FA. Human interferon regulatory factor-1 gene and its promoter sequences revealed by population-based complete gene sequencing. DNA Seq 2008;19:326−31.

[41] Liao HX, Montefiori DC, Patel DD, Lee DM, Scott WK, Pericak-Vance M, et al. Linkage of the CCR5 delta 32 mutation with a functional polymorphism of CD45RA. J Immunol 2000;165:148−57.

[42] Libert F, Cochaux P, Beckman G, Samson M, Aksenova M, Cao A, et al. The deltaCCR5 mutation conferring protection against HIV-1 in Caucasian populations has a single and recent origin in Northeastern Europe. Hum Mol Genet 1998;7:399−406.

[43] Lin A, Yan WH, Xu HH, Tang LJ, Chen XF, Zhu M, et al. 14 bp deletion polymorphism in the HLA-G gene is a risk factor for idiopathic dilated cardiomyopathy in a Chinese Han population. Tissue Antigens 2007;70:427−31.

[44] Martin MP, Carrington M, Dean M, O'Brien SJ, Sheppard HW, Wegner SA, et al. CXCR4 polymorphisms and HIV-1 pathogenesis. J Acquir Immune Defic Syndr Hum Retrovirol 1998;19:430.

[45] Martin MP, Lederman MM, Hutcheson HB, Goedert JJ, Nelson GW, van Kooyk Y, et al. Association of DC-SIGN promoter polymorphism with increased risk for parenteral, but not mucosal, acquisition of human immunodeficiency virus type 1 infection. J Virol 2004;78:14053−6.

[46] Matt C, Roger M. Genetic determinants of pediatric HIV-1 infection: Vertical transmission and disease progression among children. Mol Med 2001;7:583−9.

[47] McDermott DH, Colla JS, Kleeberger CA, Plankey M, Rosenberg PS, Smith ED, et al. Genetic polymorphism in CX3CR1 and risk of HIV disease. Science 2000;290:2031.

[48] McDermott DH, Zimmerman PA, Guignard F, Kleeberger CA, Leitman SF, Murphy PM. CCR5 promoter polymorphism and HIV-1 disease progression. Multicenter AIDS Cohort Study (MACS). Lancet 1998;352:866−70.

[49] McDermott DH, Beecroft MJ, Kleeberger CA, Al-Sharif FM, Ollier WE, Zimmerman PA, et al. Chemokine RANTES promoter polymorphism affects risk of both HIV infection and disease progression in the Multicenter AIDS Cohort Study. AIDS 2000;14:2671−8.

[50] Pelak K, Goldstein DB, Walley NM, Fellay J, Ge D, Shianna KV, et al. Host determinants of HIV-1 control in African Americans. J Infect Dis 201:1141−9.

[51] Petersen DC, Glashoff RH, Shrestha S, Bergeron J, Laten A, Gold B, et al. Risk for HIV-1 infection associated with a common CXCL12 (SDF1) polymorphism and CXCR4 variation in an African population. J Acquir Immune Defic Syndr 2005;40:521−6.

[52] Price H, Lacap P, Tuff J, Wachihi C, Kimani J, Ball TB, et-al. A TRIM5alpha exon 2 polymorphism is associated with protection from HIV-1 infection in the Pumwani Sex Worker cohort. AIDS 24:1813−21.

[53] One copy of mutation may help resistance. study. AIDS Alert 2002;17:23−4. 14.

[54] An P, Martin MP, Nelson GW, Carrington M, Smith MW, Gong K, et al. Influence of CCR5 promoter haplotypes on AIDS progression in African-Americans. AIDS 2000;14:2117−22.

[55] Arenzana-Seisdedos F, Virelizier JL, Rousset D, Clark-Lewis I, Loetscher P, Moser B, et al. HIV blocked by chemokine antagonist. Nature 1996;383:400.

[56] Blanpain C, Libert F, Vassart G, Parmentier M. CCR5 and HIV infection. Receptors Channels 2002;8:19−31.

[57] Chalmet K, Van Wanzeele F, Demecheleer E, Dauwe K, Pelgrom J, Van Der Gucht B, et al. Impact of delta 32-CCR5 heterozygosity on HIV-1 genetic evolution and variability—a study of 4 individuals infected with closely related HIV-1 strains. Virology 2008;379:213−22.

[58] Bratt G, Sandstrom E, Albert J, Samson M, Wahren B. The influence of MT-2 tropism on the prognostic implications of the delta32 deletion in the CCR-5 gene. AIDS 1997;11:1415−9.

[59] Diaz FJ, Vega JA, Patino PJ, Bedoya G, Nagles J, Villegas C, et al. Frequency of CCR5 delta-32 mutation in human immunodeficiency virus (HIV)-seropositive and HIV-exposed seronegative individuals and in general population of Medellin, Colombia. Mem Inst Oswaldo Cruz 2000;95:237−42.

[60] Gonzalez E, Bamshad M, Sato N, Mummidi S, Dhanda R, Catano G, et al. Race-specific HIV-1 disease-modifying effects associated with CCR5 haplotypes. Proc Natl Acad Sci USA 1999;96:12004−9.

[61] Huang Y, Paxton WA, Wolinsky SM, Neumann AU, Zhang L, He T, et al. The role of a mutant CCR5 allele in HIV-1 transmission and disease progression. Nat Med 1996;2:1240−3.

[62] Hummel S, Schmidt D, Kremeyer B, Herrmann B, Oppermann M. Detection of the CCR5-delta32 HIV resistance gene in Bronze Age skeletons. Genes Immun 2005;6:371−4.

[63] Kokkotou E, Philippon V, Gueye-Ndiaye A, Mboup S, Wang WK, Essex M, et al. Role of the CCR5 delta 32 allele in resistance to HIV-1 infection in West Africa. J Hum Virol 1998;1:469−74.

[64] Hedrick PW, Verrelli BC. "Ground truth" for selection on CCR5-delta32. Trends Genet 2006;22:293−6.

[65] Speelmon EC, Livingston-Rosanoff D, Li SS, Vu Q, Bui J, Geraghty DE, et al. Genetic association of the antiviral restriction factor TRIM5alpha with human immunodeficiency virus type 1 infection. J Virol 2006;80:2463—71.

[66] Diaz-Griffero F, Perron M, McGee-Estrada K, Hanna R, Maillard PV, Trono D, et al. A human TRIM5alpha B30.2/SPRY domain mutant gains the ability to restrict and prematurely uncoat B-tropic murine leukemia virus. Virology 2008;378:233—42.

[67] Takeuchi H, Matano T. Host factors involved in resistance to retroviral infection. Microbiol Immunol 2008;52:318—25.

[68] Su RC, Sivro A, Kimani J, Jaoko W, Plummer FA, Ball TB. Epigenetic control of IRF1 responses in HIV-exposed seronegative versus HIV-susceptible individuals. Blood 117: 2649—57.

[69] Hardie RA, Knight E, Bruneau B, Semeniuk C, Gill K, Nagelkerke N, et al. A common human leucocyte antigen-DP genotype is associated with resistance to HIV-1 infection in Kenyan sex workers. AIDS 2008;22:2038—42.

[70] Hardie RA, Luo M, Bruneau B, Knight E, Nagelkerke NJ, Kimani J, et al. Human leukocyte antigen-DQ alleles and haplotypes and their associations with resistance and susceptibility to HIV-1 infection. AIDS 2008;22:807—16.

[71] Lacap PA, Huntington JD, Luo M, Nagelkerke NJ, Bielawny T, Kimani J, et al. Associations of human leukocyte antigen DRB with resistance or susceptibility to HIV-1 infection in the Pumwani Sex Worker cohort. AIDS 2008;22:1029—38.

[72] MacDonald KS, Fowke KR, Kimani J, Dunand VA, Nagelkerke NJ, Ball TB, et al. Influence of HLA supertypes on susceptibility and resistance to human immunodeficiency virus type 1 infection. J Infect Dis 2000;181:1581—9.

[73] Magierowska M, Theodorou I, Debre P, Sanson F, Autran B, Riviere Y, et al. Combined genotypes of CCR5, CCR2, SDF1, and HLA genes can predict the long-term nonprogressor status in human immunodeficiency virus-1-infected individuals. Blood 1999;93:936—41.

[74] Kreiss JK, Kiviat NB, Plummer FA, Roberts PL, Waiyaki P, Ngugi E, et al. Human immunodeficiency virus, human papillomavirus, and cervical intraepithelial neoplasia in Nairobi prostitutes. Sex Transm Dis 1992;19:54—9.

[75] Kreiss JK, Koech D, Plummer FA, Holmes KK, Lightfoote M, Piot P, et al. AIDS virus infection in Nairobi prostitutes. Spread of the epidemic to East Africa. N Engl J Med 1986;314:414—8.

[76] Ndinya-achola JO, Plummer FA, Ronald AR, Piot P. Acquired immunodeficiency syndrome: Epidemiology in Africa and its implications for health services. Afr J Sex Transmi Dis 1986;2:77—80.

[77] Piot P, Colebunders R, Laga M, Ndinya-Achola JO, van der Groen G, Plummer FA. AIDS in Africa: A public health priority. J Virol Methods 1987;17:1—10.

[78] Piot P, Kreiss JK, Ndinya-Achola JO, Ngugi EN, Simonsen JN, Cameron DW, et al. Heterosexual transmission of HIV. AIDS 1987;1:199—206.

[79] Piot P, Plummer FA, Mhalu FS, Lamboray JL, Chin J, Mann JM. AIDS: An international perspective. Science 1988;239:573—9.

[80] Piot P, Plummer FA, Rey MA, Ngugi EN, Rouzioux C, Ndinya-Achola JO, et al. Retrospective seroepidemiology of AIDS virus infection in Nairobi populations. J Infect Dis 1987;155:1108—12.

[81] Nagelkerke NJ, Plummer FA, Holton D, Anzala AO, Manji F, Ngugi EN, et al. Transition dynamics of HIV disease in a cohort of African prostitutes: A Markov model approach. AIDS 1990;4:743—7.

[82] Ngugi EN, Plummer FA, Simonsen JN, Cameron DW, Bosire M, Waiyaki P, et al. Prevention of transmission of human immunodeficiency virus in Africa: Effectiveness of condom promotion and health education among prostitutes. Lancet 1988;2: 887–90.

[83] Ngugi EN, Plummer FA. Health outreach and control of HIV infection in Kenya. J Acquir Immune Defic Syndr 1988;1:566–70.

[84] Plummer FA, Ndinya-Achola JO. Sexually transmitted diseases and HIV-1: Interactions in transmission and role in control programs. East Afr Med J 1990;67:457–60.

[85] Ronald AR, Ndinya-Achola JO, Plummer FA, Simonsen JN, Cameron DW, Ngugi EN, et al. A review of HIV-1 in Africa. Bull NY Acad Med 1988;64:480–90.

[86] Simonsen JN, Cameron DW, Gakinya MN, Ndinya-Achola JO, D'Costa LJ, Karasira P, et al. Human immunodeficiency virus infection among men with sexually transmitted diseases. Experience from a center in Africa. N Engl J Med 1988;319:274–8.

[87] UNAIDS. http://www.unaids.org: http://www.unaids.org.

[88] Tersmette M, van Dongen JJ, Clapham PR, de Goede RE, Wolvers-Tettero IL, Geurts van Kessel A, et al. Human immunodeficiency virus infection studied in CD4-expressing human-murine T-cell hybrids. Virology 1989;168:267–73.

[89] Weiner DB, Huebner K, Williams WV, Greene MI. Human genes other than CD4 facilitate HIV-1 infection of murine cells. Pathobiology 1991;59:361–71.

[90] Cocchi F, DeVico AL, Garzino-Demo A, Arya SK, Gallo RC, Lusso P. Identification of RANTES, MIP-1 alpha, and MIP-1 beta as the major HIV-suppressive factors produced by CD8+ T cells. Science 1995;270:1811–5.

[91] Alkhatib G, Combadiere C, Broder CC, Feng Y, Kennedy PE, Murphy PM, et al. CC CKR5: A RANTES, MIP-1alpha, MIP-1beta receptor as a fusion cofactor for macrophage-tropic HIV-1. Science 1996;272:1955–8.

[92] Bleul CC, Farzan M, Choe H, Parolin C, Clark-Lewis I, Sodroski J, et al. The lymphocyte chemoattractant SDF-1 is a ligand for LESTR/fusin and blocks HIV-1 entry. Nature 1996;382:829–33.

[93] Choe H, Farzan M, Sun Y, Sullivan N, Rollins B, Ponath PD, et al. The beta-chemokine receptors CCR3 and CCR5 facilitate infection by primary HIV-1 isolates. Cell 1996;85:1135–48.

[94] Deng H, Liu R, Ellmeier W, Choe S, Unutmaz D, Burkhart M, et al. Identification of a major co-receptor for primary isolates of HIV-1. Nature 1996;381:661–6.

[95] Dragic T, Litwin V, Allaway GP, Martin SR, Huang Y, Nagashima KA, et al. HIV-1 entry into CD4+ cells is mediated by the chemokine receptor CC-CKR-5. Nature 1996;381:667–73.

[96] Feng Y, Broder CC, Kennedy PE, Berger EA. HIV-1 entry cofactor: Functional cDNA cloning of a seven-transmembrane, G protein-coupled receptor. Science 1996;272: 827–37.

[97] Dean M, Carrington M, Winkler C, Huttley GA, Smith MW, Allikmets R, et al. Genetic restriction of HIV-1 infection and progression to AIDS by a deletion allele of the CKR5 structural gene. Hemophilia Growth and Development Study, Multicenter AIDS Cohort Study, Multicenter Hemophilia Cohort Study, San Francisco City Cohort, ALIVE Study. Science 1996;273:1856–62.

[98] Samson M, Libert F, Doranz BJ, Rucker J, Liesnard C, Farber CM, et al. Resistance to HIV-1 infection in Caucasian individuals bearing mutant alleles of the CCR-5 chemokine receptor gene. Nature 1996;382:722–5.

[99] O'Brien SJ, Dean M. In search of AIDS-resistance genes. Sci Am 1997;277:44–51.

[100] Theodorou I, Meyer L, Magierowska M, Katlama C, Rouzioux C. HIV-1 infection in an individual homozygous for CCR5 delta 32. Seroco Study Group. Lancet 1997;349:1219–20.

[101] O'Brien SJ, Nelson GW. Human genes that limit AIDS. Nat Genet 2004;36:565–74.

[102] Stephens JC, Reich DE, Goldstein DB, Shin HD, Smith MW, Carrington M, et al. Dating the origin of the CCR5-delta32 AIDS-resistance allele by the coalescence of haplotypes. Am J Hum Genet 1998;62:1507–15.

[103] Sabeti PC, Walsh E, Schaffner SF, Varilly P, Fry B, Hutcheson HB, et al. The case for selection at CCR5-delta32. PLoS Biol 2005;3:e387.

[104] Hutter G, Nowak D, Mossner M, Ganepola S, Mussig A, Allers K, et al. Long-term control of HIV by CCR5 delta32/delta32 stem-cell transplantation. N Engl J Med 2009;360:692–8.

[105] Carrington M, Kissner T, Gerrard B, Ivanov S, O'Brien SJ, Dean M. Novel alleles of the chemokine-receptor gene CCR5. Am J Hum Genet 1997;61:1261–7.

[106] Quillent C, Oberlin E, Braun J, Rousset D, Gonzalez-Canali G, Metais P, et al. HIV-1-resistance phenotype conferred by combination of two separate inherited mutations of CCR5 gene. Lancet 1998;351:14–8.

[107] Mangano A, Gonzalez E, Dhanda R, Catano G, Bamshad M, Bock A, et al. Concordance between the CC chemokine receptor 5 genetic determinants that alter risks of transmission and disease progression in children exposed perinatally to human immunodeficiency virus. J Infect Dis 2001;183:1574–85.

[108] Capoulade-Metay C, Ma L, Truong LX, Dudoit Y, Versmisse P, Nguyen NV, et al. New CCR5 variants associated with reduced HIV coreceptor function in southeast Asia. AIDS 2004;18:2243–52.

[109] Ma L, Dudoit Y, Tran T, Xing H, Chen J, Pancino G, et al. Biochemical and HIV-1 coreceptor properties of K26R, a new CCR5 Variant in China's Sichuan population. J Acquir Immune Defic Syndr 2005;39:38–43.

[110] Saez-Cirion A, Versmisse P, Truong LX, Chakrabarti LA, Carpentier W, Barre-Sinoussi F, et al. Persistent resistance to HIV-1 infection in CD4 T cells from exposed uninfected Vietnamese individuals is mediated by entry and post-entry blocks. Retrovirology 2006;3:81.

[111] MacDonald KS, Embree J, Njenga S, Nagelkerke NJ, Ngatia I, Mohammed Z, et al. Mother–child class I HLA concordance increases perinatal human immunodeficiency virus type 1 transmission. J Infect Dis 1998;177:551–6.

[112] Mackelprang RD, John-Stewart G, Carrington M, Richardson B, Rowland-Jones S, Gao X, et al. Maternal HLA homozygosity and mother–child HLA concordance increase the risk of vertical transmission of HIV-1. J Infect Dis 2008;197:1156–61.

[113] Polycarpou A, Ntais C, Korber BT, Elrich HA, Winchester R, Krogstad P, et al. Association between maternal and infant class I and II HLA alleles and of their concordance with the risk of perinatal HIV type 1 transmission. AIDS Res Hum Retroviruses 2002;18:741–6.

[114] Thobakgale CF, Prendergast A, Crawford H, Mkhwanazi N, Ramduth D, Reddy S, et al. Impact of HLA in mother and child on disease progression of pediatric human immuno-deficiency virus type 1 infection. J Virol 2009;83:10234–44.

[115] Dorak MT, Tang J, Penman-Aguilar A, Westfall AO, Zulu I, Lobashevsky ES, et al. Transmission of HIV-1 and HLA-B allele-sharing within serodiscordant heterosexual Zambian couples. Lancet 2004;363:2137–9.

[116] Lockett SF, Robertson JR, Brettle RP, Yap PL, Middleton D, Leigh Brown AJ. Mismatched human leukocyte antigen alleles protect against heterosexual HIV transmission. J Acquir Immune Defic Syndr 2001;27:277–80.

[117] Liu C, Carrington M, Kaslow RA, Gao X, Rinaldo CR, Jacobson LP, et al. Association of polymorphisms in human leukocyte antigen class I and transporter associated with antigen processing genes with resistance to human immunodeficiency virus type 1 infection. J Infect Dis 2003;187:1404−10.

[118] Rohowsky-Kochan C, Skurnick J, Molinaro D, Louria D. HLA antigens associated with susceptibility/resistance to HIV-1 infection. Hum Immunol 1998;59:802−15.

[119] MacDonald KS, Embree JE, Nagelkerke NJ, Castillo J, Ramhadin S, Njenga S, et al. The HLA A2/6802 supertype is associated with reduced risk of perinatal human immunodeficiency virus type 1 transmission. J Infect Dis 2001;183:503−6.

[120] Fabio G, Scorza R, Lazzarin A, Marchini M, Zarantonello M, D'Arminio A, et al. HLA-associated susceptibility to HIV-1 infection. Clin Exp Immunol 1992;87:20−3.

[121] Sriwanthana B, Hodge T, Mastro TD, Dezzutti CS, Bond K, Stephens HA, et al. HIV-specific cytotoxic T lymphocytes, HLA-A11, and chemokine-related factors may act synergistically to determine HIV resistance in CCR5 delta32-negative female sex workers in Chiang Rai, northern Thailand. AIDS Res Hum Retroviruses 2001;17:719−34.

[122] Mackelprang RD, Carrington M, John-Stewart G, Lohman-Payne B, Richardson BA, Wamalwa D, et al. Maternal human leukocyte antigen A*2301 is associated with increased mother-to-child HIV-1 transmission. J Infect Dis 202:1273−7.

[123] Winchester R, Chen Y, Rose S, Selby J, Borkowsky W. Major histocompatibility complex class II DR alleles DRB1*1501 and those encoding HLA-DR13 are preferentially associated with a diminution in maternally transmitted human immunodeficiency virus 1 infection in different ethnic groups: Determination by an automated sequence-based typing method. Proc Natl Acad Sci USA 1995;92:12374−8.

[124] Winchester R, Pitt J, Charurat M, Magder LS, Goring HH, Landay A, et al. Mother-to-child transmission of HIV-1: Strong association with certain maternal HLA-B alleles independent of viral load implicates innate immune mechanisms. J Acquir Immune Defic Syndr 2004;36:659−70.

[125] Martin MP, Gao X, Lee JH, Nelson GW, Detels R, Goedert JJ, et al. Epistatic interaction between KIR3DS1 and HLA-B delays the progression to AIDS. Nat Genet 2002;31:429−34.

[126] Martin MP, Nelson G, Lee JH, Pellett F, Gao X, Wade J, et al. Cutting edge: Susceptibility to psoriatic arthritis: Influence of activating killer Ig−like receptor genes in the absence of specific HLA-C alleles. J Immunol 2002;169:2818−22.

[127] Martin MP, Qi Y, Gao X, Yamada E, Martin JN, Pereyra F, et al. Innate partnership of HLA-B and KIR3DL1 subtypes against HIV-1. Nat Genet 2007;39:733−40.

[128] Jennes W, Verheyden S, Demanet C, Adje-Toure CA, Vuylsteke B, Nkengasong JN, et al. Cutting edge: Resistance to HIV-1 infection among African female sex workers is associated with inhibitory KIR in the absence of their HLA ligands. J Immunol 2006;177: 6588−92.

[129] Boulet S, Kleyman M, Kim JY, Kamya P, Sharafi S, Simic N, et al. A combined genotype of KIR3DL1 high expressing alleles and HLA-B*57 is associated with a reduced risk of HIV infection. AIDS 2008;22:1487−91.

[130] Boulet S, Sharafi S, Simic N, Bruneau J, Routy JP, Tsoukas CM, et al. Increased proportion of KIR3DS1 homozygotes in HIV-exposed uninfected individuals. AIDS 2008;22:595−9.

[131] Urban TJ, Weintrob AC, Fellay J, Colombo S, Shianna KV, Gumbs C, et al. CCL3L1 and HIV/AIDS susceptibility. Nat Med 2009;15:1112−5.

[132] Field SF, Howson JM, Maier LM, Walker S, Walker NM, Smyth DJ, et al. Experimental aspects of copy number variant assays at CCL3L1. Nat Med 2009;15:1115−7.

[133] Gardner L, Patterson AM, Ashton BA, Stone MA, Middleton J. The human Duffy antigen binds selected inflammatory but not homeostatic chemokines. Biochem Biophys Res Commun 2004;321:306−12.

[134] Lachgar A, Jaureguiberry G, Le Buenac H, Bizzini B, Zagury JF, Rappaport J, et al. Binding of HIV-1 to RBCs involves the Duffy antigen receptors for chemokines (DARC). Biomed Pharmacother 1998;52:436−9.

[135] Horuk R, Chitnis CE, Darbonne WC, Colby TJ, Rybicki A, Hadley TJ, et al. A receptor for the malarial parasite *Plasmodium vivax*: The erythrocyte chemokine receptor. Science 1993;261:1182−4.

[136] He W, Neil S, Kulkarni H, Wright E, Agan BK, Marconi VC, et al. Duffy antigen receptor for chemokines mediates trans-infection of HIV-1 from red blood cells to target cells and affects HIV-AIDS susceptibility. Cell Host Microbe 2008;4:52−62.

[137] Horne KC, Li X, Jacobson LP, Palella F, Jamieson BD, Margolick JB, et al. Duffy antigen polymorphisms do not alter progression of HIV in African Americans in the MACS cohort. Cell Host Microbe 2009;5:415−7.

[138] Winkler CA, An P, Johnson R, Nelson GW, Kirk G. Expression of Duffy antigen receptor for chemokines (DARC) has no effect on HIV-1 acquisition or progression to AIDS in African Americans. Cell Host Microbe 2009;5:411−3.

[139] Walley NM, Julg B, Dickson SP, Fellay J, Ge D, Walker BD, et al. The Duffy antigen receptor for chemokines null promoter variant does not influence HIV-1 acquisition or disease progression. Cell Host Microbe 2009;5:408−10.

[140] Geijtenbeek TB, van Kooyk Y. DC-SIGN: A novel HIV receptor on DCs that mediates HIV-1 transmission. Curr Top Microbiol Immunol 2003;276:31−54.

[141] Bashirova AA, Geijtenbeek TB, van Duijnhoven GC, van Vliet SJ, Eilering JB, Martin MP, et al. A dendritic cell-specific intercellular adhesion molecule 3-grabbing nonintegrin (DC-SIGN)-related protein is highly expressed on human liver sinusoidal endothelial cells and promotes HIV-1 infection. J Exp Med 2001;193:671−8.

[142] Mitchell DA, Fadden AJ, Drickamer K. A novel mechanism of carbohydrate recognition by the C-type lectins DC-SIGN and DC-SIGNR. Subunit organization and binding to multivalent ligands. J Biol Chem 2001;276:28939−45.

[143] Zhang J, Zhang X, Fu J, Bi Z, Arheart KL, Barreiro LB, et al. Protective role of DC-SIGN (CD209) neck-region alleles with <5 repeat units in HIV-1 transmission. J Infect Dis 2008;198:68−71.

[144] Lichterfeld M, Nischalke HD, van Lunzen J, Sohne J, Schmeisser N, Woitas R, et al. The tandem-repeat polymorphism of the DC-SIGNR gene does not affect the susceptibility to HIV infection and the progression to AIDS. Clin Immunol 2003;107:55−9.

[145] Liu H, Carrington M, Wang C, Holte S, Lee J, Greene B, et al. Repeat-region polymorphisms in the gene for the dendritic cell-specific intercellular adhesion molecule-3-grabbing non-integrin-related molecule: Effects on HIV-1 susceptibility. J Infect Dis 2006;193:698−702.

[146] Wichukchinda N, Kitamura Y, Rojanawiwat A, Nakayama EE, Song H, Pathipvanich P, et al. The polymorphisms in DC-SIGNR affect susceptibility to HIV type 1 infection. AIDS Res Hum Retroviruses 2007;23:686−92.

[147] Rathore A, Chatterjee A, Sivarama P, Yamamoto N, Dhole TN. Role of homozygous DC-SIGNR 5/5 tandem repeat polymorphism in HIV-1 exposed seronegative North Indian individuals. J Clin Immunol 2008;28:50−7.

[148] Vallinoto AC, Menezes-Costa MR, Alves AE, Machado LF, de Azevedo VN, Souza LL, et al. Mannose-binding lectin gene polymorphism and its impact on human immunodeficiency virus 1 infection. Mol Immunol 2006;43:1358−62.

[149] Pastinen T, Liitsola K, Niini P, Salminen M, Syvanen AC. Contribution of the CCR5 and MBL genes to susceptibility to HIV type 1 infection in the Finnish population. AIDS Res Hum Retroviruses 1998;14:695−8.

[150] Garred P, Madsen HO, Balslev U, Hofmann B, Pedersen C, Gerstoft J, et al. Susceptibility to HIV infection and progression of AIDS in relation to variant alleles of mannose-binding lectin. Lancet 1997;349:236−40.

[151] Boniotto M, Braida L, Pirulli D, Arraes L, Amoroso A, Crovella S. MBL2 polymorphisms are involved in HIV-1 infection in Brazilian perinatally infected children. AIDS 2003;17:779−80.

[152] Boniotto M, Crovella S, Pirulli D, Scarlatti G, Spano A, Vatta L, et al. Polymorphisms in the MBL2 promoter correlated with risk of HIV-1 vertical transmission and AIDS progression. Genes Immun 2000;1:346−8.

[153] Catano G, Agan BK, Kulkarni H, Telles V, Marconi VC, Dolan MJ, et al. Independent effects of genetic variations in mannose-binding lectin influence the course of HIV disease: The advantage of heterozygosity for coding mutations. J Infect Dis 2008;198:72−80.

[154] Winkler C, Modi W, Smith MW, Nelson GW, Wu X, Carrington M, et al. Genetic restriction of AIDS pathogenesis by an SDF-1 chemokine gene variant. ALIVE Study, Hemophilia Growth and Development Study (HGDS), Multicenter AIDS Cohort Study (MACS), Multicenter Hemophilia Cohort Study (MHCS), San Francisco City Cohort (SFCC). Science 1998;279:389−93.

[155] Wang C, Song W, Lobashevsky E, Wilson CM, Douglas SD, Mytilineos J, et al. Cytokine and chemokine gene polymorphisms among ethnically diverse North Americans with HIV-1 infection. J Acquir Immune Defic Syndr 2004;35:446−54.

[156] Tiensiwakul P. Stromal cell-derived factor (SDF) 1-3′A polymorphism may play a role in resistance to HIV-1 infection in seronegative high-risk Thais. Intervirology 2004;47: 87−92.

[157] Reiche EM, Ehara Watanabe MA, Bonametti AM, Kaminami Morimoto H, Akira Morimoto A, Wiechmann SL, et al. The effect of stromal cell-derived factor 1 (SDF1/ CXCL12) genetic polymorphism on HIV-1 disease progression. Intl J Mol Med 2006;18: 785−93.

[158] Royo JL, Ruiz A, Borrego S, Rubio A, Sanchez B, Nunez-Roldan A, et al. Fluorescence resonance energy transfer analysis of CCR-V64I and SDF1-3′a polymorphisms: Prevalence in southern Spain HIV type 1+ cohort and noninfected population. AIDS Res Hum Retroviruses 2001;17:663−6.

[159] Suresh P, Wanchu A, Sachdeva RK, Bhatnagar A. Gene polymorphisms in CCR5, CCR2, CX3CR1, SDF-1 and RANTES in exposed but uninfected partners of HIV-1 infected individuals in North India. J Clin Immunol 2006;26:476−84.

[160] Tan XH, Zhang JY, Di CH, Hu AR, Yang L, Qu S, et al. Distribution of CCR5-delta32, CCR5m303A, CCR2-64I and SDF1-3′A in HIV-1 infected and uninfected high-risk Uighurs in Xinjiang, China. Infect Genet Evol 10:268−72.

[161] Soriano A, Martinez C, Garcia F, Plana M, Palou E, Lejeune M, et al. Plasma stromal cell-derived factor (SDF)-1 levels, SDF1-3′A genotype, and expression of CXCR4 on T lymphocytes: Their impact on resistance to human immunodeficiency virus type 1 infection and its progression. J Infect Dis 2002;186:922−31.

[162] Stremlau M, Owens CM, Perron MJ, Kiessling M, Autissier P, Sodroski J. The cytoplasmic body component TRIM5alpha restricts HIV-1 infection in Old World monkeys. Nature 2004;427:848−53.

[163] Sheehy AM, Gaddis NC, Choi JD, Malim MH. Isolation of a human gene that inhibits HIV-1 infection and is suppressed by the viral Vif protein. Nature 2002;418:646–50.

[164] Valcke HS, Bernard NF, Bruneau J, Alary M, Tsoukas CM, Roger M. APOBEC3G genetic variants and their association with risk of HIV infection in highly exposed Caucasians. AIDS 2006;20:1984–6.

[165] An P, Johnson R, Phair J, Kirk GD, Yu XF, Donfield S, et al. APOBEC3B deletion and risk of HIV-1 acquisition. J Infect Dis 2009;200:1054–8.

[166] Javanbakht H, An P, Gold B, Petersen DC, O'Huigin C, Nelson GW, et al. Effects of human TRIM5alpha polymorphisms on antiretroviral function and susceptibility to human immunodeficiency virus infection. Virology 2006;354:15–27.

[167] Franke EK, Yuan HE, Luban J. Specific incorporation of cyclophilin A into HIV-1 virions. Nature 1994;372:359–62.

[168] Luban J, Bossolt KL, Franke EK, Kalpana GV, Goff SP. Human immunodeficiency virus type 1 Gag protein binds to cyclophilins A and B. Cell 1993;73:1067–78.

[169] An P, Wang LH, Hutcheson-Dilks H, Nelson G, Donfield S, Goedert JJ, et al. Regulatory polymorphisms in the cyclophilin A gene, PPIA, accelerate progression to AIDS. PLoS Pathog 2007;3:e88.

[170] Cardoso CB, Uthida-Tanaka AM, Magalhaes RF, Magna LA, Kraemer MH. Association between psoriasis vulgaris and MHC-DRB, -DQB genes as a contribution to disease diagnosis. Eur J Dermatol 2005;15:159–63.

[171] Plummer FA, Laga M, Brunham RC, Piot P, Ronald AR, Bhullar V, et al. Postpartum upper genital tract infections in Nairobi, Kenya: Epidemiology, etiology, and risk factors. J Infect Dis 1987;156:92–8.

[172] Plummer FA, Nagelkerke NJ, Moses S, Ndinya-Achola JO, Bwayo J, Ngugi E. The importance of core groups in the epidemiology and control of HIV-1 infection. AIDS 1991;5(Suppl 1):S169–76.

[173] Ronald AR, Plummer F. Chancroid. A newly important sexually transmitted disease. Arch Dermatol 1989;125:1413–4.

[174] Ronald AR, Plummer FA. Chancroid and *Haemophilus ducreyi*. Ann Intern Med 1985;102:705–7.

[175] Plummer FA, D'Costa LJ, Nsanze H, Dylewski J, Karasira P, Ronald AR. Epidemiology of chancroid and *Haemophilus ducreyi* in Nairobi, Kenya. Lancet 1983;2:1293–5.

[176] Plummer FA, Brunham RC. Gonococcal recidivism, diversity, and ecology. Rev Infect Dis 1987;9:846–50.

[177] Plummer FA, Simonsen JN, Chubb H, Slaney L, Kimata J, Bosire M, et al. Epidemiologic evidence for the development of serovar-specific immunity after gonococcal infection. J Clin Invest 1989;83:1472–6.

[178] Plummer FA, Maggwa N, D'Costa LJ, Nsanze H, Karasira P, Maclean IW, et al. Cefotaxime treatment of *Haemophilus ducreyi* infection in Kenya. Sex Transm Dis 1984;11:304–7.

[179] Plummer FA, D'Costa LJ, Nsanze H, Karasira P, MacLean IW, Piot P, et al. Clinical and microbiologic studies of genital ulcers in Kenyan women. Sex Transm Dis 1985;12:193–7.

[180] Datta P, Laga M, Plummer FA, Ndinya-Achola JO, Piot P, Maitha G, et al. Infection and disease after perinatal exposure to *Chlamydia trachomatis* in Nairobi, Kenya. J Infect Dis 1988;158:524–8.

[181] D'Costa LJ, Plummer FA, Bowmer I, Fransen L, Piot P, Ronald AR, et al. Prostitutes are a major reservoir of sexually transmitted diseases in Nairobi, Kenya. Sex Transm Dis 1985;12:64–7.

[182] Simonsen JN, Plummer FA, Ngugi EN, Black C, Kreiss JK, Gakinya MN, et al. HIV infection among lower socioeconomic strata prostitutes in Nairobi. AIDS 1990;4:139—44.

[183] Miura T, Brockman MA, Schneidewind A, Lobritz M, Pereyra F, Rathod A, et al. HLA-B57/B*5801 human immunodeficiency virus type 1 elite controllers select for rare Gag variants associated with reduced viral replication capacity and strong cytotoxic T-lymphocyte recognition. J Virol 2009;83:2743—55.

[184] McNeil AJ, Yap PL, Gore SM, Brettle RP, McColl M, Wyld R, et al. Association of HLA types A1-B8-DR3 and B27 with rapid and slow progression of HIV disease. Q J Med 1996;89:177—85.

[185] Costello C, Tang J, Rivers C, Karita E, Meizen-Derr J, Allen S, et al. HLA-B*5703 independently associated with slower HIV-1 disease progression in Rwandan women. AIDS 1999;13:1990—1.

[186] Wang SS, Hildesheim A, Gao X, Schiffman M, Herrero R, Bratti MC, et al. Comprehensive analysis of human leukocyte antigen class I alleles and cervical neoplasia in 3 epidemiologic studies. J Infect Dis 2002;186:598—605.

[187] Moore CB, John M, James IR, Christiansen FT, Witt CS, Mallal SA. Evidence of HIV-1 adaptation to HLA-restricted immune responses at a population level. Science 2002;296:1439—43.

[188] Carrington M, O'Brien SJ. The influence of HLA genotype on AIDS. Annu Rev Med 2003;54:535—51.

[189] Kawashima Y, Pfafferott K, Frater J, Matthews P, Payne R, Addo M, et al. Adaptation of HIV-1 to human leukocyte antigen class I. Nature 2009;458:641—5.

[190] Cassinotti A, Birindelli S, Clerici M, Trabattoni D, Lazzaroni M, Ardizzone S, et al. HLA and autoimmune digestive disease: A clinically oriented review for gastroenterologists. Am J Gastroenterol 2009;104:195—217.

[191] Sanz L, Gonzalez-Escribano F, de Pablo R, Nunez-Roldan A, Kreisler M, Vilches C. HLA-Cw*1602: A new susceptibility marker of Behcet's disease in southern Spain. Tissue Antigens 1998;51:111—4.

[192] Hendel H, Caillat-Zucman S, Lebuanec H, Carrington M, O'Brien S, Andrieu JM, et al. New class I and II HLA alleles strongly associated with opposite patterns of progression to AIDS. J Immunol 1999;162:6942—6.

[193] Ngumbela KC, Day CL, Mncube Z, Nair K, Ramduth D, Thobakgale C, et al. Targeting of a CD8 T cell env epitope presented by HLA-B*5802 is associated with markers of HIV disease progression and lack of selection pressure. AIDS Res Hum Retroviruses 2008;24:72—82.

[194] Jin X, Gao X, Ramanathan Jr M, Deschenes GR, Nelson GW, O'Brien SJ, et al. Human immunodeficiency virus type 1 (HIV-1)-specific CD8+-T-cell responses for groups of HIV-1-infected individuals with different HLA-B*35 genotypes. J Virol 2002;76:12603—10.

[195] Farquhar C, Rowland-Jones S, Mbori-Ngacha D, Redman M, Lohman B, Slyker J, et al. Human leukocyte antigen (HLA) B*18 and protection against mother-to-child HIV type 1 transmission. AIDS Res Hum Retroviruses 2004;20:692—7.

[196] Beyrer C, Artenstein AW, Rugpao S, Stephens H, VanCott TC, Robb ML, et al. Epidemiologic and biologic characterization of a cohort of human immunodeficiency virus type 1 highly exposed, persistently seronegative female sex workers in northern Thailand. Chiang Mai HEPS Working Group. J Infect Dis 1999;179:59—67.

[197] Carrington M, Nelson GW, Martin MP, Kissner T, Vlahov D, Goedert JJ, et al. HLA and HIV-1: Heterozygote advantage and B*35-Cw*04 disadvantage. Science 1999;283:1748—52.

[198] Borghans JA, Molgaard A, de Boer RJ, Kesmir C. HLA alleles associated with slow progression to AIDS truly prefer to present HIV-1 p24. PLoS One 2007;2:e920.

[199] Emu B, Sinclair E, Hatano H, Ferre A, Shacklett B, Martin JN, et al. HLA class I-restricted T-cell responses may contribute to the control of human immunodeficiency virus infection, but such responses are not always necessary for long-term virus control. J Virol 2008;82:5398−407.

[200] Gao X, Nelson GW, Karacki P, Martin MP, Phair J, Kaslow R, et al. Effect of a single amino acid change in MHC class I molecules on the rate of progression to AIDS. N Engl J Med 2001;344:1668−75.

[201] Kiepiela P, Leslie AJ, Honeyborne I, Ramduth D, Thobakgale C, Chetty S, et al. Dominant influence of HLA-B in mediating the potential co-evolution of HIV and HLA. Nature 2004;432:769−75.

[202] Rousseau CM, Daniels MG, Carlson JM, Kadie C, Crawford H, Prendergast A, et al. HLA class I-driven evolution of human immunodeficiency virus type 1 subtype c proteome: Immune escape and viral load. J Virol 2008;82:6434−46.

[203] Steel CM, Ludlam CA, Beatson D, Peutherer JF, Cuthbert RJ, Simmonds P, et al. HLA haplotype A1 B8 DR3 as a risk factor for HIV-related disease. Lancet 1988;1:1185−8.

[204] Trachtenberg E, Korber B, Sollars C, Kepler TB, Hraber PT, Hayes E, et al. Advantage of rare HLA supertype in HIV disease progression. Nat Med 2003;9:928−35.

[205] de Sorrentino AH, Marinic K, Motta P, Sorrentino A, Lopez R, Illiovich E. HLA class I alleles associated with susceptibility or resistance to human immunodeficiency virus type 1 infection among a population in Chaco Province, Argentina. J Infect Dis 2000;182:1523−6.

[206] Ndung'u T, Gaseitsiwe S, Sepako E, Doualla-Bell F, Peter T, Kim S, et al. Major histocompatibility complex class II (HLA-DRB and -DQB) allele frequencies in Botswana: Association with human immunodeficiency virus type 1 infection. Clin Diagn Lab Immunol 2005;12:1020−8.

[207] Tang J, Penman-Aguilar A, Lobashevsky E, Allen S, Kaslow RA. HLA-DRB1 and -DQB1 alleles and haplotypes in Zambian couples and their associations with heterosexual transmission of HIV type 1. J Infect Dis 2004;189:1696−704.

[208] Selvaraj P, Swaminathan S, Alagarasu K, Raghavan S, Narendran G, Narayanan P. Association of human leukocyte antigen-A11 with resistance and B40 and DR2 with susceptibility to HIV-1 infection in south India. J Acquir Immune Defic Syndr 2006;43:497−9.

[209] Sun JC, Bevan MJ. Defective CD8 T cell memory following acute infection without CD4 T cell help. Science 2003;300:339−42.

[210] Sun JC, Williams MA, Bevan MJ. CD4+ T cells are required for the maintenance, not programming, of memory CD8+ T cells after acute infection. Nat Immunol 2004;5:927−33.

[211] Shedlock DJ, Shen H. Requirement for CD4 T cell help in generating functional CD8 T cell memory. Science 2003;300:337−9.

[212] Shedlock DJ, Whitmire JK, Tan J, MacDonald AS, Ahmed R, Shen H. Role of CD4 T cell help and costimulation in CD8 T cell responses during *Listeria monocytogenes* infection. J Immunol 2003;170:2053−63.

[213] Bourgeois C, Veiga-Fernandes H, Joret AM, Rocha B, Tanchot C. CD8 lethargy in the absence of CD4 help. Eur J Immunol 2002;32:2199−207.

[214] Bourgeois C, Tanchot C. Mini-review CD4 T cells are required for CD8 T cell memory generation. Eur J Immunol 2003;33:3225−31.

[215] Ogg GS, Jin X, Bonhoeffer S, Dunbar PR, Nowak MA, Monard S, et al. Quantitation of HIV-1-specific cytotoxic T lymphocytes and plasma load of viral RNA. Science 1998;279: 2103−6.

[216] Koup RA, Safrit JT, Cao Y, Andrews CA, McLeod G, Borkowsky W, et al. Temporal association of cellular immune responses with the initial control of viremia in primary human immunodeficiency virus type 1 syndrome. J Virol 1994;68:4650−5.

[217] Harrer T, Harrer E, Kalams SA, Barbosa P, Trocha A, Johnson RP, et al. Cytotoxic T lymphocytes in asymptomatic long-term nonprogressing HIV-1 infection. Breadth and specificity of the response and relation to *in vivo* viral quasispecies in a person with prolonged infection and low viral load. J Immunol 1996;156:2616−23.

[218] Harrer T, Harrer E, Kalams SA, Elbeik T, Staprans SI, Feinberg MB, et al. Strong cytotoxic T cell and weak neutralizing antibody responses in a subset of persons with stable nonprogressing HIV type 1 infection. AIDS Res Hum Retroviruses 1996;12:585−92.

[219] Kapustin SI, Popova TI, Lyschov AA, Togo AV, Abdulkadyrov KM, Blinov MN. HLA-DR2 frequency increase in severe aplastic anemia patients is mainly attributed to the prevalence of DR15 subtype. Pathol Oncol Res 1997;3:106−8.

[220] Prat E, Tomaru U, Sabater L, Park DM, Granger R, Kruse N, et al. HLA-DRB5*0101 and -DRB1*1501 expression in the multiple sclerosis-associated HLA-DR15 haplotype. J Neuroimmunol 2005;167:108−19.

[221] Kapitany A, Zilahi E, Szanto S, Szucs G, Szabo Z, Vegvari A, et al. Association of rheumatoid arthritis with HLA-DR1 and HLA-DR4 in Hungary. Ann NY Acad Sci 2005;1051:263−70.

[222] Zsilak S, Gal J, Hodinka L, Rajczy K, Balog A, Sipka S, et al. HLA-DR genotypes in familial rheumatoid arthritis: Increased frequency of protective and neutral alleles in a multicase family. J Rheumatol 2005;32:2299−302.

[223] Debaz H, Olivo A, Vazquez Garcia MN, de la Rosa G, Hernandez A, Lino L, et al. Relevant residues of DRbeta1 third hypervariable region contributing to the expression and to severity of rheumatoid arthritis (RA) in Mexicans. Hum Immunol 1998;59:287−94.

[224] Matsuki K, Grumet FC, Lin X, Gelb M, Guilleminault C, Dement WC, et al. DQ (rather than DR) gene marks susceptibility to narcolepsy. Lancet 1992;339:1052.

[225] Fogdell A, Hillert J, Sachs C, Olerup O. The multiple sclerosis- and narcolepsy-associated HLA class II haplotype includes the DRB5*0101 allele. Tissue Antigens 1995;46:333−6.

[226] Baisch JM, Weeks T, Giles R, Hoover M, Stastny P, Capra JD. Analysis of HLA-DQ genotypes and susceptibility in insulin-dependent diabetes mellitus. N Engl J Med 1990;322:1836−41.

[227] Todd JA, Bell JI, McDevitt HO. A molecular basis for genetic susceptibility to insulin-dependent diabetes mellitus. Trends Genet 1988;4:129−34.

[228] Yang S, Wang JY, Gao M, Liu HS, Sun LD, He PP, et al. Association of HLA-DQA1 and DQB1 genes with vitiligo in Chinese Hans. Int J Dermatol 2005;44:1022−7.

[229] Geng L, Wang Y, Zhai N, Lu YN, Song FJ, Chen HD. Association between pemphigus vulgaris and human leukocyte antigen in Han nation of northeast China. Chin Med Sci J 2005;20:166−70.

[230] Cinek O, Kolouskova S, Snajderova M, Sumnik Z, Sedlakova P, Drevinek P, et al. HLA class II genetic association of type 1 diabetes mellitus in Czech children. Pediatr Diabetes 2001;2:98−102.

[231] Bieniasz PD. Intrinsic immunity: A front-line defense against viral attack. Nat Immunol 2004;5:1109−15.

[232] Yap MW, Nisole S, Lynch C, Stoye JP. Trim5alpha protein restricts both HIV-1 and murine leukemia virus. Proc Natl Acad Sci USA 2004;101:10786−91.

[233] Perron MJ, Stremlau M, Song B, Ulm W, Mulligan RC, Sodroski J. TRIM5alpha mediates the postentry block to N-tropic murine leukemia viruses in human cells. Proc Natl Acad Sci USA 2004;101:11827−32.

[234] Lee K, KewalRamani VN. In defense of the cell: TRIM5alpha interception of mammalian retroviruses. Proc Natl Acad Sci USA 2004;101:10496−7.

[235] Sokolskaja E, Berthoux L, Luban J. Cyclophilin A and TRIM5alpha independently regulate human immunodeficiency virus type 1 infectivity in human cells. J Virol 2006;80:2855−62.

[236] van Manen D, Rits MA, Beugeling C, van Dort K, Schuitemaker H, Kootstra NA. The effect of Trim5 polymorphisms on the clinical course of HIV-1 infection. PLoS Pathog 2008;4:e18.

[237] Nakayama EE, Carpentier W, Costagliola D, Shioda T, Iwamoto A, Debre P, et al. Wild type and H43Y variant of human TRIM5alpha show similar anti-human immunodeficiency virus type 1 activity both *in vivo* and *in vitro*. Immunogenetics 2007;59:511−5.

[238] Stremlau M, Perron M, Lee M, Li Y, Song B, Javanbakht H, et al. Specific recognition and accelerated uncoating of retroviral capsids by the TRIM5alpha restriction factor. Proc Natl Acad Sci USA 2006;103:5514−9.

[239] Perez-Caballero D, Hatziioannou T, Yang A, Cowan S, Bieniasz PD. Human tripartite motif 5alpha domains responsible for retrovirus restriction activity and specificity. J Virol 2005;79:8969−78.

[240] Mische CC, Javanbakht H, Song B, Diaz-Griffero F, Stremlau M, Strack B, et al. Retroviral restriction factor TRIM5alpha is a trimer. J Virol 2005;79:14446−50.

[241] Javanbakht H, Diaz-Griffero F, Stremlau M, Si Z, Sodroski J. The contribution of RING and B-box 2 domains to retroviral restriction mediated by monkey TRIM5alpha. J Biol Chem 2005;280:26933−40.

[242] Li X, Sodroski J. The TRIM5alpha B-box 2 domain promotes cooperative binding to the retroviral capsid by mediating higher-order self-association. J Virol 2008;82:11495−502.

[243] Song B, Gold B, O'Huigin C, Javanbakht H, Li X, Stremlau M, et al. The B30.2(SPRY) domain of the retroviral restriction factor TRIM5alpha exhibits lineage-specific length and sequence variation in primates. J Virol 2005;79:6111−21.

[244] Taniguchi T, Ogasawara K, Takaoka A, Tanaka N. IRF family of transcription factors as regulators of host defense. Annu Rev Immunol 2001;19:623−55.

[245] Taki S, Sato T, Ogasawara K, Fukuda T, Sato M, Hida S, et al. Multistage regulation of Th1-type immune responses by the transcription factor IRF-1. Immunity 1997;6:673−9.

[246] Lohoff M, Ferrick D, Mittrucker HW, Duncan GS, Bischof S, Rollinghoff M, et al. Interferon regulatory factor-1 is required for a T helper 1 immune response *in vivo*. Immunity 1997;6:681−9.

[247] Battistini A, Marsili G, Sgarbanti M, Ensoli B, Hiscott J. IRF regulation of HIV-1 long terminal repeat activity. J Interferon Cytokine Res 2002;22:27−37.

[248] Marsili G, Borsetti A, Sgarbanti M, Remoli AL, Ridolfi B, Stellacci E, et al. On the role of interferon regulatory factors in HIV-1 replication. Ann NY Acad Sci 2003;1010:29−42.

[249] Ji H, Ball TB, Ao Z, Kimani J, Yao X, Plummer FA. Reduced HIV-1 long terminal repeat transcription in subjects with protective interferon regulatory factor-1 genotype: A potential mechanism mediating resistance to infection by HIV-1. Scand J Infect Dis 42:389−94.

[250] Bach MA, Phan-Dinh-Tuy F, Bach JF, Wallach D, Biddison WE, Sharrow SO, et al. Unusual phenotypes of human inducer T cells as measured by OKT4 and related monoclonal antibodies. J Immunol 1981;127:980−2.

[251] Lederman S, DeMartino JA, Daugherty BL, Foeldvari I, Yellin MJ, Cleary AM, et al. A single amino acid substitution in a common African allele of the CD4 molecule ablates binding of the monoclonal antibody, OKT4. Mol Immunol 1991;28:1171−81.

[252] Hodge TW, Sasso DR, McDougal JS. Humans with OKT4-epitope deficiency have a single nucleotide base change in the CD4 gene, resulting in substitution of TRP240 for ARG240. Hum Immunol 1991;30:99−104.

[253] Maddon PJ, Littman DR, Godfrey M, Maddon DE, Chess L, Axel R. The isolation and nucleotide sequence of a cDNA encoding the T cell surface protein T4: A new member of the immunoglobulin gene family. Cell 1985;42:93−104.

[254] Matthias LJ, Yam PT, Jiang XM, Vandegraaff N, Li P, Poumbourios P, et al. Disulfide exchange in domain 2 of CD4 is required for entry of HIV-1. Nat Immunol 2002;3:727−32.

[255] Fleury S, Lamarre D, Meloche S, Ryu SE, Cantin C, Hendrickson WA, et al. Mutational analysis of the interaction between CD4 and class II MHC: Class II antigens contact CD4 on a surface opposite the gp120-binding site. Cell 1991;66:1037−49.

[256] Fuller TC, Trevithick JE, Fuller AA, Colvin RB, Cosimi AB, Kung PC. Antigenic polymorphism of the T4 differentiation antigen expressed on human T helper/inducer lymphocytes. Hum Immunol 1984;9:89−102.

[257] Oyugi J, Vouriot FCM, Alimonti J, Stephen Wayne S, Luo M, Land AM, et al. A common CD4 gene variant is associated with increased risk of HIV-1 infection in Kenyan female sex workers. J Infect Dis 2009;199:1327−34.

[258] Kitano H. Systems biology: A brief overview. Science 2002;295:1662−4.

[259] Songok EM, Osero B, McKinnon L, Rono MK, Apidi W, Matey EJ, et al. CD26/dipeptidyl peptidase IV (CD26/DPPIV) is highly expressed in peripheral blood of HIV-1 exposed uninfected female sex workers. Virol J 7:343.

[260] Burgener A, Boutilier J, Wachihi C, Kimani J, Carpenter M, Westmacott G, et al. Identification of differentially expressed proteins in the cervical mucosa of HIV-1-resistant sex workers. J Proteome Res 2008;7:4446−54.

[261] Boonacker E, Van Noorden CJ. The multifunctional or moonlighting protein CD26/DPPIV. Eur J Cell Biol 2003;82:53−73.

[262] Gorrell MD. Dipeptidyl peptidase IV and related enzymes in cell biology and liver disorders. Clin Sci (Lond) 2005;108:277−92.

[263] Ohtsuki T, Tsuda H, Morimoto C. Good or evil: CD26 and HIV infection. J Dermatol Sci 2000;22:152−60.

[264] Ohtsuki T, Hosono O, Kobayashi H, Munakata Y, Souta A, Shioda T, et al. Negative regulation of the anti-human immunodeficiency virus and chemotactic activity of human stromal cell-derived factor 1alpha by CD26/dipeptidyl peptidase IV. FEBS Lett 1998;431:236−40.

[265] Proost P, Menten P, Struyf S, Schutyser E, De Meester I, Van Damme J. Cleavage by CD26/dipeptidyl peptidase IV converts the chemokine LD78beta into a most efficient monocyte attractant and CCR1 agonist. Blood 2000;96:1674−80.

[266] De Meester I, Korom S, Van Damme J, Scharpe S. CD26, let it cut or cut it down. Immunol Today 1999;20:367−75.

[267] Schols D, Proost P, Struyf S, Wuyts A, De Meester I, Scharpe S, et al. CD26-processed RANTES(3-68), but not intact RANTES, has potent anti-HIV-1 activity. Antiviral Res 1998;39:175−87.

Chapter 7

The Immune System and Resisting HIV Infection

Keith R. Fowke [1,2], Catherine M. Card [1] and Rupert Kaul [3]

[1] *Laboratory of Viral Immunology, Department of Medical Microbiology, University of Manitoba, Winnipeg, Manitoba, Canada,* [2] *Department of Community Health Sciences, University of Manitoba, Winnipeg, Manitoba, Canada,* [3] *Departments of Medicine and Immunology, University of Toronto, Toronto, Canada*

INTRODUCTION

The challenges of HIV vaccine and microbicide design have led to a renewed emphasis on elucidating the natural correlates of protection to HIV. The phenomenon of resistance to HIV infection, observed in multiple cohorts of HIV-exposed seronegative (HESN) individuals, provides a unique opportunity to study the factors that mediate protection against HIV infection. As described here and in other chapters, multiple genetic and immune factors have been associated with HIV resistance. This chapter will focus on some of the major immune mechanisms that correlate with resistance against HIV infection.

CELL-MEDIATED IMMUNITY

Multiple lines of evidence suggest that HIV-specific T cell responses correlate with resistance against HIV infection. Peripheral and mucosal

Models of Protection Against HIV/SIV. DOI: 10.1016/B978-0-12-387715-4.00007-1

HIV-specific T cell responses have been detected in numerous cases of HESN individuals, including commercial sex workers (CSW) [1−15], men who have sex with men (MSM) [16−19], discordant couples [17,18,20−36], occupationally exposed healthcare workers [17,37−39], intravenous drug users [18,40] and perinatally exposed infants [41−48]. In addition, molecular epidemiological studies have demonstrated a strong association between resistance to HIV infection and certain HLA class I and class II alleles [49−55], which function to present antigen to cognate T cells, stimulating a T cell response. The notion that the T cell responses elicited by these "protective" HLA molecules may mediate resistance to infection has been explored in studies examining the specificity of the epitopes targeted by HIV-specific T cells and the functional nature of the T cell response. Both CD4+ T helper (Th) and CD8+ cytotoxic T lymphocyte (CTL) responses have been linked with resistance to HIV infection in HESNs.

CD4+ T Cells

HIV-specific CD4+ T cell responses in the absence of HIV seropositivity were first described in HIV-exposed uninfected MSM [16] whose peripheral blood mononuclear cells (PBMCs) produced IL-2 in response to stimulation with HIV envelope peptides. This observation was subsequently confirmed in independent cohorts of HESNs [5,22,38], and was expanded to demonstrate HIV-specific proliferation [12,21,23,29,36] and IFNγ production [12,30,35] by CD4+ T cells directed against multiple HIV proteins. Similarly, HIV envelope-specific production of IL-2 has been observed in CD4+ T cells from cord blood in uninfected children born to HIV-infected mothers [42] and in peripheral blood of occupationally exposed healthcare workers [37,39], demonstrating that such responses could be mounted in the absence of repeated exposure or productive infection. However, these responses waned over time, consistent with studies indicating that HIV-specific CD4+ T cell responses in HESNs are related to the frequency of exposure to HIV [10,33].

CD8+ T Cells

HIV-specific CTLs in the absence of an antibody response were first described in HIV-exposed uninfected infants [41,43,44]. The responses detected in these infants varied in their duration but eventually waned, consistent with evidence of a requirement for persistent exposure in maintenance of memory CTL responses in HESNs [8−11,33,56]. Early studies characterized HIV-specific CTLs from HESNs capable of lyzing target cells expressing multiple HIV proteins [1,2,5,17,23,25,38,39,41,43−45], and identified elevated precursor frequency of HIV-specific CTLs as a correlate of protection in HESNs relative to low-risk controls [20,23], indicating that the potential to protect against subsequent exposure to HIV exists.

Quality of Response

The majority of early studies in HESNs sought to determine whether these individuals were able to mount HIV-specific T cell responses. As described above, HIV-specific CD4+ and CD8+ T cells were detectable in numerous examples of HESNs. However, not all HIV-specific T cell responses are necessarily associated with protection against infection. Indeed, there are multiple examples of seroconversion in the presence of natural [8,9,11,14] or vaccine-induced HIV-specific T cell responses [57]. Likewise, the majority of HIV-infected individuals mount HIV-specific T cell responses that are insufficient to control virus replication and prevent disease progression. Models of protective responses in HIV-infected individuals suggest that the quality of the HIV-specific T cell responses is important in differentiating protective responses from non-protective responses [58].

The qualitative nature of HIV-specific T cell responses has been investigated in order to determine the drivers of protection. Investigation of the relative contribution of CD4+ T cell subsets to the HIV-specific response demonstrated that Env-stimulated PBMCs from uninfected partners in serodiscordant relationships produced more IL-2 and less IL-10 than those from HIV-infected partners, suggesting qualitative differences in HIV-specific responses in HESNs [22]. Consistent with these observations, a comparison of HIV-specific CD4+ T cell responses between HESNs and HIV-infected CSW from the Pumwani cohort revealed that HESNs tended to mount much stronger proliferation responses to HIV gag p24 peptides than HIV-infected women, whereas the magnitude of IFNγ responses to the same peptides were comparable between the two groups [12]. HIV-specific proliferation was later shown to be associated with reduced subsequent HIV acquisition in HESNs, providing further evidence that proliferation may be a qualitative indicator of protective responses [14].

Initial studies of HIV-specific CTLs demonstrated that these cells were capable of cytotoxic lysis of infected target cells [1,2,5,17,23,25,38,39,41, 43−45]. Production of perforin and granzyme B by HIV-specific CTL supports a role for cytotoxic killing of infected cells in HESNs [33]. CD8+ T cells from HESNs may also be able to suppress HIV replication in a non-cytotoxic manner [24,26,27,29,46]. Consistent with a role for a non-cytotoxic CTL response to HIV in HESNs, multiple studies have identified HIV-specific CTLs producing antiviral cytokines such as IFNγ [2,6−8,13,18,28−31,35,40,59] and β-chemokines such as MIP-1α, MIP-1β and RANTES [26,29,34,35]. HIV-specific CD4+ T cells from HESNs have also been shown to produce β-chemokines [21,34], which associate with suppression of HIV replication *in vitro* [21]. In this context, β-chemokine production by HIV-specific T cells may directly inhibit HIV infection through competitive binding to the HIV coreceptor CCR5.

HIV-specific CD8+ [19,34,35,47,60] and CD4+ [34] T cells co-producing multiple cytokines have also been identified in HESNs, suggesting poly-functionality of HIV-specific T cells may be protective. These results parallel studies implicating polyfunctional HIV-specific CTLs in the control of virus replication in HIV-infected subjects [58], but further studies are needed to determine if polyfunctional T cells provide similar protection against infection as they do against disease progression.

Differential CD8+ Epitope Specificity in HESNs

The phenomena of both relative HIV resistance (RHR) and long-term HIV non-progressive infection (LTNP) have been associated with specific class I HLA alleles, although these associations are much better defined in the latter context. For instance, LTNP has been consistently and strongly associated with the alleles HLA-B*27, B*5701 and B*5703 [61]; RHR has been associated with A11 and B57 in some studies [62,63]. Host CD8+ T cell responses are directed against epitope peptides 8−10 amino acids long, derived from newly transcribed cellular proteins [64]. Since these epitopes are presented to host CD8+ T cells in conjunction with class I HLA molecules, this implies that CD8+ T cell responses might play a role in both RHR and LTNP. In keeping with this, the presence of HIV-specific CD8+ T cell responses has been described in many studies of HESN individuals [1,2,5−8,11,13−15,18−20,23,25−28,33,35,38−40,43,48,59,63], although some studies have not found them [65,66], or have found them at a very low frequency [67,68]. Furthermore, the association of LTNP and RHR with specific HLA alleles suggests that these alleles may restrict CD8+ T cell responses that target specific protective epitopes—a concept with clear relevance for the HIV vaccine field.

The concept of differential epitope recognition and HIV protection is borne out by studies in LTNP individuals, especially those carrying the B*27 allele. These individuals consistently demonstrate delayed disease progression, and this protection is clearly linked to B*27-restricted CD8+ T cell responses directed against the KK10 epitope located at amino acids 263−272 within HIV-1 p24 Gag. Although mutational escape at this epitope requires a complex series of sequential mutations in order to maintain viral fitness, eventual escape is the rule and is associated with subsequent disease progression [69]; if a virus containing this escape mutation is transmitted to a second individual carrying the B*27 allele, no B*27-mediated disease amelioration is seen [70,71]. The concept of differential "protective" epitope recognition is also supported by the observation that protective class I MHC alleles in HIV-infected humans and SIV-infected macaques tend to focus on homologous conserved areas of the retroviral genome [72].

Although epitope specificity of the host CD8+ T cell response is clearly important in the maintenance of a LTNP phenotype, its importance is less clear in the RHR context. CD8+ T cell responses in RHR—when they are detected—are generally low frequency and often intermittent [8,18], making formal epitope mapping difficult, albeit not impossible [19]. Despite this, it has been described that RHR individuals are less likely to respond to HIV Env-derived epitopes than are HIV-infected individuals [31]. Furthermore, when responses were screened against a panel of 54 epitopes restricted by common class I HLA alleles within the Nairobi Pumwani RHR cohort, there was evidence of differential epitope targeting by HIV-infected and RHR individuals sharing the same class I HLA allele [7]. For instance, HLA A*0201+ RHR individuals were much more likely to recognize the Pol epitope IV9, while infected individuals generally targeted the immunodominant p17 Gag epitope SL9; a similar pattern of differential epitope recognition was seen in a European cohort of HESN individuals, where IV9 recognition was confirmed using class I HLA peptide tetramers [59]. Interestingly, when late HIV sero-conversion was observed in initially "resistant" female sex workers, epitope "switching" generally occurred from IV9 to SL9 [7].

Overall, mapping of CD8+ T cell responses to the epitope level has rarely been done in the HESN context. When it has, or when responses have been screened to a panel of predefined epitopes, there is a suggestion that different epitopes and HIV genes may be targeted compared to HIV-infected individuals. However, the reasons for and implications of this observation are not at all clear. Targeting of epitopes that are derived from genes other than *env* has been associated with improved host HIV immune control in some studies of HIV-infected individuals [73] but not in others [74]. Certainly this region of the virus is more variable than others, but many HESN studies have found frequent Env-specific responses in HESN individuals. The Pol IV9 epitope, and others preferentially recognized by HESNs in one study, are not more conserved than those recognized in HIV-infected participants; furthermore, there was little evidence that pre-existing CD8+ responses placed any evolutionary pressure on viruses responsible for subsequent infection, which generally contained wild-type epitope and flanking sequences [8]. Therefore, the impact of differential HESN epitope recognition on selection of epitopes for HIV vaccines remains unclear.

HIV-Specific Responses in HESNs—Phenotype or Artifact?

It is important to step back and consider whether the HIV-specific CD8+ T cell responses that have been described in HESN individuals are real or simply a lab artifact. Methodological weaknesses are certainly apparent in the studies that have described these responses. These studies are often cross-sectional in nature, with a relatively small number of participants, and control (putatively "unexposed") groups are lacking or may be poorly described. The responses are low level and often intermittent, which means that responses may not be confirmed in the same individual at a later time point, and confirmation using alternative immunological techniques is often not performed. Perhaps most important, assays have frequently not been performed by blinded researchers; given the low frequency of the CD8+ T cell responses and the sometimes subjective nature of defining a positive response (for instance, defining a "spot" in the IFNg ELISPOT assay), this could introduce bias.

Nonetheless, several factors suggest that these HESN CD8+ T cell responses are real. While not definitive proof, the sheer number of studies that have observed these responses in HESN individuals [1,2,5−8,11,13−15, 18−20,23,25−28,33,35,38−40,43,48,59,63] suggests that the phenomenon must have some validity. Furthermore, a variety of techniques have been used to demonstrate CD8+ T cell responses in these studies, including the interferon gamma ELISPOT [2,6−8,14,18,28,40,48,59,63], target lysis with ^{51}Cr release [1,5,11,20,25, 38, 39, 43, 63], class I HLA tetramers [59], intracellular cytokine staining [13,15,19,33,35], production of the cellular antiviral factor [27] and T cell proliferation [14]. In some cases CD8+ T cell responses have been confirmed by multiple techniques, and even mapped to the epitope level [19,59].

While many of the studies are cross-sectional, the presence of HESN CD8+ responses against HIV has been associated with reduced HIV acquisition in several prospective studies [11,14,40,48]; in these studies the baseline assays were generally performed by investigators prior to or blinded to the subsequent HIV acquisition event, using predefined assay protocols. In an additional study of HESN women who went on to acquire HIV at a later date, the presence of HIV-specific CD8+ T cell responses prior to acquisition was associated with a reduced HIV viral load and enhanced HIV-specific CD8+ T cell proliferation after infection [15]. The fact that these studies were blinded and prospective provides strong protection against possible investigator bias, and demonstrates that HESN HIV-specific CD8+ T cell responses are likely to be a real phenomenon.

Marker of Exposure or Protective Mechanism?

Although the prospective, blinded studies described above provide the strongest evidence that HIV-specific CD8+ T cell responses in HESN individuals are real, they do not prove that these CD8+ responses are actually protecting individuals against HIV acquisition. As always in observational studies, the direction of causation cannot be determined: two possible models apply. In the first model, the priming of HIV-specific T cell responses—perhaps by exposure to a low dose of HIV that caused a mucosal focus of infection but was insufficient to expand and cause systemic infection, or by exposure to replication-incompetent virus—provides some protection against HIV in the context of subsequent exposures, albeit not complete protection [8]. The fact that HESN responses tend to be enhanced in the genital mucosa compared to HIV-infected individuals [6] supports this hypothesis, although if the CD8+ T cell responses are truly protective then it is not clear why later infection would occur in the absence of any viral escape from the pre-existing CTL responses [8].

An alternative explanation for the phenomenon is that exposure to HIV in the absence of infection induces low-level HIV-specific CD8+ T cell responses that are not protective, but are simply a marker for non-productive HIV exposure. These exposed individuals might have been protected against HIV infection by another mechanism, such as a genetic polymorphism [75−77], mucosal antibody [14,22,78,79] or enhanced innate immune function [80]; if this were the case, then individuals with an HIV-specific CD8+ T cell response would demonstrate a reduced HIV incidence when followed prospectively. In addition, if the same protective mechanism modulated HIV immunopathogenesis after subsequent infection, then these individuals might manifest an altered viral load and/or HIV-specific immune response. Alternatively, since approximately 999/1000 (99.9%) of sexual exposures to HIV do not result in HIV infection, individuals with an exposure-induced HIV-specific CD8+ T cell response may not be protected against HIV at all, and in this case their subsequent risk of HIV acquisition would be the same as individuals without CD8+ responses.

In all three of these scenarios one might expect to see "boosting" of virus-specific CD8+ T cell responses after a recent HIV exposure, whether that exposure is sexual or parenteral, and that is what has been described by several investigators [8,38,59]. However, prospective studies have shown a reduced HIV incidence in participants with a virus-specific CD8+ T cell response [11,14,40], as well as enhanced HIV host immune control in those who do acquire HIV [15]. This suggests either that these responses themselves are protective, or at least that they are markers of exposure while HIV protection is being mediated through an alternate mechanism. Small studies have not been powered to examine the protective role of CD8+ T cell responses after controlling for behavioral covariates and other potential protective immune factors, but the largest prospective study performed to date found that both HIV-specific CD8+ T cell proliferation and mucosal HIV-neutralizing IgA were independently associated with HIV non-acquisition [14]. While this is the strongest evidence to date that CD8+ T cell responses are causally linked to HIV protection, even here the observational nature of the study means that confounding (by other unknown protective immune responses, for instance) cannot be completely ruled out.

INNATE IMMUNITY IN HESN INDIVIDUALS

In addition to the potential contribution of adaptive immune mechanisms to resistance against infection, described above, innate immunity is also likely to confer protection against HIV in HESNs. The innate immune system consists of a complex network of anatomical barriers, soluble factors and innate immune cells that coordinate to fight infection at the earliest stages following exposure. These mechanisms are likely to be particularly important upon primary exposure to the virus, before adaptive responses have developed. Infection upon subsequent exposure to HIV may also be limited by innate immune responses, which may block tissue infiltration entirely or attenuate cellular infection until adaptive HIV-specific T cells can target low-level infection [81,82]. Some of these mechanisms will be discussed in detail in Chapter 5. However, a brief discussion of evidence supporting a role for natural killer cells in resistance to infection will be presented here.

Natural Killer Cells

Accumulating genetic and functional evidence supports a role for natural killer (NK) cells in resistance to HIV infection. NK cells represent the first line of defense against virally infected cells. Their function is modulated by the combined signals of inhibitory and activating NK cell receptors on the cell surface. Of particular interest, killer immunoglobulin-like receptors (KIRs) are highly polymorphic and bind to HLA class I molecules. The expression of particular KIR/HLA-B combinations has been associated with varying outcomes of HIV disease [83], as well as resistance to HIV infection [80,84,85]. In particular, the activating receptor KIR3DS1 has been associated with HIV-exposed seronegativity [84,85], suggesting activated NK cells may be involved in resisting infection.

Functional studies support a role for activated NK cells in resistance to HIV infection. NK cells from HESN injection drug users (IDUs) have been shown to exhibit elevated NK cytotoxic activity [86] and antiviral cytokine production [86,87]. Phenotypic analyses demonstrate that NK cells from HESNs tend to have an activated phenotype, as demonstrated by elevated expression of CD69 [88,89] and reduced expression of inhibitory receptors [88,90], and exhibit high degranulation activity, as indicated by expression of CD107a [88–90]. Collectively, these studies support a role for enhanced NK activity in protection against HIV infection.

IMMUNE QUIESCENCE OR IMMUNE ACTIVATION?

As described in other sections, resistance to HIV infection is associated with multiple genetic and immune factors, both innate and adaptive. However, none of the correlates of protection described account for all cases of HIV-exposed seronegativity. HIV preferentially establishes productive infection in activated T cells due to its dependency on host proteins for viral entry and replication [91,92]. Indeed, multiple genome-wide siRNA screens identified a wide array of host dependency factors required for efficient HIV replication [93–95], which are primarily expressed in activated cells. It is therefore reasonable to hypothesize that low levels of T cell activation may protect against infection by limiting substrates available for HIV replication and reducing the pool of target cells available for infection. Consistent with this hypothesis, monkey studies have demonstrated that limiting inflammation at the site of SIV exposure can reduce infiltration of activated target cells and prevent infection [96]. The role of immune activation in resistance and susceptibility to HIV infection in HESNs is therefore a relevant avenue of investigation.

Systems biology approaches provide the opportunity to study immune function using an unbiased approach, identifying new candidate mechanisms of protection against HIV. These approaches were employed to investigate potential mechanisms of resistance to infection in the Pumwani CSW cohort. Interrogation of gene expression using microarray technology showed that unstimulated CD4+ T cells from HESNs have a characteristically lower level of generalized gene expression than controls, suggesting a resting or quiescent cellular state. Further analysis revealed that genes involved in T cell receptor signaling and host factors required for HIV replication were among the genes expressed at lower levels in HESNs [97]. Consistent with these observations of low activation, unstimulated cells from HESNs produced lower levels of multiple cytokines *ex vivo* than controls. However, the production of cytokines in response to stimulation with a mitogen or recall antigen was comparable between HESNs and controls, indicating that HESNs are not immunosuppressed, but demonstrate a lower level of cellular activation than controls at baseline. This phenotype has been termed "immune quiescence" [97].

Additional studies from the Pumwani CSW cohort also provide evidence for immune quiescence as a mechanism of resistance to HIV infection. Phenotyping analyses revealed that HESNs have lower frequencies of activated CD4+ and CD8+ T cells relative to controls, as demonstrated by CD69 expression. This was associated with elevated frequencies of regulatory T cells, which function to moderate levels of activation and may be one driver of immune quiescence [98]. An additional potential driver of the quiescent phenotype was described in a proteomic screen of cervicovaginal lavage samples, which identified over-expression of anti-proteases from the serpin B family in HESNs. Serpins have anti-inflammatory activity, and their presence in the mucosa may serve to limit inflammation [99].

Evidence for immune quiescence is not limited to HESNs from the Pumwani CSW cohort. Independent studies of uninfected hemophiliacs who were exposed to HIV-contaminated blood products and of high-risk MSM both found less spontaneous or mitogen-induced lymphoproliferation in HESNs compared to healthy controls [100,101]. In addition to low lymphoproliferative responses, the study of high-risk MSM also identified low frequencies of CD4+ and CD8+ T cells expressing activation markers HLA-DR, CD38, CD70 and Ki67 to associate with resistance to infection in HESNs [101]. Consistent with these data, analysis of T cell activation in discordant couples from the Central African Republic found reduced expression of HLA DR and CCR5 on CD4+ T cells in HESNs [102]. Accordingly, unstimulated PBMCs from HESNs were found to have reduced susceptibility to *in vitro* HIV infection, an effect that disappeared when the PBMCs were stimulated with mitogen prior to infection. These results indicate that differences in cellular susceptibility to infection that exist due to varying levels of activation may be masked by assays that measure infectibility following polyclonal activation with a mitogen [102]. Additional evidence for immune quiescence is provided by the finding that expression of CD69 and pro-inflammatory cytokines and chemokines by allostimulated lymphocytes was lower in HESN CSW from Abidjan, Côte d'Ivoire compared to controls. Interestingly, the suppressed allostimulated response was found to associate with higher levels of unprotected sex [103], suggesting that frequent sexual exposure to multiple partners may induce regulation of inflammation in HESNs. Lower baseline activation was shown in uninfected partners of discordant couples from Senegal, who expressed lower levels of CD38 on CD4+ T cells, though differences in immune activation may have been attributed to concurrent differences in the use of condoms in this study [104], underscoring the need to investigate differences in sexual behavior characteristics when analyzing potential correlates of protection.

In contrast to reports suggesting that immune quiescence is associated with protection, some conflicting studies actually identify elevated immune activation as a correlate of resistance to HIV infection. Elevated levels of T cell activation [30,35,105] and pro-inflammatory cytokine production [106] have been found in multiple cohorts of HESNs. In some reports, differences in mucosal, but not systemic, immune activation characterized HESNs [30,106], emphasizing the need to confirm potential correlates of protection at the site of HIV exposure. Increased responsiveness to Toll-like receptor agonists among HESN subjects has also been observed, perhaps suggesting hypersensitivity of the innate arm of the immune system in HESNs [107]. The conflicting data from the above studies may be reconciled by differences in the site and/or intensity of HIV exposure, exposure to other immunogenic factors, and differences in assays used to characterize immune activation. It may also be possible that these states are not incompatible. A hypersensitive innate system that quickly activates but then just as quickly returns to baseline has been observed for the immune regulating molecule IRF-1 in the Pumwani cohort [108]. It may be possible that an innate system with rapid on/off kinetics minimizes the duration of inflammation, thereby limiting immune activation leading to an immune quiescent phenotype as observed in T cells. Future studies should aim to address these discrepancies and confirm potential correlates of protection in independent cohorts.

CONCLUSION

Since the phenomenon of relative HIV resistance was first identified, efforts have focused on identifying correlates of immune protection against infection. The correlates discussed here are summarized in Table 7.1. HIV-specific T cell

TABLE 7.1 Summary of putative immune mechanisms of resistance to HIV infection identified in HESNs

Putative mechanism	References
Cell-mediated immunity	
HIV-specific CD8+ T cells	
Target cell cytolysis	1, 2, 5, 17, 23, 25, 38, 39, 41, 43–45
Production of perforin and granzyme B	33
Non-cytotoxic CTL activity	24, 26, 27, 29, 46
Production of IFNγ	2, 6–8, 13, 18, 28–31, 35, 40, 59
Production of β-chemokines	26, 29, 34, 35
Differential quality of response	14, 19, 34, 35, 47, 60
Differential epitope specificity	7, 59
Associations with HLA class I alleles	49–53, 62, 63
HIV-specific CD4+ T cells	
Production of IL-2	5, 16, 22, 37–39, 42
Production of IFNγ	12, 30, 35
Proliferation	12, 21, 23, 29, 36
Production of β-chemokines	21, 26, 29, 34, 35
Associations with HLA class II alleles	49, 52, 54, 55
Differential quality of response	12, 14, 22, 34
Innate immunity	
NK cells	
Associations with KIR alleles	80, 84, 85
Elevated cytotoxicity	86
Elevated antiviral cytokine production	86, 87
Elevated activation and degranulation	88–90
Elevated Toll-like receptor responsiveness	107
Immune quiescence	
Low level of gene expression in CD4+ T cells	97
Under-expression of genes involved in T cell activation and HIV replication	97

Continued

TABLE 7.1 Summary of putative immune mechanisms of resistance to HIV infection identified in HESNs—cont'd

Putative mechanism	References
Low levels of cytokine expression at baseline or following stimulation	97, 103
Reduced frequencies of activated T cells	98, 101–104
Elevated frequencies of regulatory T cells	98
Elevated mucosal expression of anti-inflammatory serpins	99
Reduced spontaneous or antigen-induced lymphoproliferation	100, 101
Reduced susceptibility of unstimulated cells to in vitro HIV-1 infection	102
Differential kinetics of IRF-1	108

responses have been identified in numerous cohorts and have been correlated with reduced subsequent HIV acquisition, supporting the hypothesis that adaptive immunity plays a role in protection. While some studies have addressed the quality and epitope-specificity of HIV-specific T cell responses in HESNs, further work is needed to differentiate "protective" T cell responses from those that do not provide protection.

In addition to adaptive immunity, there is accumulating evidence that innate immunity plays a role in resistance to HIV infection. Differential NK cell activation and Toll-like receptor responsiveness in HESNs suggests robust innate defenses against HIV. However, low levels of immune activation have also been observed in multiple cohorts of HESNs, suggesting a role for immune quiescence in resistance to infection. It is an intriguing hypothesis that HESNs resist infection by limiting the pool of activated target cells, thereby limiting substrates available for HIV replication.

No single factor appears to account for all cases of resistance to HIV infection. It is likely that the adaptive immune system works in conjunction with innate defenses. However, simultaneous assessment of multiple potential correlates of protection has often been precluded by limited sample material, but with the rapid advancement of technology and systems biology techniques we may be able to address these questions in the future. In addition, an important direction of research in the field will be to confirm putative correlates of resistance in independent cohorts of HESNs. More prospective studies are also needed to address causality, as the majority of studies to date have been cross-sectional in design.

We know that resistance to HIV infection is complex, as is the virus itself. Thus, our approach to vaccine and microbicide design may need to adjust accordingly to incorporate new methods of immunomodulation. By elucidating the correlates of protection against infection in HESNs, we can educate the design of vaccines and microbicides to mimic protection in nature.

REFERENCES

[1] Rowland-Jones S, Sutton J, Ariyoshi K, Dong T, Gotch F, McAdam S, et al. HIV-specific cytotoxic T-cells in HIV-exposed but uninfected Gambian women. Nat Med 1995;1:59−64.

[2] Rowland-Jones SL, Dong T, Fowke KR, Kimani J, Krausa P, Newell H, et al. Cytotoxic T cell responses to multiple conserved HIV epitopes in HIV-resistant prostitutes in Nairobi. J Clin Invest 1998;102:1758−65.

[3] Plummer FA, Blake Ball T, Kimania J, Fowke KR. Resistance to HIV-1 infection among highly exposed sex workers in Nairobi: What mediates protection and why does it develop? Immunol Lett 1999;66:27−34.

[4] Rowland-Jones SL, Dong T, Dorrell L, Ogg G, Hansasuta P, Krausa P, et al. Broadly cross-reactive HIV-specific cytotoxic T-lymphocytes in highly-exposed persistently seronegative donors. Immunol Lett 1999;66:9−14.

[5] Fowke KR, Nagelkerke NJ, Kimani J, Simonsen JN, Anzala AO, Bwayo JJ, et al. HIV-1-specific cellular immune responses among HIV-1-resistant sex workers. Immunol Cell Biol 2000;78:586−95.

[6] Kaul R, Plummer FA, Kimani J, Dong T, Kiama P, Rostron T, et al. HIV-1-specific mucosal CD8+ lymphocyte responses in the cervix of HIV-1-resistant prostitutes in Nairobi. J Immunology 2000;164:1602−11.

[7] Kaul R, Dong T, Plummer FA, Kimani J, Rostron T, Kiama P, et al. CD8(+) lymphocytes respond to different HIV epitopes in seronegative and infected subjects. J Clin Invest 2001;107:1303−10.

[8] Kaul R, Rowland-Jones SL, Kimani J, Dong T, Yang HB, Kiama P, et al. Late seroconversion in HIV-resistant Nairobi prostitutes despite pre-existing HIV-specific CD8+ responses. J Clin Invest 2001;107:341−9.

[9] Kaul R, Rowland-Jones SL, Kimani J, Fowke K, Dong T, Kiama P, et al. New insights into HIV-1 specific cytotoxic T-lymphocyte responses in exposed, persistently seronegative Kenyan sex workers. Immunol Lett 2001;79:3−13.

[10] Jennes W, Vuylsteke B, Borget M-Y, Traore-Ettiegne V, Maurice C, Nolan M, et al. HIV-specific T helper responses and frequency of exposure among HIV-exposed seronegative female sex workers in Abidjan, Cote d'Ivoire. J Infect Dis 2004;189:602−10.

[11] Kaul R, Rutherford J, Rowland-Jones SL, Kimani J, Onyango JI, Fowke K, et al. HIV-1 Env-specific cytotoxic T-lymphocyte responses in exposed, uninfected Kenyan sex workers: A prospective analysis. AIDS 2004;18:2087−9.

[12] Alimonti JB, Koesters SA, Kimani J, Matu L, Wachihi C, Plummer FA, et al. CD4+ T cell responses in HIV-exposed seronegative women are qualitatively distinct from those in HIV-infected women. J Infect Dis 2005;191:20−4.

[13] Alimonti JB, Kimani J, Matu L, Wachihi C, Kaul R, Plummer FA, et al. Characterization of CD8 T-cell responses in HIV-1-exposed seronegative commercial sex workers from Nairobi, Kenya. Immunol Cell Biol 2006;84:482−5.

[14] Hirbod T, Kaul R, Reichard C, Kimani J, Ngugi E, Bwayo JJ, et al. HIV-neutralizing immunoglobulin A and HIV-specific proliferation are independently associated with reduced HIV acquisition in Kenyan sex workers. AIDS 2008;22:727−35.

[15] Kaul R, MacDonald KS, Nagelkerke NJ, Kimani J, Fowke K, Ball TB, et al. HIV viral set point and host immune control in individuals with HIV-specific CD8+ T-cell responses prior to HIV acquisition. AIDS 2010;24:1449−54.

[16] Clerici M, Giorgi JV, Chou CC, Gudeman VK, Zack JA, Gupta P, et al. Cell-mediated immune response to human immunodeficiency virus (HIV) type 1 in seronegative homosexual men with recent sexual exposure to HIV-1. J Infect Dis 1992;165: 1012−9.

[17] Bernard NF, Yannakis CM, Lee JS, Tsoukas CM. Human immunodeficiency virus (HIV)-specific cytotoxic T lymphocyte activity in HIV-exposed seronegative persons. J Infect Dis 1999;179:538−47.

[18] Makedonas G, Bruneau J, Alary M, Tsoukas CM, Lowndes CM, Lamothe F, et al. Comparison of HIV-specific CD8 T-cell responses among uninfected individuals exposed to HIV parenterally and mucosally. AIDS 2005;19:251−9.

[19] Erickson AL, Willberg CB, McMahan V, Liu A, Buchbinder SP, Grohskopf LA, et al. Potentially exposed but uninfected individuals produce cytotoxic and polyfunctional human immunodeficiency virus type 1-specific CD8+ T-cell responses which can be defined to the epitope level. Clin Vacc Immunol 2008;15:1745−8.

[20] Langlade-Demoyen P, Ngo-Giang-Huong N, Ferchal F, Oksenhendler E. Human immuno-deficiency virus (HIV) nef-specific cytotoxic T lymphocytes in noninfected heterosexual contact of HIV-infected patients. J Clin Invest 1994;93:1293−7.

[21] Furci L, Scarlatti G, Burastero S, Tambussi G, Colognesi C, Quillent C, et al. Antigen-driven C-C chemokine-mediated HIV-1 suppression by CD4(+) T cells from exposed uninfected individuals expressing the wild-type CCR-5 allele. J Exp Med 1997;186:455−60.

[22] Mazzoli S, Trabattoni D, Lo Caputo S, Piconi S, Blé C, Meacci F, et al. HIV-specific mucosal and cellular immunity in HIV-seronegative partners of HIV-seropositive individuals. Nat Med 1997;3:1250−7.

[23] Goh W, Markee J, Akridge R, Meldorf M, Musey L, Karchmer T, et al. Protection against human immunodeficiency virus type 1 infection in persons with repeated exposure: Evidence for T cell immunity in the absence of inherited CCR5. J Infect Dis 1999;179: 548−547.

[24] Stranford SA, Skurnick J, Louria D, Osmond D, Chang SY, Sninsky J, et al. Lack of infection in HIV-exposed individuals is associated with a strong CD8(+) cell noncytotoxic anti-HIV response. Proc Natl Acad Sci USA 1999;96:1030−5.

[25] Bienzle D, MacDonald KS, Smaill FM, Kovacs C, Baqi M, Courssaris B, et al. Factors contributing to the lack of human immunodeficiency virus type 1 (HIV-1) transmission in HIV-1-discordant partners. J Infect Dis 2000;182:123−32.

[26] Nicastri E, Ercoli L, Sarmati L, d'Ettorre G, Iudicone P, Massetti P, et al. Human immu-nodeficiency virus-1 specific and natural cellular immunity in HIV seronegative subjects with multiple sexual exposures to virus. J Med Virol 2001;64:232−7.

[27] Furci L, Lopalco L, Loverro P, Sinnone M, Tambussi G, Lazzarin A, et al. Non-cytotoxic inhibition of HIV-1 infection by unstimulated CD8+ T lymphocytes from HIV-exposed-uninfected individuals. AIDS 2002;16:1003−8.

[28] Shacklett BL, Means RE, Larsson M, Wilkens DT, Beadle TJ, Merritt MJ, et al. Dendritic cell amplification of HIV type 1-specific CD8+ T cell responses in exposed, seronegative heterosexual women. AIDS Res Hum Retroviruses 2002;18:805−15.

[29] Skurnick JH, Palumbo P, Devico AL, Shacklett BL, Valentine FT, Merges M, et al. Correlates of nontransmission in US women at high risk of human immunodeficiency virus type 1 infection through sexual exposure. J Infect Dis 2002;185: 428–38.

[30] Lo Caputo S, Trabattoni D, Vichi F, Piconi S, Lopalco L, Villa ML, et al. Mucosal and systemic HIV-1-specific immunity in HIV-1-exposed but uninfected heterosexual men. AIDS 2003;17:531–9.

[31] Promadej N, Costello C, Wernett MM, Kulkarni PS, Robison VA, Nelson KE, et al. Broad human immunodeficiency virus (HIV)-specific T cell responses to conserved HIV proteins in HIV-seronegative women highly exposed to a single HIV-infected partner. J Infect Dis 2003;187:1053–63.

[32] Kebba A, Kaleebu P, Rowland S, Ingram R, Whitworth J, Imami N, et al. Distinct patterns of peripheral HIV-1-specific interferon-gamma responses in exposed HIV-1-seronegative individuals. J Infect Dis 2004;189:1705–13.

[33] Pallikkuth S, Wanchu A, Bhatnagar A, Sachdeva RK, Sharma M. Human immunodeficiency virus (HIV) gag antigen-specific T-helper and granule-dependent CD8 T-cell activities in exposed but uninfected heterosexual partners of HIV type 1-infected individuals in North India. Clini Vaccine Immunol 2007;14:1196–202.

[34] Pérez CL, Hasselrot K, Bratt G, Broliden K, Karlsson AC. Induction of systemic HIV-1-specific cellular immune responses by oral exposure in the uninfected partner of discordant couples. AIDS 2010;24:969–74.

[35] Restrepo C, Rallón NI, del Romero J, Rodríguez C, Hernando V, López M, et al. Low-level exposure to HIV induces virus-specific T cell responses and immune activation in exposed HIV-seronegative individuals. J Immunol 2010;185:982–9.

[36] Kelker HC, Seidlin M, Vogler M, Valentine FT. Lymphocytes from some long-term seronegative heterosexual partners of HIV-infected individuals proliferate in response to HIV antigens. AIDS Res Hum Retroviruses 1992;8:1355–9.

[37] Clerici M, Levin JM, Kessler HA, Harris A, Berzofsky JA, Landay AL, et al. HIV-specific T-helper activity in seronegative health care workers exposed to contaminated blood. J Am Med Assoc 1994;271:42–6.

[38] Pinto LA, Sullivan J, Berzofsky JA, Clerici M, Kessler HA, Landay AL, et al. ENV-specific cytotoxic T lymphocyte responses in HIV seronegative health care workers occupationally exposed to HIV-contaminated body fluids. J Clin Invest 1995;96:867.

[39] Pinto LA, Landay AL, Berzofsky JA, Kessler HA, Shearer GM. Immune response to human immunodeficiency virus (HIV) in healthcare workers occupationally exposed to HIV-contaminated blood. Am J Med 1997;102:21–4.

[40] Makedonas G, Bruneau J, Lin H, Sékaly R-P, Lamothe F, Bernard NF. HIV-specific CD8 T-cell activity in uninfected injection drug users is associated with maintenance of seronegativity. AIDS 2002;16:1595–602.

[41] Cheynier R, Langlade-Demoyen P, Marescot MR, Blanche S, Blondin G, Wain-Hobson S, et al. Cytotoxic T lymphocyte responses in the peripheral blood of children born to human immunodeficiency virus-1-infected mothers. Eur J Immunol 1992;22:2211–7.

[42] Clerici M, Sison AV, Berzofsky JA, Rakusan TA, Brandt CD, Ellaurie M, et al. Cellular immune factors associated with mother-to-infant transmission of HIV. AIDS 1993;7: 1427–33.

[43] Rowland-Jones SL, Nixon DF, Aldhous MC, Gotch F, Ariyoshi K, Hallam N, et al. HIV-specific cytotoxic T-cell activity in an HIV-exposed but uninfected infant. Lancet 1993;341:860–1.

[44] Aldhous MC, Watret KC, Mok JY, Bird AG, Froebel KS. Cytotoxic T lymphocyte activity and CD8 subpopulations in children at risk of HIV infection. Clin Exp Immunol 1994;97:61−7.

[45] De Maria A, Cirillo C, Moretta L. Occurrence of human immunodeficiency virus type 1 (HIV-1)-specific cytolytic T cell activity in apparently uninfected children born to HIV-1-infected mothers. J Infect Dis 1994;170:1296−9.

[46] Levy JA, Hsueh F, Blackbourn DJ, Wara D, Weintrub PS. CD8 cell noncytotoxic antiviral activity in human immunodeficiency virus-infected and -uninfected children. J Infect Dis 1998;177:470−2.

[47] Legrand FA, Nixon DF, Loo CP, Ono E, Chapman JM, Miyamoto M, et al. Strong HIV-1-specific T cell responses in HIV-1-exposed uninfected infants and neonates revealed after regulatory T cell removal. PLoS ONE 2006;1:e102.

[48] John-Stewart GC, Mbori-Ngacha D, Payne BL, Farquhar C, Richardson BA, Emery S, et al. HV-1-specific cytotoxic T lymphocytes and breast milk HIV-1 transmission. J Infect Dis 2009;199:889−98.

[49] Rohowsky-Kochan C, Skurnick J, Molinaro D, Louria D. HLA antigens associated with susceptibility/resistance to HIV-1 infection. Human Immunol 1998;59:802−15.

[50] Beyrer C, Artenstein AW, Rugpao S, Stephens H, VanCott TC, Robb ML, et al. Epidemiologic and biologic characterization of a cohort of human immunodeficiency virus type 1 highly exposed, persistently seronegative female sex workers in northern Thailand. Chiang Mai HEPS Working Group. J Infect Dis 1999;179:59−67.

[51] MacDonald KS, Fowke KR, Kimani J, Dunand VA, Nagelkerke NJ, Ball TB, et al. Influence of HLA supertypes on susceptibility and resistance to human immunodeficiency virus type 1 infection. J Infect Dis 2000;181:1581−9.

[52] Lockett SF, Robertson JR, Brettle RP, Yap PL, Middleton D, Leigh Brown AJ. Mismatched human leukocyte antigen alleles protect against heterosexual HIV transmission. J Acquir Immune Defic Syndr 2001;27:277−80.

[53] Sriwanthana B, Hodge T, Mastro TD, Dezzutti CS, Bond K, Stephens HA, et al. HIV-specific cytotoxic T lymphocytes, HLA-A11, and chemokine-related factors may act synergistically to determine HIV resistance in CCR5 delta32-negative female sex workers in Chiang Rai, northern Thailand. AIDS Res Hum Retroviruses 2001;17:719−34.

[54] Hardie RA, Knight E, Bruneau B, Semeniuk C, Gill K, Nagelkerke N, et al. A common human leucocyte antigen-DP genotype is associated with resistance to HIV-1 infection in Kenyan sex workers. AIDS 2008;22:2038−42.

[55] Hardie RA, Luo M, Bruneau B, Knight E, Nagelkerke NJ, Kimani J, et al. Human leukocyte antigen-DQ alleles and haplotypes and their associations with resistance and susceptibility to HIV-1 infection. AIDS 2008;22:807−16.

[56] Rowland-Jones SL, Pinheiro S, Kaul R, Hansasuta P, Gillespie G, Dong T, et al. How important is the 'quality' of the cytotoxic T lymphocyte (CTL) response in protection against HIV infection? Immunol Lett 2001;79:15−20.

[57] McElrath MJ, de Rosa SC, Moodie Z, Dubey S, Kierstead L, Janes H, et al. HIV-1 vaccine-induced immunity in the test-of-concept Step Study: A case-cohort analysis. Lancet 2008;372:1894−905.

[58] Betts MR, Harari A. Phenotype and function of protective T cell immune responses in HIV. Curr Opin HIV AIDS 2008;3:349−55.

[59] Missale G, Papagno L, Penna A, Pilli M, Zerbini A, Vitali P, et al. Parenteral exposure to high HIV viremia leads to virus-specific T cell priming without evidence of infection. Eur J Immunol 2004;34:3208−15.

[60] Suresh P, Wanchu A, Bhatnagar A, Sachdeva RK, Sharma M. Spontaneous and antigen-induced chemokine production in exposed but uninfected partners of HIV type 1-infected individuals in North India. AIDS Res Hum Retroviruses 2007;23:261−8.

[61] Kiepiela P, Leslie AJ, Honeyborne I, Ramduth D, Thobakgale C, Chetty S, et al. Dominant influence of HLA-B in mediating the potential co-evolution of HIV and HLA. Nature 2004;432:769−75.

[62] Boulet S, Kleyman M, Kim JY, Kamya P, Sharafi S, Simic N, et al. A combined genotype of KIR3DL1 high expressing alleles and HLA-B*57 is associated with a reduced risk of HIV infection. AIDS 2008;22:1487−91.

[63] McNicholl JM, Promadej N. Insights into the role of host genetic and T-cell factors in resistance to HIV transmission from studies of highly HIV-exposed Thais. Immunol Res 2004;29:161−74.

[64] McMichael AJ, Rowland-Jones SL. Cellular immune responses to HIV. Nature 2001;410:980−7.

[65] Addo MM, Altfeld M, Brainard DM, Rathod A, Piechocka-Trocha A, Fideli U, et al. Lack of detectable HIV-1-specific CD8+ T cell responses in Zambian HIV-1-exposed seronegative partners of HIV-1-positive individuals. J Infect Dis 2011;203:258−62.

[66] Nguyen M, Pean P, Lopalco L, Nouhin J, Phoung V, Ly N, et al. HIV-specific antibodies but not T-cell responses are associated with protection in seronegative partners of HIV-1-infected individuals in Cambodia. J Acquir Immune Def Syndr 1999;42:412−9. 2006.

[67] Hladik F, Desbien A, Lang J, Wang L, Ding Y, Holte S, et al. Most highly exposed seronegative men lack HIV-1-specific, IFN-gamma-secreting T cells. J Immunol 2003;171:2671−83.

[68] Suy A, Castro P, Nomdedeu M, García F, López A, Fumero E, et al. Immunological profile of heterosexual highly HIV-exposed uninfected individuals: Predominant role of CD4 and CD8 T-cell activation. J Infect Dis 2007;196:1191−201.

[69] Kelleher AD, Long C, Holmes EC, Allen RL, Wilson J, Conlon C, et al. Clustered mutations in HIV-1 gag are consistently required for escape from HLA-B27-restricted cytotoxic T lymphocyte responses. J Exp Med 2001;193:375−86.

[70] Goulder PJ, Brander C, Tang Y, Tremblay C, Colbert RA, Addo MM, et al. Evolution and transmission of stable CTL escape mutations in HIV infection. Nature 2001;412:334−8.

[71] Goulder PJ, Phillips RE, Colbert RA, McAdam S, Ogg G, Nowak MA, et al. Late escape from an immunodominant cytotoxic T-lymphocyte response associated with progression to AIDS. Nat Med 1997;3:212−7.

[72] de Groot NG, Heijmans CM, Zoet YM, de Ru AH, Verreck FA, van Veelen PA, et al. AIDS-protective HLA-B*27/B*57 and chimpanzee MHC class I molecules target analogous conserved areas of HIV-1/SIVcpz. Proc Natl Acad Sci USA 2010;107:15175−80.

[73] Kiepiela P, Ngumbela K, Thobakgale C, Ramduth D, Honeyborne I, Moodley E, et al. CD8+ T-cell responses to different HIV proteins have discordant associations with viral load. Nat Med 2007;13:46−53.

[74] McKinnon LR, Kaul R, Kimani J, Nagelkerke NJ, Wachihi C, Fowke KR, et al. HIV-specific CD8(+) T-cell proliferation is prospectively associated with delayed disease progression. Immunol Cell Biol 2011. in press.

[75] Ball TB, Ji H, Kimani J, McLaren P, Marlin C, Hill AVS, et al. Polymorphisms in IRF-1 associated with resistance to HIV-1 infection in highly exposed uninfected Kenyan sex workers. AIDS 2007;21:1091−101.

[76] Ji H, Ball TB, Ao Z, Kimani J, Yao X, Plummer FA. Reduced HIV-1 long terminal repeat transcription in subjects with protective interferon regulatory factor-1 genotype: A potential

mechanism mediating resistance to infection by HIV-1. Scand J Infect Dis 2010; 42:389—94.

[77] Price H, Lacap P, Tuff J, Wachihi C, Kimani J, Ball TB, et al. A TRIM5alpha exon 2 polymorphism is associated with protection from HIV-1 infection in the Pumwani Sex Worker cohort. AIDS 2010;24:1813—21.

[78] Devito C, Hinkula J, Kaul R, Kimani J, Kiama P, Lopalco L, et al. Cross-clade HIV-1-specific neutralizing IgA in mucosal and systemic compartments of HIV-1-exposed, persistently seronegative subjects. J Acquir Immune Defic Syndr 2002;30:413—20.

[79] Kaul R, Trabattoni D, Bwayo JJ, Arienti D, Zagliani A, Mwangi FM, et al. HIV-1-specific mucosal IgA in a cohort of HIV-1-resistant Kenyan sex workers. AIDS 1999;13:23—9.

[80] Jennes W, Verheyden S, Demanet C, Adjé-Touré CA, Vuylsteke B, Nkengasong JN, et al. Cutting edge: Resistance to HIV-1 infection among African female sex workers is associated with inhibitory KIR in the absence of their HLA ligands. J Immunol 2006; 177:6588—92.

[81] Biasin M, Clerici M, Piacentini L. Innate immunity in resistance to HIV infection. J Infect Dis 2010;202(Suppl 3):S361—5.

[82] Tomescu C, Abdulhaqq S, Montaner LJ. Evidence for the innate immune response as a correlate of protection in human immunodeficiency virus (HIV)-1 highly exposed sero-negative subjects (HESN). Clin Exp Immunol 2011. in press.

[83] Carrington M, Martin M, Vanbergen J. KIR—HLA intercourse in HIV disease. Trends Microbiol 2008;16:620—7.

[84] Boulet S, Sharafi S, Simic N, Bruneau J, Routy J-P, Tsoukas CM, et al. Increased proportion of KIR3DS1 homozygotes in HIV-exposed uninfected individuals. AIDS 2008;22: 595—9.

[85] Guerini FR, Lo Caputo S, Gori A, Bandera A, Mazzotta F, Uglietti A, et al. Under-representation of the inhibitory KIR3DL1 molecule and the KIR3DL1+/BW4+ complex in HIV exposed seronegative individuals. J Infect Dis 2011;203:1235—9.

[86] Scott-Algara D, Truong LX, Versmisse P, David A, Luong TT, Nguyen NV, et al. Cutting edge: Increased NK cell activity in HIV-1-exposed but uninfected Vietnamese intravascular drug users. J Immunol 2003;171:5663—7.

[87] Montoya C, Velilla PA, Chougnet CA, Landay A, Rugeles M. Increased IFN-γ production by NK and CD3+/CD56+ cells in sexually HIV-1-exposed but uninfected individuals. Clin Immunol 2006;120:138—46.

[88] Ravet S, Scott-Algara D, Bonnet E, Tran HK, Tran T, Nguyen N, et al. Distinctive NK-cell receptor repertoires sustain high-level constitutive NK-cell activation in HIV-exposed uninfected individuals. Blood 2007;109:4296—305.

[89] Tomescu C, Duh F-M, Lanier MA, Kapalko A, Mounzer KC, Martin MP, et al. Increased plasmacytoid dendritic cell maturation and natural killer cell activation in HIV-1 exposed, uninfected intravenous drug users. AIDS 2010;24:2151—60.

[90] Ballan WM, Vu B-AN, Long BR, Loo CP, Michaëlsson J, Barbour JD, et al. Natural killer cells in perinatally HIV-1-infected children exhibit less degranulation compared to HIV-1-exposed uninfected children and their expression of KIR2DL3, NKG2C, and NKp46 correlates with disease severity. J Immunol 2007;179:3362—70.

[91] Zhang Z, Schuler T, Zupancic M, Wietgrefe S, Staskus KA, Reimann KA, et al. Sexual transmission and propagation of SIV and HIV in resting and activated CD4+ T cells. Science 1999;286:1353—7.

[92] Zhang Z-Q, Wietgrefe SW, Li Q, Shore MD, Duan L, Reilly C, et al. Roles of substrate availability and infection of resting and activated CD4+ T cells in transmission and

acute simian immunodeficiency virus infection. Proc Natl Acad Sci USA 2004;101: 5640−5.

[93] Brass AL, Dykxhoorn DM, Benita Y, Yan N, Engelman A, Xavier RJ, et al. Identification of host proteins required for HIV infection through a functional genomic screen. Science 2008;319:921−6.

[94] König R, Zhou Y, Elleder D, Diamond TL, Bonamy GMC, Irelan JT, et al. Global analysis of host−pathogen interactions that regulate early-stage HIV-1 replication. Cell 2008;135:49−60.

[95] Zhou H, Xu M, Huang Q, Gates AT, Zhang XD, Castle JC, et al. Genome-scale RNAi screen for host factors required for HIV replication. Cell Host Microbe 2008;4:495−504.

[96] Li Q, Estes JD, Schlievert PM, Duan L, Brosnahan AJ, Southern PJ, et al. Glycerol mon-olaurate prevents mucosal SIV transmission. Nature 2009;458:1034−8.

[97] McLaren P, Ball T, Wachihi C, Jaoko W, Kelvin D, Danesh A, et al. HIV-exposed sero-negative commercial sex workers show a quiescent phenotype in the CD4+ T cell compartment and reduced expression of HIV-dependent host factors. J Infect Dis 2010;202(Suppl 3):S339−44.

[98] Card CM, McLaren PJ, Wachihi C, Kimani J, Plummer FA, Fowke KR. Decreased immune activation in resistance to HIV-1 infection is associated with an elevated frequency of CD4(+)CD25(+)FOXP3(+) regulatory T cells. J Infect Dis 2009;199:1318−22.

[99] Burgener A, Boutilier J, Wachihi C, Kimani J, Carpenter M, Westmacott G, et al. Identi-fication of differentially expressed proteins in the cervical mucosa of HIV-1-resistant sex workers. J Proteome Res 2008;7:4446−54.

[100] Salkowitz JR, Purvis SF, Meyerson H, Zimmerman P, O'Brien TR, Aledort L, et al. Characterization of high-risk HIV-1 seronegative hemophiliacs. Clin Immunol 2001;98:200−11.

[101] Koning FA, Otto SA, Hazenberg MD, Dekker L, Prins M, Miedema F, et al. Low-level CD4+ T cell activation is associated with low susceptibility to HIV-1 infection. J Immunol 2005;175:6117−22.

[102] Begaud E, Chartier L, Marechal V, Ipero J, Leal J, Versmisse P, et al. Reduced CD4 T cell activation and *in vitro* susceptibility to HIV-1 infection in exposed uninfected Central Africans. Retrovirology 2006;3:35.

[103] Jennes W, Evertse D, Borget M-Y, Vuylsteke B, Maurice C, Nkengasong JN, et al. Sup-pressed cellular alloimmune responses in HIV-exposed seronegative female sex workers. Clin Exp Immunol 2006;143:435−44.

[104] Camara M, Dieye TN, Seydi M, Diallo AA, Fall M, Diaw PA, et al. Low-level CD4+ T cell activation in HIV-exposed seronegative subjects: Influence of gender and condom use. J Infect Dis 2010;201:835−42.

[105] Tran HK, Chartier L, Troung LX, Nguyen NN, Fontanet A, Barre-Sinoussi FE, et al. Systemic immune activation in HIV-1-exposed uninfected Vietnamese intravascular drug users. AIDS Res Hum Retroviruses 2006;22:255−61.

[106] Biasin M, Caputo SL, Speciale L, Colombo F, Racioppi L, Zagliani A, et al. Mucosal and systemic immune activation is present in human immunodeficiency virus-exposed sero-negative women. J Infect Dis 2000;182:1365−74.

[107] Biasin M, Piacentini L, lo Caputo S, Naddeo V, Pierotti P, Borelli M, et al. TLR activation pathways in HIV-1-exposed seronegative individuals. J Immunol 2010;184:2710−7.

[108] Su R-C, Sivro A, Kimani J, Jaoko W, Plummer FA, Ball TB. A transient IRF1 response in HIV-exposed, seronegative individuals differs from that in HIV-susceptible controls and is governed by epigenetic mechanisms. Blood 2011. in press.

HIV-1 Controllers

Chapter 8

Definition, Natural History and Heterogeneity of HIV Controllers

Asier Sáez-Cirión[1], Gianfranco Pancino[1] and Olivier Lambotte[2,3], for the ANRS CO18 Cohort

[1] Institut Pasteur, Unité de Régulation des Infections Rétrovirales, Paris, France, [2] Inserm U1012, Le Kremlin-Bicêtre, France, [3] AP-HP, Hôpital Bicêtre, Service de Médecine Interne et Maladies Infectieuses, Le Kremlin-Bicêtre, France

Chapter Outline

HISTORY, IDENTIFICATION AND DEFINITION OF HIV CONTROLLERS

Non-Progression to Infection

As the years after the beginning of the AIDS pandemic passed, it became evident that a small number of HIV-infected patients experienced a mild course of infection. These patients, who represented approximately 5 percent of infected persons [1–3], were able to maintain high CD4+ T cell counts for unusually long periods of time in the absence of antiretroviral therapy, and were therefore referred to as "long-term non-progressors" (LTNPs).

LTNPs were thus defined according to an immunological definition. Numerous studies have been focused on these individuals, aiming to determine the factors associated with non-progression. The presence of attenuated viruses

Models of Protection Against HIV/SIV. DOI: 10.1016/B978-0-12-387715-4.00008-3

such as the Nef mutated viruses found in the Sydney cohort [4] could explain some cases. Genetic factors such as CCR5-Δ32 polymorphisms [5] or certain HLA class I alleles (such as HLA B27 and B57) have been reported. The immune response was also involved with high titers of neutralizing antibodies, especially with anti-HIV IgG2a isotype [1,6], HIV-specific CD4+ and CD8+ T immune response [6,7] and the enhanced production of antiviral soluble factors [8], which were described in different groups of LTNPs. However, data were heterogeneous, and a clear consensus about the most relevant mechanisms has not been reached.

Part of this complexity may arise from the fact that definitions of LTNPs in the different studies varied depending on the level of CD4+ T cell and the time of required follow-up [9]. On a clinical basis, outcomes among LTNPs were also variable. A large number of the individuals enrolled in the LTNPs cohorts eventually showed, although delayed, a drop in their CD4+ T cell counts and progressed to immunosuppression [2,6,10]. The treatment with antiretroviral drugs of a large part of the viremic LTNPs who experienced a negative CD4 T cell slope probably explains the reduced prevalence of LTNPs in the studies recently published [11]. In 2009, Okulicz and colleagues found 3.32 and 2.04 percent of individuals from the US Military HIV Natural History Study (NHS) classified as LTNPs with a CD4 T cell count > 500 cells/µl during 7 and 10 years of follow-up, respectively [3]. Their frequency was lower in a French study [11] which found 0.4 percent of LTNPs with a CD4 T cell count > 500 cells/µl and a positive slope between 2000 and 2005 among 46,880 patients in the French Hospital Database.

With the advent of widespread plasma viral load (VL) testing in the mid-1990s, it was observed that a major cause of heterogeneity among LTNPs was the level of HIV replication. Some LTNPs are able to maintain low immune activation and asymptomatic infection despite an extremely high VL [12], a phenotype that resembles the non-pathogenic SIV infection in African non-human primates (see Chapter 1). However, in general terms, the patients who remain asymptomatic with high CD4+ T cell counts in the LTNP cohorts are usually those with the lowest VLs (Box 8.1) [2,13−17].

The Identification of HIV Controllers

The availability of routine VL testing made it possible to identify a few HIV-infected individuals who were characterized by undetectable plasma viral loads for extended periods of time. We have termed these patients "HIV controllers" (HICs), but they are also known as "elite controllers", "elite suppressors" or "natural viral suppressors" [18−21]. The definition of the controller status varies among the different studies, mostly in terms of duration of control and level of viral replication allowed. In the French National HIV Controller cohort set up by the National Agency for Research on HIV and Viral Hepatitis (ANRS), an "HIV controller" is defined as

BOX 8.1 Overlap Between HICs and LTNPs

Since prolonged virologic control has been associated with elevated CD4 cell counts [3,23], there is some overlap between HIC and LTNP groups despite the differing definitions. For example, recent analyses in the US Military HIV Natural History Study (NHS) and SEROCO/HEMOCO cohorts found the percentages of LNTPs also meeting HIC criteria to be 4 and 12 percent, respectively [3,91]. In a study of the French Hospital database [11], 12 percent of the patients share the French definitions of LTNPs and HICs. This incomplete overlap is interesting, because it suggests that mechanisms leading to the control of HIV replication and those leading to keeping a high CD4 T cell count are not necessarily the same.

a patient infected by HIV-1 for more than 5 years and having the five most recent consecutive plasmatic viral RNA measurements below 400 RNA copies/ml, without any antiretroviral treatment (ART). This extends the initial definition of the HIV controller by the National Observatoire in 2005, which included patients infected for more than 10 years, with more than 90 percent of the VL determinations below 400 RNA copies/ml [22]. The threshold of 400 copies was chosen because it was the threshold of detection in the first commercial VL assays in 1995–1996. Actually, 76 percent of HICs in the French cohort have a median VL < 50 copies/ml. In the United States, the International HIV Controller Study and other groups define elite controllers as having had three or more VL determinations below the limit of assay detection (generally < 50 copies/ml) spanning a period greater than 12 months in the absence of ART for ≥ 1 year before and during the period of virologic control [20]. Viremic controllers form a separate group, defined as having three or more VL determinations between 50 and 2,000 copies/ml spanning a period greater than 12 months in the absence of ART for ≥ 1 year [20]. The University of California, San Francisco (UCSF) cohort, defines controllers as patients maintaining undetectable plasma HIV RNA levels (< 75 copies/ml) for ≥ 5 years in the absence of ART, with at least two plasma HIV RNA determinations in a 1-year period [23]. Other groups require undetectable VLs for at least 2 years [24]. Allowances for some quantity and/or degree of detectable VLs are usually made, given the possibility of transient viremia due to concurrent illnesses, vaccinations, variation in VL testing, or other unexplained causes. Some groups also enroll patients who were previously treated with ART but in whom viral replication remains undetectable after ART stops [3,25], though specific considerations should be made regarding controllers after therapy interruption (see Box 8.2).

Despite the common characteristic among the controllers from the different cohorts—maintenance of undetectable viremia when using standard techniques to measure plasma VLs—it is important to notice that in nearly all

BOX 8.2 HIV Controllers After Post-Treatment Interruption

Although treatment interruption is usually accompanied by a rapid rebound in the VL, a special group of patients are able to control viremia for long periods of time after stopping HAART. In most cases, these patients were treated early during their primary infection. Although it is not possible to exclude that ART may have masked spontaneous control of infection in some cases, these controllers post-therapy seem in general to be different from HICs (ANRS Visconti Study). Their HIV-specific CD8+ T cell responses are extremely weak, and their genetic background is different from that of HICs [92]. It is thus possible that a prolonged period of ART in primary infection may allow some patients to develop mechanisms to control the virus off therapy.

HICs viral replication does occur, albeit at an extremely low level. In addition, several studies employing ultrasensitive single-copy VL assays have found detectable viremia in the majority of HICs. One study examining a median of five longitudinal time-points found detectable VLs in 45 of 46 elite controllers [26]. Another longitudinal study showed that in HICs with VLs below the limit of detection by single-copy assay, only 6 of 11 had VLs < 1 copy/ml at all time-points measured [27]. It is uncertain whether a small subset of HICs remains persistently aviremic, as these individuals may have detectable VLs if studied over longer periods. In contrast to HAART-treated individuals in whom residual viremia is thought to be due to release of virus from the viral reservoirs, in HICs there is evidence of continuous viral replication and evolution [28,29] (see Chapter 9).

The prevalence of HICs among the HIV-infected population has been estimated in several studies. Transient control of viremia in the absence of therapy is not uncommon. For example, 6.7 percent of patients in one study had two consecutive HIV RNA values below 500 copies/ml [14]. The median period of undetectable viremia in that study was 11.2 months. Prolonged control of viremia, however, is far rarer. In one clinic-based cohort and in the French SEROCO cohort, only 0.6 percent of the patients maintained HIV RNA below 400 copies/ml for more than 10 years [19]. Of 46,880 patients followed in the French Hospital Database in 2005, 0.2 percent had more than 90 percent of plasma VL values below 500 copies/ml for greater than 10 years [11]. Similar results were obtained in the French HIC National Observatoire (2007−2008) [22] and in the United States, with a reported prevalence of 0.55 percent for elite controllers in the HIV NHS cohort [3]. Taken together, these studies suggest that durable control of HIV viremia generally occurs in less than 0.6 percent of HIV-1-infected patients. Nevertheless, the prevalence might be different in other regions of the world, such as Asia, Africa or South America, where information about HICs is extremely scarce.

EPIDEMIOLOGIC AND CLINICAL CHARACTERISTICS OF HIV CONTROLLERS

Comparison between some of the main cohorts of HICs studied today leads to one conclusion: HIC patients have common characteristics among the cohorts, although there is not a unique phenotype for HICs. The median age at HIV diagnosis is between 25 and 30 years [3,22], and the median age at enrolment is between 45 and 50 years [3,22–24]. This highlights the prolonged duration of HIV infection in these patients, with a persistent undetectable viremia and no disease progression during 5.5–17 years of infection, depending on the cohort (Table 8.1). Both male and female HICs are included, but ratios depend on the cohort studied (Table 8.1). Females seem to be more frequently presented in several HIC cohorts when compared to general matched-populations of HIV-1-infected individuals. Whether this is due to the general capacity of women to maintain lower VLs than men [30] or to other factors [22] remains unclear. Racial and ethnic differences in HIC prevalence have not been generally found, with the exception of the exclusive presence of African Americans in one cohort [24] and higher frequencies of patients of African origin in the ANRS cohort [22] and the International HIC Initiative.

All modes of transmission have been reported among HICs: heterosexual and homosexual transmission, intravenous drug use, blood transfusions and mother-to-child transmission. In the French HIC Observatoire, intravenous drug users (IDUs) seem to be significantly more frequently present among HICs than in the general HIV-1-infected population [22]. Conversely, homosexuals are significantly under-represented among HIC males in the same group. Although these observations are provocative, they need to be considered with caution because cohorts are prone to include some biases during inclusions due to time period, socio-demographics or other factors. For instance, the low frequency of homosexual men in the French Observatoire might be due to the widespread treatment of homosexual men when ART was first available.

HICs have been the subject of several studies to determine possible genetic factors that may explain their capacity to control HIV-1 infection. This aspect will be treated in greater detail in Chapter 12. In a general way, it is important to point out that over-representation of some "protective" HLA alleles (B5701, which is present in 45–86 percent of the patients according to the cohort, and B2705) which contain the Bw4 [31] motif have been found in all HIC cohorts [19,20,32]. In contrast, there is no over-representation of CCR5-Δ32 hetero-zygous patients among HICs [20], which had been associated with slow progression or protection against infection.

In contrast to LTNPs, the CD4+ T cell count is not included in the definition of HIC. In general, most HICs maintain high CD4+ T cell counts: the median CD4+ T cell counts of seven cohorts range from 644 to 935 and none in the first interquartile range in these cohorts is below 500 cells/mm^3. Interestingly, a transversal study on a group of HICs with stable blood CD4+

TABLE 8.1 Summary of the characteristics of HIV controllers in large published cohorts

	Baltimore natural viral suppressors [21]		International HIV controller consortium [20]		ANRS EP36 observatoire [22]		Military HIV NHS [3]		SCOPE SFC [23,26,71]	
	NVSs	Reference population	ECs	Reference population	HICs	Reference population	ECs	Reference population	HICs	Reference population
n	40	46	66	30	81	528	25[a]	4,290	46	187
Females	48%	35%	36%	20%	43%	32%	20%	15%	39%	17%
Race:										
White	0%	15%	54%	57%	84%	94%	52%	44%	35%	44%
Black	100%	85%	29%	10%	16%	4%	44%	44%	37%	44%
Asiatic	NA		NA	NA	NA	NA	0%	2%	7%	7%
Hispanic			14%	27%	NA	NA	0%	8%	11%	2%
Other/unknown			3%	6%	0%	2%	4%	2%	7%	NA
HLA-B57	44%	NA	44%	NA	45%	6%	NA	NA	37%	NA
HLA-B27	NA	NA	15%	NA	15%	7%	NA	NA	NA	NA

Transmission route:								
Sexual	45%	41%	NA	NA	52%	65%	NA	NA
IDU	55%	59%	NA	NA	31%	8%	NA	NA
Other			NA	NA	17%	27%	NA	NA
Sexual preference men:								
Homosexual	33%	NA	NA	NA	26%	54%	NA	NA
Heterosexual	66%	NA	NA	NA	74%	46%	NA	NA
Year of HIV diagnosis	1994 [1991–1997]	NA	NA	NA	1989 [1988–1990]	1989 [1987–1994]	NA	NA
Duration of diagnosis (years)	15 [9–22]	5.5 [1–17]	NA	NA	17 [13–19.1]	7.8 [5.6–11.7]	—	13 [8–17]
Duration of control (years)[b]	6.6 [4.6–9.0]	NA	—	NA	8.2 [6.2–9.4]	2.3 [1.5–4.8]	—	NA

[a]17/25 were naive of antiretroviral therapy before the period of control; [b]time since first available undetectable viral load.

T cell counts found an intact size of CD4+ T cell populations, similar to that of uninfected individuals, also in the gut mucosa [33]. Long-term follow-up of CD4+ T cell counts is available for several cohorts. In general, these analyses indicate that HICs, as a whole, show no overall decrease in CD4+ T cell counts over a period spanning 10–18 years of follow-up [3,34] (see example in Figure 8.1A). Nevertheless, a significant proportion of HICs show a clear, although modest, decline of CD4+ T cell counts over time [22,27,34] (see Figure 8.1B). The evolution of CD4+ T cell counts was analyzed in HICs included in the French HIC National Observatoire. Three HIC subsets were defined according to having maintained all their available VLs between diagnosis and inclusion in the observatory below the limit of detection, or showing periodic or frequent episodes of detectable viremia (blips between 50 and 400 copies of HIV-1 RNA/ml of plasma) in this period of time: no blippers, rare blippers and frequent blippers [22]. The median CD4+ T cell count at diagnosis was similar in all the subgroups. However, whereas in HICs in whom detectable viremia was never found the CD4+ T cell slope was 0 with no decrease of the CD4+ T cell count over the time, in the other HICs ("blippers") the CD4+ T cell count slope was negative with a slow loss of CD4+ T cells of between 10 and 20 cells/year. These results are in agreement with another study which analyzed the magnitude of virologic control in HICs using a single-copy VL assay and the corresponding CD4+ T cell trajectories. This study showed that significant CD4+ T cell loss was more common in patients with detectable low level viremia (VL ≥ 1 copy/ml) compared to those with undetectable viremia (< 1 copy/ml) [27]. Studies comparing both elite and viremic controllers are also informative in this regard. Although the VL thresholds differed by less than one-half log between elites and viremic controllers in a study by the NHS [3], the ability to control VL below the limit of detection by standard assays was associated with more favorable outcomes in the elite group, including the magnitude and stability of CD4+ T cell counts, and the development of AIDS and death. All these studies suggest that the maintenance of high and stable CD4+ T cell counts in HICs is associated with the control of viral replication.

A few cases of severe depletion of CD4+ T cells (below 350 cells/mm^3, and in rarer cases even below 200 cells/mm^3) have been reported among HICs. Actually, AIDS events have been described in HICs, either related to CD4+ T cell criteria or to development of AIDS-defining events, such as pulmonary tuberculosis and Kaposi's sarcoma in two patients from the UCSF cohort [3,23]. Antiretroviral therapy is therefore prescribed in some rare HICs, although data are scarce in the literature. For example, six HICs from the US Military HIV NHS have been treated [35], one at the Johns Hopkins Hospital [34] in Baltimore, Maryland, and five in France. Treatment responses have been heterogeneous. Some HICs seem to benefit from ART, although they exhibit smaller CD4+ T cell gains compared to non-controllers [35]. However, other patients do not experience any increase in their CD4+ T cell counts despite

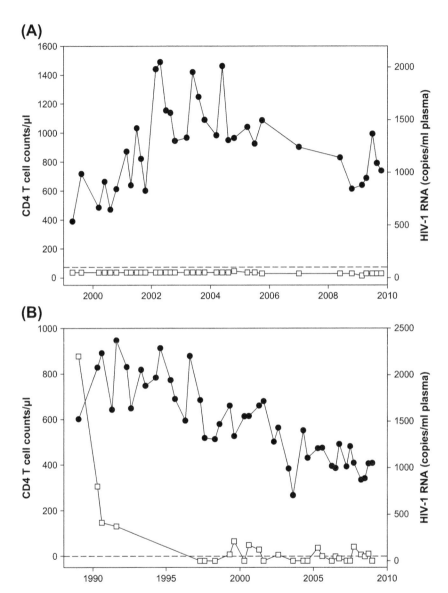

FIGURE 8.1 Evolution over time of CD4+ T cell counts (filled circles) and plasma HIV-1 RNA load (open squares) in two representative HIV controllers (HICs) from the ANRS CO18 cohort. The first (top panel) shows a very tight control of infection and stable number of CD4+ T cells. The second (bottom panel) was followed from primary infection, and experienced some small blips in the viral load after achieving control of infection. In this HIC, these blips are accompanied by a decay in the number of CD4+ T cells. The dashed line represents the limit of detection for the viral load tests (i.e., 50 RNA copies/ml of plasma).

strictly undetectable viremia ([34] and observations in the French cohort). Therefore, factors different from the viral load may be driving the loss of CD4+ T cells in some HICs.

One such factor may be immune activation. Indeed, despite controlled viremia, a relative high activation of blood CD4+ and CD8+ T cell compartments—higher than in HAART-treated patients—is generally found among HICs [23,36], and is associated with the decline in CD4+ T cell counts in these individuals [23]. Although the precise mechanisms underlying the decline of CD4+ T cells are not known, immune activation might cause the exhaustion of lymphopoiesis and impair the replenishment of the lost CD4+ T cells. Along these lines, qualitative and quantitative alterations of the hematopoietic progenitor cells have been reported in HICs with decreasing CD4+ T cell counts [37]. Immune activation could be related to low-level residual replication [26] but also to a low regulatory T cell response [38,39], which may facilitate the development of a robust T cell response at the expense of generalized immune activation [38], or to translocation of bacterial products from the gut mucosa [23,40]. Besides a supposed role in the loss of CD4+ T cells, the long-term consequences of this abnormal activation of the immune system in HICs are unknown. Among possible consequences, an increase in cardiovascular risk has been evoked. Supporting this hypothesis, Hsue and colleagues have reported an increase in atherosclerosis, with higher carotid intima-media thickness, in HICs [41]. The question of an increase in cancer risk is also present (three cases of cancer among HICs having periodical blips in VL have been described in the French cohort [22]) and should be addressed by international studies involving a large number of patients to reach sufficient statistical power. Therefore, the long-term clinical follow-up of HICs is of paramount importance to identify the long-term impact of HIV infection in hosts without the ART confounding factor.

MECHANISMS OF CONTROL AND OPEN QUESTIONS

As mentioned above, short-term spontaneous control of infection among HIV-1-infected patients is not such a rare event. However, most of these patients lose control of viremia within a few months. Although control of infection seems tighter in long-term HICs, loss of virologic control has also been rarely described ([42], and unpublished observations from the French cohort). Interestingly, CD4+ T cell decline and loss of control of viremia seem to occur separately in most patients. Current experience suggests that this loss of control of infection may be related to superinfection, or to the development of comorbidities, such as cancer (O. Lambotte's observation). It is, however, interesting to note that although loss of control of viremia following superinfection has been reported in HICs ([42,43]), evidence of the ability of HICs to control several HIV strains has been documented [28,44,45]. It is not clear whether the extraordinary capacity of HICs to control HIV-1 infection extends to other viral infections. The prevalence of hepatitis C virus (HCV) infection in HICs varies among cohorts depending on the mode of contamination; however, a couple of studies have suggested that HICs could clear HCV infection more frequently [46] or that HCV RNA VLs are lower in HICs [47] in the absence of treatment. The capacity to control HCV infection might be also related to the presence of the protective HLA alleles HLA-B27 and HLA-B57, over-represented in HICs, which have also been associated with better control of HCV [48−50], and/or to the capacity of HICs to develop an efficient adaptive response [38,51].

The immune system is a major actor in explaining the HIC phenotype (see Chapter 10). In combination with genetic background, some commonalities have been found. A large group of HICs has strong HIV-specific CD8+ T cell responses [52,53]. This is a significant characteristic, since the magnitude of the HIV-specific CD8+ T cell response is generally associated with the level of VL and is thus very weak in individuals receiving ART [54]. In contrast, the frequency of HIV-specific CD8+ T cell responses in these HICs is comparable to and even higher than the frequency found in viremic progressors. However, the cells from HIC are qualitatively different from those of viremic individuals which are impaired functionally due to exhaustion [55−58]. In HICs, HIV-specific CD8+ T cells are able to produce several cytokines [59,60] and, in response to antigen, have the capacity to proliferate, rapidly upregulate granzyme and perforine [61−63], and degranulate, which traduces in an impressive capacity to suppress HIV-1 infection of autologous CD4+ T cells [53]. In addition, probably linked to the overwhelming presence of protective HLA alleles, the responses against Gag are predominant in HICs [64−66], which may confer an additional advantage in controlling HIV-1 infection [66−68]. Robust HIV-specific CD4 T cell responses are also found in a large group of HICs [20,64]. As in the case of CD8+ T cell responses, the HIV-specific CD4+ T cells are qualitatively different from those from non-controllers, and are able to produce multiple cytokines [36,64] and react to limited amounts of antigen [69]. The reasons underlying the strong and effective T cell response in HICs are not yet fully understood. Myeloid dendritic cells, which are responsible for the priming of the T specific response, have been shown to have enhanced antigen-presenting capacities in HICs, and also to produce a different set of cytokines than the cells from progressors [51]. These factors may be of critical relevance for inducing an effective T cell response in a setting of limited antigen availability. In addition, the HIV-specific CD8+ T cells have longer telomeres due to high constitutive telomerase activity in these cells, which may protect them from antigen-driven exhaustion and contribute to preserving their functional capacities [70].

All this evidence points to an important role for the HIV-specific T cell response in maintaining long-lasting control of infection. However, the frequencies of HIV-specific CD4+ and CD8+ T cells, their phenotype, the number of cytokines that they produce and even their ability to block viral replication are really heterogeneous among HICs [20,64,66]. Some of this heterogeneity may be partially associated to the level of residual viremia in HICs [66,71], especially in the case of the HIV-specific CD4+ T cell response [71]. Low-level viral replication may be necessary to boost the T cell response, or, as recently reported, the HIV-specific CD4+ T cells themselves may be sustaining some degree of viral replication serving as privileged targets for infection [71]. In contrast, the lowest levels of HIV-specific T cells in HICs are generally found in individuals with an extremely well controlled VL. Moreover, HICs have been found to be able to keep controlling the virus despite the emergence of CTL-escaping mutants [18]. The contribution of the humoral response to control of infection in HICs is not clear. The antibody-dependent cell cytotoxicity response has been reported to be higher in HICs than in viremic patients [72], although this observation requires further exploration. In contrast, the levels of neutralizing antivirus are relatively weak in HICs [27,72]. As in the case of the T cell response, the levels of both humoral responses are very heterogeneous [20,72], and also linked to the level of viremia [27]. This suggests that other mechanisms, different from adaptive immunity, may contribute to control of HIV infection in HIC.

Information on the kinetics of viral control after infection and studies on the early phases of this control are obviously crucial to comprehending such mechanisms. However, most HICs have been studied after long-term infection. Although very little information is therefore available on the acute phase of infection in these individuals, existing data suggest that control of viral replication occurs early in most controllers. Partial and delayed seroconversion has been reported in some HICs [73]. Eight patients from the Primary Infection French Cohort (PRIMO) spontaneously controlled viral replication in the months following the primary infection [74], and they had significantly lower VLs at first testing. The same results have been found in the NHS, where most HICs had spontaneous virologic control in the year following primary infection [3]. Both viral and host determinants may underlie this early control of viral replication.

Most HICs are infected with replication-competent viruses that do not present significant genetic defects [45,66,75,76]. However, the fitness cost associated with some escape mutations driven by the T cell response may limit viral replication. Indeed, different studies suggest that B*57 and B*27-restricted CD8+ T cell responses target epitopes that are located within structurally important sequences of the virus, where variations would come at a cost to viral fitness [77–79]. Moreover, one study has shown that most patients who become controllers harbor, during the early stages of infection, viruses with reduced replication capacity, which is likely associated with transmitted or acquired CTL escape mutations or transmitted drug resistance mutations [80]. These data suggest that viral dynamics, especially during acute infection, may have an impact on HIV disease outcome and control of viremia.

Host innate immune responses and/or intrinsic mechanisms of cell resistance to infection may also play an important role in the control of viremia very early in infection, when adaptive immunity is not yet developed. Early activation of innate immunity, and in particular natural killer (NK) cells, might not only contribute to control infection but also provide a favorable cytokine environment for the development of an effective adaptive response. Innate immunity has been linked to control of infection through genetic association of some killer immunoglobulin-like receptors with the HLA-Bw04 alleles [81] which, as already mentioned, are over-represented in HICs. However, information about the functionality of NK cells in HICs is still scarce and concerns especially their antiviral activity *in vitro* [82,83].

Although some studies suggested that intrinsic CD4+ T cell resistance to infection does not play a role in control of infection in HICs [53,84], recent evidence has indicated that the cells from HICs are actually less susceptible to infection than those from healthy donors or other HIV-infected patients. One study has shown that CD4+ T cells from HICs carry, *in vivo*, an excess of unintegrated viral DNA in relation to the reduced levels of integrated virus found in these cells [85]. This observation points to an inefficient integration of HIV-1 into the cells from HICs, although an intrinsic resistance to HIV-1 could not be evidenced *in vitro* in this study. In contrast, another group has found *in vitro* restriction of HIV-1 replication before and after viral integration in CD4+ T cells from HICs [86]. These blocks were associated with a higher constitutive expression of p21$^{waf1/cip1}$, a kinase-dependent cycline inhibitor which has been shown to block HIV-1 in macrophages and hematopoietic stem cells [87,88]. A parallel study of the French cohort showed that both CD4+ T cells and macrophages from HICs present a pre-integrative block of HIV replication [89]. Although, in this study, p21 was also found to be more strongly expressed in CD4+ T cells *ex vivo* from HICs, the block was not associated to p21 expression but attributed to a saturable factor, which is still unknown. The implication of a saturable restriction factor may explain the apparent contradictory data in the literature, and the difficulty of exposing these mechanisms *in vitro*. In addition, in this latter study an association was found between the reduced susceptibility of CD4+ T cells from HICs to infection *in vitro* and the low levels of viral DNA that these cells carried *in vivo*. This implies that intrinsic cell resistance to infection may play an important role in controlling the size of the viral reservoir in HICs. Indeed, a reduced viral reservoir is found in HICs from different cohorts when compared to progressors and even to HAART-treated patients [19,21,85]. A limited viral reservoir may not only contribute to attenuating the dynamics of viral replication, but also favor the development and maturation of the optimal adaptive response, which could overcome later viral replication.

Although considerable advances have been made in our understanding of the factors and mechanisms associated with the spontaneous control of HIV-1 infection in HICs, many questions remain still unanswered. It is likely that spontaneous control of infection is the result of concurrence of several of the mechanisms described above (Figure 8.2). Although it is possible that several

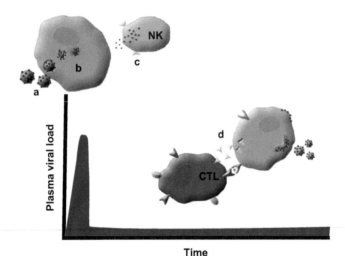

Time

FIGURE 8.2   **It is likely that the long-term control of viremia in HIV controllers is due to the interplay between several mechanisms.** In particular, infection with a less fitted virus (a), the reduced susceptibility of cells from HIC to HIV-1 infection (b), or innate immunity (c) may help to decrease the dynamics of viral replication during primary infection, reducing the viral reservoir and facilitating the development of an efficient adaptive T cell response (d) and the control of infection.

subgroups of HICs exist according to the mechanisms involved in the control of HIV [66,90], it is also possible that all these mechanisms are interlinked and regulated by factors such as residual viremia and immune activation. From a clinical point of view, several questions remain outstanding. It will be important to determine which is the source of viral replication at the origin of the residual viral replication observed in HICs, and of the blips in the plasma VL that are observed in some of these patients. These punctual fluctuations in the VL may also have consequences regarding the risk of HIV-1 transmission. Finally, it is important to gather further information about how HICs respond to HAART or to alternative therapies. Immune activation appears to be a suitable target for these therapies, as the relatively strong levels of activation observed in HICs may have negative consequences in the long term.

REFERENCES

[1] Cao Y, Qin L, Zhang L, Safrit J, Ho DD. Virologic and immunologic characterization of long-term survivors of human immunodeficiency virus type 1 infection. N Engl J Med 1995; 332:201–8.

[2] Lefrere JJ, Morand-Joubert L, Mariotti M, Bludau H, Burghoffer B, Petit JC, et al. Even individuals considered as long-term nonprogressors show biological signs of progression after 10 years of human immunodeficiency virus infection. Blood 1997;90:1133–40.

[3] Okulicz JF, Marconi VC, Landrum ML, Wegner S, Weintrob A, Ganesan A, et al. Clinical outcomes of elite controllers, viremic controllers, and long-term nonprogressors in the US Department of Defense HIV Natural History Study. J Infect Dis 2009;200:1714–23.

[4] Deacon NJ, Tsykin A, Solomon A, Smith K, Ludford-Menting M, Hooker DJ, et al. Genomic structure of an attenuated quasi species of HIV-1 from a blood transfusion donor and recipients. Science 1995;270:988−91.

[5] Magierowska M, Theodorou I, Debre P, Sanson F, Autran B, Riviere Y, et al. Combined genotypes of CCR5, CCR2, SDF1, and HLA genes can predict the long-term nonprogressor status in human immunodeficiency virus-1-infected individuals. Blood 1999;93:936−41.

[6] Martinez V, Costagliola D, Bonduelle O, N'go N, Schnuriger A, Theodorou I, et al. Combination of HIV-1-specific CD4 Th1 cell responses and IgG2 antibodies is the best predictor for persistence of long-term nonprogression. J Infect Dis 2005;191:2053−63.

[7] Greenough TC, Brettler DB, Kirchhoff F, Alexander L, Desrosiers RC, O'Brien SJ, et al. Long-term nonprogressive infection with human immunodeficiency virus type 1 in a hemophilia cohort. J Infect Dis 1999;180:1790−802.

[8] Scala E, D'Offizi G, Rosso R, Turriziani O, Ferrara R, Mazzone AM, et al. C-C chemokines, IL-16, and soluble antiviral factor activity are increased in cloned T cells from subjects with long-term nonprogressive HIV infection. J Immunol 1997;158:4485−92.

[9] Strathdee SA, Veugelers PJ, Page-Shafer KA, McNulty A, Moss AR, Schechter MT, et al. Lack of consistency between five definitions of nonprogression in cohorts of HIV-infected seroconverters. AIDS 1996;10:959−65.

[10] Learmont JC, Geczy AF, Mills J, Ashton LJ, Raynes-Greenow CH, Garsia RJ, et al. Immunologic and virologic status after 14 to 18 years of infection with an attenuated strain of HIV-1. A report from the Sydney Blood Bank Cohort. N Engl J Med 1999;340:1715−22.

[11] Grabar S, Selinger-Leneman H, Abgrall S, Pialoux G, Weiss L, Costagliola D. Prevalence and comparative characteristics of long-term nonprogressors and HIV controller patients in the French Hospital Database on HIV. AIDS 2009;23:1163−9.

[12] Choudhary SK, Vrisekoop N, Jansen CA, Otto SA, Schuitemaker H, Miedema F, et al. Low immune activation despite high levels of pathogenic human immunodeficiency virus type 1 results in long-term asymptomatic disease. J Virol 2007;81:8838−42.

[13] Goudsmit J, Bogaards JA, Jurriaans S, Schuitemaker H, Lange JM, Coutinho RA, et al. Naturally HIV-1 seroconverters with lowest viral load have best prognosis, but in time lose control of viraemia. AIDS 2002;16:791−3.

[14] Madec Y, Boufassa F, Rouzioux C, Delfraissy JF, Meyer L. Undetectable viremia without antiretroviral therapy in patients with HIV seroconversion: An uncommon phenomenon? Clin Infect Dis 2005;40:1350−4.

[15] O'Brien TR, Blattner WA, Waters D, Eyster E, Hilgartner MW, Cohen AR, et al. Serum HIV-1 RNA levels and time to development of AIDS in the Multicenter Hemophilia Cohort Study. J Am Med Assoc 1996;276:105−10.

[16] Rinaldo C, Huang XL, Fan ZF, Ding M, Beltz L, Logar A, et al. High levels of anti-human immunodeficiency virus type 1 (HIV-1) memory cytotoxic T-lymphocyte activity and low viral load are associated with lack of disease in HIV-1-infected long-term nonprogressors. J Virol 1995;69:5838−42.

[17] Rodes B, Toro C, Paxinos E, Poveda E, Martinez-Padial M, Benito JM, et al. Differences in disease progression in a cohort of long-term non-progressors after more than 16 years of HIV-1 infection. AIDS 2004;18:1109−16.

[18] Bailey JR, Williams TM, Siliciano RF, Blankson JN. Maintenance of viral suppression in HIV-1-infected HLA-B*57+ elite suppressors despite CTL escape mutations. J Exp Med 2006;203:1357−69.

[19] Lambotte O, Boufassa F, Madec Y, Nguyen A, Goujard C, Meyer L, et al. HIV controllers: A homogeneous group of HIV-1-infected patients with spontaneous control of viral replication. Clin Infect Dis 2005;41:1053−6.

[20] Pereyra F, Addo MM, Kaufmann DE, Liu Y, Miura T, Rathod A, et al. Genetic and immunologic heterogeneity among persons who control HIV infection in the absence of therapy. J Infect Dis 2008;197:563−71.

[21] Sajadi MM, Heredia A, Le N, Constantine NT, Redfield RR. HIV-1 natural viral suppressors: Control of viral replication in the absence of therapy. AIDS 2007;21:517−9.

[22] Boufassa F, Saez-Cirion A, Lechenadec J, Zucman D, Avettand-Fenoel V, Venet A, et al. CD4 dynamics over a 15 year period among HIV controllers enrolled in the ANRS French Observatory. PLoS ONE 2011;6:e18726.

[23] Hunt PW, Brenchley J, Sinclair E, McCune JM, Roland M, Page-Shafer K, et al. Relationship between T cell activation and CD4+ T cell count in HIV-seropositive individuals with undetectable plasma HIV RNA levels in the absence of therapy. J Infect Dis 2008;197:126−33.

[24] Sajadi MM, Constantine NT, Mann DL, Charurat M, Dadzan E, Kadlecik P, et al. Epidemiologic characteristics and natural history of HIV-1 natural viral suppressors. J Acquir Immune Defic Syndr 2009;50:403−8.

[25] Ruiz-Mateos E, Ferrando-Martinez S, Machmach K, Viciana P, Pacheco YM, Nogales N, et al. High levels of CD57+CD28- T-cells, low T-cell proliferation and preferential expansion of terminally differentiated CD4+ T-cells in HIV-elite controllers. Curr HIV Res 2010;8:471−81.

[26] Hatano H, Delwart EL, Norris PJ, Lee TH, Dunn-Williams J, Hunt PW, et al. Evidence for persistent low-level viremia in individuals who control human immunodeficiency virus in the absence of antiretroviral therapy. J Virol 2009;83:329−35.

[27] Pereyra F, Palmer S, Miura T, Block BL, Wiegand A, Rothchild AC, et al. Persistent low-level viremia in HIV-1 elite controllers and relationship to immunologic parameters. J Infect Dis 2009;200:984−90.

[28] Mens H, Kearney M, Wiegand A, Shao W, Schonning K, Gerstoft J, et al. HIV-1 continues to replicate and evolve in patients with natural control of HIV infection. J Virol 2010;84:12971−81.

[29] O'Connell KA, Brennan TP, Bailey JR, Ray SC, Siliciano RF, Blankson JN. Control of HIV-1 in elite suppressors despite ongoing replication and evolution in plasma virus. J Virol 2010;84:7018−28.

[30] Farzadegan H, Hoover DR, Astemborski J, Lyles CM, Margolick JB, Markham RB, et al. Sex differences in HIV-1 viral load and progression to AIDS. Lancet 1998;352:1510−4.

[31] Flores-Villanueva PO, Yunis EJ, Delgado JC, Vittinghoff E, Buchbinder S, Leung JY, et al. Control of HIV-1 viremia and protection from AIDS are associated with HLA-Bw4 homozygosity. Proc Natl Acad Sci USA 2001;98:5140−5.

[32] Migueles SA, Sabbaghian MS, Shupert WL, Bettinotti MP, Marincola FM, Martino L, et al. HLA B*5701 is highly associated with restriction of virus replication in a subgroup of HIV-infected long term nonprogressors. Proc Natl Acad Sci USA 2000;97:2709−14.

[33] Ciccone EJ, Greenwald JH, Lee PI, Biancotto A, Read SW, Yao MA, et al. CD4+ T cells, including Th17 and cycling subsets, are intact in the gut mucosa of HIV-1 infected long-term non-progressors. J Virol 2011;85:5880−8.

[34] Sedaghat AR, Rastegar DA, O'Connell KA, Dinoso JB, Wilke CO, Blankson JN. T cell dynamics and the response to HAART in a cohort of HIV-1-infected elite suppressors. Clin Infect Dis 2009;49:1763−6.

[35] Okulicz JF, Grandits GA, Weintrob AC, Landrum ML, Ganesan A, Crum-Cianflone NF, et al. CD4 T cell count reconstitution in HIV controllers after highly active antiretroviral therapy. Clin Infect Dis 2010;50:1187−91.

[36] Potter SJ, Lacabaratz C, Lambotte O, Perez-Patrigeon S, Vingert B, Sinet M, et al. Preserved central memory and activated effector memory CD4+ T cell subsets in HIV controllers: An ANRS EP36 study. J Virol 2007;81:13904−15.

[37] Sauce D, Larsen M, Fastenackels S, Pauchard M, Ait-Mohand H, Schneider L, et al. HIV disease progression despite suppression of viral replication is associated with exhaustion of lymphopoiesis. Blood 2011;117:5142−51.

[38] Hunt PW, Landay AL, Sinclair E, Martinson JA, Hatano H, Emu B, et al. A low T regulatory cell response may contribute to both viral control and generalized immune activation in HIV controllers. PLoS ONE 2011;6:e15924.

[39] Schulze Zur Wiesch J, Thomssen A, Hartjen P, Toth I, Lehmann C, Meyer-Olson D, et al. Comprehensive analysis of frequency and phenotype of T regulatory cells in HIV infection: CD39 expression of FoxP3+ T regulatory cells correlates with progressive disease. J Virol 2011;85:1287−97.

[40] Brenchley JM, Price DA, Schacker TW, Asher TE, Silvestri G, Rao S, et al. Microbial translocation is a cause of systemic immune activation in chronic HIV infection. Nat Med 2006;12:1365−71.

[41] Hsue PY, Hunt PW, Sinclair E, Bredt B, Franklin A, Killian M, et al. Increased carotid intima-media thickness in HIV patients is associated with increased cytomegalovirus-specific T-cell responses. AIDS 2006;20:2275−83.

[42] Rachinger A, Navis M, van Assen S, Groeneveld PH, Schuitemaker H. Recovery of viremic control after superinfection with pathogenic HIV type 1 in a long-term elite controller of HIV type 1 infection. Clin Infect Dis 2008;47:e86−89.

[43] Clerc O, Colombo S, Yerly S, Telenti A, Cavassini M. HIV-1 elite controllers: Beware of super-infections. J Clin Virol 2010;47:376−8.

[44] Casado C, Pernas M, Alvaro T, Sandonis V, Garcia S, Rodriguez C, et al. Coinfection and super-infection in patients with long-term, nonprogressive HIV-1 disease. J Infect Dis 2007;196:895−9.

[45] Lamine A, Caumont-Sarcos A, Chaix ML, Sáez-Cirión A, Rouzioux C, Delfraissy JF, et al. Replication-competent HIV strains infect HIV controllers despite undetectable viremia (ANRS EP36 study). AIDS 2007;21:1043−5.

[46] Sajadi MM, Shakeri N, Talwani R, Redfield RR. Hepatitis C infection in HIV-1 natural viral suppressors. AIDS 2010;24:1689−95.

[47] Ruiz-Mateos E, Machmach K, Romero-Sanchez MC, Ferrando-Martinez S, Viciana P, Del Val M, et al. Hepatitis C virus replication in Caucasian HIV controllers. J Viral Hepatitis 2011;18:e350−357.

[48] Chuang WC, Sarkodie F, Brown CJ, Owusu-Ofori S, Brown J, Li C, et al. Protective effect of HLA-B57 on HCV genotype 2 infection in a West African population. J Med Virol 2007;79:724−33.

[49] Kim AY, Kuntzen T, Timm J, Nolan BE, Baca MA, Reyor LL, et al. Spontaneous control of HCV is associated with expression of HLA-B 57 and preservation of targeted epitopes. Gastroenterology 2011;140:686−96.

[50] Neumann-Haefelin C, McKiernan S, Ward S, Viazov S, Spangenberg HC, Killinger T, et al. Dominant influence of an HLA-B27 restricted CD8+ T cell response in mediating HCV clearance and evolution. Hepatology 2006;43:563−72.

[51] Huang J, Burke PS, Cung TD, Pereyra F, Toth I, Walker BD, et al. Leukocyte immuno-globulin-like receptors maintain unique antigen-presenting properties of circulating myeloid dendritic cells in HIV-1-infected elite controllers. J Virol 2010;84:9463−71.

[52] Gea-Banacloche JC, Migueles SA, Martino L, Shupert WL, McNeil AC, Sabbaghian MS, et al. Maintenance of large numbers of virus-specific CD8+ T cells in HIV-infected progressors and long-term nonprogressors. J Immunol 2000;165:1082−92.

[53] Sáez-Cirión A, Lacabaratz C, Lambotte O, Versmisse P, Urrutia A, Boufassa F, et al. HIV controllers exhibit potent CD8 T cell capacity to suppress HIV infection *ex vivo* and peculiar CTL activation phenotype. Proc Natl Acad Sci USA 2007;104:6776−81.

[54] Lacabaratz-Porret C, Urrutia A, Doisne JM, Goujard C, Deveau C, Dalod M, et al. Impact of antiretroviral therapy and changes in virus load on human immunodeficiency virus (HIV)-specific T cell responses in primary HIV infection. J Infect Dis 2003;187:748−57.

[55] Day CL, Kaufmann DE, Kiepiela P, Brown JA, Moodley ES, Reddy S, et al. PD-1 expression on HIV-specific T cells is associated with T-cell exhaustion and disease progression. Nature 2006;443:350−4.

[56] Petrovas C, Casazza JP, Brenchley JM, Price DA, Gostick E, Adams WC, et al. PD-1 is a regulator of virus-specific CD8+ T cell survival in HIV infection. J Exp Med 2006;203:2281−92.

[57] Trautmann L, Janbazian L, Chomont N, Said EA, Gimmig S, Bessette B, et al. Upregulation of PD-1 expression on HIV-specific CD8+ T cells leads to reversible immune dysfunction. Nat Med 2006;12:1198−202.

[58] Zhang JY, Zhang Z, Wang X, Fu JL, Yao J, Jiao Y, et al. PD-1 up-regulation is correlated with HIV-specific memory CD8+ T-cell exhaustion in typical progressors but not in long-term nonprogressors. Blood 2007;109:4671−8.

[59] Betts MR, Nason MC, West SM, De Rosa SC, Migueles SA, et al. HIV nonprogressors preferentially maintain highly functional HIV-specific CD8+ T cells. Blood 2006;107:4781−9.

[60] Zimmerli SC, Harari A, Cellerai C, Vallelian F, Bart PA, Pantaleo G. HIV-1-specific IFN-gamma/IL-2-secreting CD8 T cells support CD4-independent proliferation of HIV-1-specific CD8 T cells. Proc Natl Acad Sci USA 2005;102:7239−44.

[61] Hersperger AR, Pereyra F, Nason M, Demers K, Sheth P, Shin LY, et al. Perforin expression directly *ex vivo* by HIV-specific CD8 T-cells is a correlate of HIV elite control. PLoS Pathog 2010;6:e1000917.

[62] Migueles SA, Laborico AC, Shupert WL, Sabbaghian MS, Rabin R, Hallahan CW, et al. HIV-specific CD8+ T cell proliferation is coupled to perforin expression and is maintained in nonprogressors. Nat Immunol 2002;3:1061−8.

[63] Migueles SA, Osborne CM, Royce C, Compton AA, Joshi RP, Weeks KA, et al. Lytic granule loading of CD8+ T cells is required for HIV-infected cell elimination associated with immune control. Immunity 2008;29:1009−21.

[64] Emu B, Sinclair E, Hatano H, Ferre A, Shacklett B, Martin JN, et al. HLA class I-restricted T-cell responses may contribute to the control of human immunodeficiency virus infection, but such responses are not always necessary for long-term virus control. J Virol 2008;82:5398−407.

[65] Kiepiela P, Ngumbela K, Thobakgale C, Ramduth D, Honeyborne I, Moodley E, et al. CD8+ T-cell responses to different HIV proteins have discordant associations with viral load. Nat Med 2007;13:46−53.

[66] Saez-Cirion A, Sinet M, Shin SY, Urrutia A, Versmisse P, Lacabaratz C, et al. Heterogeneity in HIV suppression by CD8 T cells from HIV controllers: Association with Gag-specific CD8 T cell responses. J Immunol 2009;182:7828−37.

[67] Julg B, Williams KL, Reddy S, Bishop K, Qi Y, Carrington M, et al. Enhanced anti-HIV functional activity associated with Gag-specific CD8 T-cell responses. J Virol 2010;84:5540−9.

[68] Sacha JB, Chung C, Rakasz EG, Spencer SP, Jonas AK, Bean AT, et al. Gag-specific CD8+ T lymphocytes recognize infected cells before AIDS-virus integration and viral protein expression. J Immunol 2007;178:2746−54.

[69] Vingert B, Perez-Patrigeon S, Jeannin P, Lambotte O, Boufassa F, Lemaitre F, et al. HIV controller CD4+ T cells respond to minimal amounts of Gag antigen due to high TCR avidity. PLoS Pathog 2010;6:e1000780.

[70] Lichterfeld M, Mou D, Cung TD, Williams KL, Waring MT, Huang J, et al. Telomerase activity of HIV-1-specific CD8+ T cells: Constitutive up-regulation in controllers and selective increase by blockade of PD ligand 1 in progressors. Blood 2008;112:3679−87.

[71] Hunt PW, Hatano H, Sinclair E, Lee TH, Busch MP, Martin JN, et al. HIV-specific CD4+ T cells may contribute to viral persistence in HIV controllers. Clin Infect Dis 2011;52:681−7.

[72] Lambotte O, Ferrari G, Moog C, Yates NL, Liao HX, Parks RJ, et al. Heterogeneous neutralizing antibody and antibody-dependent cell cytotoxicity responses in HIV-1 elite controllers. AIDS 2009;23:897−906.

[73] Clerc O, Cavassini M, Boni J, Schupbach J, Burgisser P. Prolonged seroconversion in an elite controller of HIV-1 infection. J Clin Virol 2009;46:371−3.

[74] Goujard C, Chaix ML, Lambotte O, Deveau C, Sinet M, Guergnon J, et al. Spontaneous control of viral replication during primary HIV infection: When is "HIV controller" status established? Clin Infect Dis 2009;49:982−6.

[75] Blankson JN, Bailey JR, Thayil S, Yang H-C, Lassen K, Lai J, et al. Isolation and characterization of replication-competent HIV-1 from a subset of elite suppressors. J Virol 2007;81:2508−18.

[76] Miura T, Brockman MA, Brumme CJ, Brumme ZL, Carlson JM, Pereyra F, et al. Genetic characterization of human immunodeficiency virus type 1 in elite controllers: Lack of gross genetic defects or common amino acid changes. J Virol 2008;82:8422−30.

[77] Leslie AJ, Pfafferott KJ, Chetty P, Draenert R, Addo MM, Feeney M, et al. HIV evolution: CTL escape mutation and reversion after transmission. Nat Med 2004;10:282−9.

[78] Martinez-Picado J, Prado JG, Fry EE, Pfafferott K, Leslie A, Chetty S, et al. Fitness cost of escape mutations in p24 Gag in association with control of human immunodeficiency virus type 1. J Virol 2006;80:3617−23.

[79] Nietfield W, Bauer M, Fevrier M, Maier R, Holzwarth B, Frank R, et al. Sequence constraints and recognition by CTL of an HLA-B27-restricted HIV-1 gag epitope. J Immunol 1995;154:2189−97.

[80] Miura T, Brumme ZL, Brockman MA, Rosato P, Sela J, Brumme CJ, et al. Impaired replication capacity of acute/early viruses in persons who become HIV controllers. J Virol 2010;84:7581−91.

[81] Martin MP, Qi Y, Gao X, Yamada E, Martin JN, Pereyra F, et al. Innate partnership of HLA-B and KIR3DL1 subtypes against HIV-1. Nat Genet 2007;39:733−40.

[82] O'Connell KA, Han Y, Williams TM, Siliciano RF, Blankson JN. Role of natural killer cells in a cohort of elite suppressors: Low frequency of the protective KIR3DS1 allele and limited inhibition of human immunodeficiency virus type 1 replication *in vitro*. J Virol 2009; 83:5028−34.

[83] Vieillard V, Fausther-Bovendo H, Samri A, Debre P. Specific phenotypic and functional features of natural killer cells from HIV-infected long-term nonprogressors and HIV controllers. J Acquir Immune Defic Syndr 2010;53:564−73.

[84] Rabi SA, O'Connell KA, Nikolaeva D, Bailey JR, Jilek BL, Shen L, et al. Unstimulated primary CD4+ T cells from HIV-1-positive elite suppressors are fully susceptible to HIV-1 entry and productive infection. J Virol 2011;85:979−86.

[85] Graf EH, Mexas AM, Yu JJ, Shaheen F, Liszewski MK, Di Mascio M, et al. Elite suppressors harbor low levels of integrated HIV DNA and high levels of 2-LTR circular HIV DNA compared to HIV+ patients on and off HAART. PLoS Pathog 2011;7:e1001300.

[86] Chen H, Li C, Huang J, Cung T, Seiss K, Beamon J, et al. CD4+ T cells from elite controllers resist HIV-1 infection by selective upregulation of p21. J Clin Invest 2011;121:1549–60.

[87] Bergamaschi A, David A, Le Rouzic E, Nisole S, Barre-Sinoussi F, Pancino G. The CDK inhibitor p21Cip1/WAF1 is induced by FcgammaR activation and restricts the replication of human immunodeficiency virus type 1 and related primate lentiviruses in human macrophages. J Virol 2009;83:12253–65.

[88] Zhang J, Scadden DT, Crumpacker CS. Primitive hematopoietic cells resist HIV-1 infection via p21. J Clin Invest 2007;117:473–81.

[89] Sáez-Cirión A, Hamimi C, Bergamaschi A, David A, Versmisse P, Melard A, et al. Restriction of HIV-1 replication in macrophages and CD4+ T cells from HIV controllers. Blood 2011;118:955–64.

[90] Vigneault F, Woods M, Buzon MJ, Li C, Pereyra F, Crosby SD, et al. Transcriptional profiling of CD4 T cells identifies distinct subgroups of HIV-1 elite controllers. J Virol 2011;85:3015–9.

[91] Madec Y, Boufassa F, Avettand-Fenoel V, Hendou S, Melard A, Boucherit S, et al. Early control of HIV-1 infection in long-term nonprogressors followed since diagnosis in the ANRS SEROCO/HEMOCO cohort. J Acquir Immune Defic Syndr 2009;50:19–26.

[92] Saez-Cirion A, Hocqueloux L, Avettand-Fenoel V, Goujard C, Prazuck T, Viard J-P, et al. For the ANRS VISCONTI Group (2011). Long-term HIV-1 control after interruption of a treatment initiated at the time of primary infection is associated to low cell-HIV DNA levels (ANRS VISCONTI Study). Abstract #515, 18th Conference on Retrovirus and Opportunistic Infections, February 27–March 2, 2011, Boston, USA.

Chapter 9

Residual Viremia and Viral Reservoirs in Elite Controllers

Robert W. Buckheit III and Joel N. Blankson

Johns Hopkins University School of Medicine, Baltimore, Maryland, USA

Chapter Outline

INTRODUCTION

Clinical outcome of HIV-1 infection varies greatly between infected individuals. Elite controllers (ECs) are HIV-1-infected individuals who maintain viral loads of less than 50 copies/ml in the absence of antiretroviral treatment. The mechanism for these patients' remarkable control of HIV-1 replication are poorly understood, and the object of debate. Initially, it was thought infection with a deficient virus could explain this clinical phenotype. Defects in key viral genes and unusual polymorphisms were documented, and hypothesized to explain elite control. However, replication-competent virus was soon after isolated from cohorts of ECs, and it rapidly became clear that infection with attenuated or defective viral strains could not exclusively account for the clinical outcome of infection. Additional studies have led to the growing

Models of Protection Against HIV/SIV. DOI: 10.1016/B978-0-12-387715-4.00009-5

appreciation for host contribution to this clinical phenotype, and provide support for the development of a therapeutic vaccine. Studies of HIV-1 transmission pairs, where a progressive patient transmits virus to an individual who subsequently develops into an EC, provide clear evidence of the importance of host factors in the clinical outcome of infection. These and other unique case studies have allowed a greater understanding of the unique strength of ECs' immune response. ECs are seen to have a lower proportion of latently infected cells, possibly as a consequence of the low magnitude of peak viremia seen in acute infection. However, continued viral evolution has been observed in residual viremia from ECs, suggesting ongoing replication continues in these patients. This indicates that even while ECs are able to maintain low viral loads, beginning early in infection, a fully pathogenic virus continues to persist in these patients at low levels. It is currently unclear whether the residual viremia seen in the plasma of ECs is due to low-level ongoing replication, or is the result of release from latently infected CD4 T cells or a novel, unidentified cellular reservoir. Elite control of HIV-1 infection may represent a tenuous balance between host and viral factors, each contributing to the clinical outcome of infection. Here we focus on viral factors that determine the clinical outcome of infection, specifically viral fitness, latency, and residual viremia in ECs. Understanding the interplay of host and viral factors, and understanding the evolution of virus from acute infection to long-term control, is important in understanding the mechanisms of elite control and how this information can be applied to a therapeutic vaccine.

VIRAL FACTORS OF ELITE CONTROL

HIV-1 infection is typically characterized by peak viral loads in acute infection. Viral replication continues at high levels in the absence of therapy, and progressive CD4 T cell decline and AIDS usually develops within 10 years after initial infection. Upon initiation of HAART therapy, viral replication is completely halted, leading to an HIV-1 viral load < 50 copies/ml, which is the limit of clinical viral load assays. A group of individuals known as long-term non-progressors (LTNPs) were identified early in the HIV-1 epidemic. These individuals are clinically defined as HIV-1-infected individuals who, in the absence of antiretroviral therapy, are able to maintain stable CD4 T cell counts exceeding 500 cells/μl for longer than 7 years. This clinical designation is based solely on CD4 T cell counts, and is independent of levels of viremia. Incredibly, a group of patients known as elite controllers (ECs) are able to control HIV-1 replication to levels below the limit of detection of standard commercial assays (< 50 copies/ml) in the absence of HAART treatment (Figure 9.1). These patients represent less than 1 percent of the HIV-1-infected population [1]. The mechanisms of elite control remain poorly understood, and the individual contributions of host and viral factors to this phenotype remain undefined. Understanding these factors could potentially contribute to the development of a therapeutic HIV-1 vaccine.

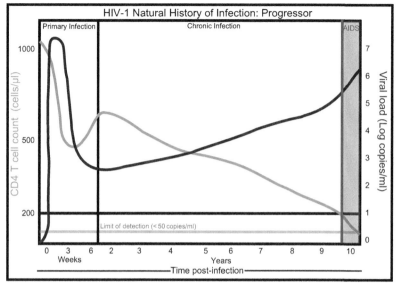

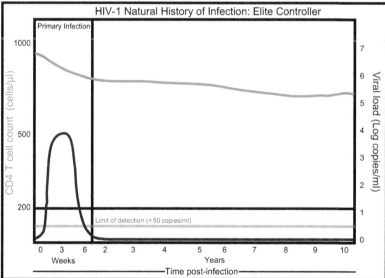

FIGURE 9.1 Comparative, representative natural histories of infection for a typical progressor and an elite controller. HIV-1 infection in a progressive patient is characterized by robust viral replication during primary infection, and a reduction in CD4 T cell counts. CD4 T cell counts recover, and viral replication declines to set-point levels which persist for the duration of chronic infection. In the absence of therapy, progressive CD4 T cell loss occurs. A patient is clinically defined as having AIDS once the CD4 T cell counts fall below 200 cells/μl, usually accompanied by an increasing viral load. Elite controllers (ECs) similarly have peak viremia in primary infection, but this has been shown to be blunted compared to progressive patients [21,22]. In the absence of therapy, the viral load falls to undetectable limits (< 50 copies/ml). No progressive CD4 T cell loss or AIDS defining symptoms occur. Utilizing ultrasensitive viral load assays, low-level viremia is still observed in many ECs [23–26].

The contribution of viral factors to the elite controller phenotype remains poorly understood, and is a much debated topic. While infection with a defective or attenuated viral strain can increase the likelihood of elite control and long-term non-progression, it is by no means the exclusive cause of control. Initial studies demonstrated the presence of gross defects in viral isolates from patients who were LTNPs and ECs, and hinted that rare, unusual polymorphisms may account for this remarkable phenotype. However, some individuals infected with similar viral isolates did not have similar clinical outcomes. Additionally, evolution of defective virus within infected hosts was still observed, indicating that the viral isolates were capable of some degree of ongoing replication. More recent studies have demonstrated that ECs and LTNPs are infected with replication-competent HIV-1, and in-depth sequence analysis of HIV-1 isolates from ECs clearly demonstrated that they are infected with pathogenic virus. Most convincingly, observational studies of transmission pairs, where both patients are infected with similar viruses, have shown remarkably different clinical outcomes of infection. This suggests the contribution of viral factors alone cannot account for elite control. Here we will discuss viral fitness, residual viremia and viral reservoirs in ECs, and how these factors influence elite control (Table 9.1). Delineating the important viral aspect of control is paramount in the development of an HIV-1 vaccine, and can guide future studies to clarify the clinical progression of HIV-1 infection.

TABLE 9.1   Viral factors of elite control

Feature	Hypothesis	Experimental evidence	Conclusions
Defective virus	Infection with defective virus leads to elite control in some patients	Deletions in *nef, vpr, vpu* are seen in some isolates amplified from ECs and LTNPs [2−7,9]	Some accessory genes may play a key role in HIV-1 pathogenesis
		Sydney Blood Bank cohort patients all progressed to either EC or LTNP phenotype [2,11]	Even with the same infecting virus, differences in clinical outcome remain
Attenuated virus	Host immune pressure induces virologic escape; escape mutants may be less fit than wild-type virus	Mutations in HLA-restricted epitopes result in diminished fitness [36,41]	Virologic escape from strong immune pressure in ECs and LTNPs may result in an attenuated phenotype
			Host-mediated immune pressure dictates viral evolution and maintains attenuated viral quasispecies

TABLE 9.1 Viral factors of elite control—cont'd

Feature	Hypothesis	Experimental evidence	Conclusions
Pathogenic virus	Some ECs are infected with fully replication-competent virus	No large deletions or frameshift insertions noted in full genome sequencing study of replication-competent virus [13] Replication-competent virus cultured from latent reservoir in ECs [14] Transmission of virus from patients with progressive disease to patients who developed elite control [40,42]	Viral defect may play a role in control in some patients, but many ECs appear to be infected with replication-competent virus
Latent reservoir	Latent reservoir is smaller in ECs than in patients on HAART	Isolation and activation of CD4 T cells from ECs resulted in reduced viral outgrowth compared to viremic controllers and progressive patients [17] Reduction in latent reservoir by 1.5 log when compared to HAART-treated patients [19]	Seeding of latent reservoir is less efficient in ECs than in patients with progressive disease
Residual viremia	ECs have residual virus in plasma	ECs and patients on HAART have similar levels of plasma viremia [23–26]	Random release from latently infected cells or ongoing replication continues in these patients
	There is ongoing viral replication and evolution in ECs	Striking discordance between proviral and plasma sequences obtained from amplification, and sequence analysis of *gag,* and *nef* and low-level evolution quantified in *pro-RT* and *env* genes [27–31]	There is ongoing viral replication in ECs; plasma virus is not solely due to simple release from the latent reservoir

EVIDENCE OF DEFECTIVE VIRUS

Early studies indicated that LTNPs and ECs were infected with defective virus, thus allowing control of viral replication. The Sydney Blood Bank cohort represents a unique group of individuals with blood-transfusion-transmitted HIV, all from the same donor between February 1981 and July 1984 [2]. Interestingly, of the seven members of the cohort, no member progressed to AIDS and none had HIV-related illness or progressive CD4 T cell decline at the time of the initial reporting. Extensive sequencing was performed, and all members were found to have been infected with an HIV-1 isolate with a large deletion in *nef* and the U3 region of the long terminal repeat region [2]. While *nef* is not required *in vitro* for viral replication, it is required for progression to AIDS in SIV models [3]. Thus, deletion of one or both of these regions was hypothesized to lead to impaired viral fitness, allowing some measure of control. Essentially, long-term control was thought be a result of a defective infecting virus [2].

Subsequently, multiple reports documented deletions and alterations in *nef* leading to a LTNP phenotype [4–6]. In one such study, HIV-1 *nef* was amplified from 5 LTNPs [4]. In the majority of patients full-length *nef* was amplified, thus defects in *nef* could not explain clinical outcome. However, in one patient all viral isolates possessed deletions in *nef* and the U3 region of LTR. Additionally, this patient was seen to have a lower viral burden compared to the other patients in the study. These data support the idea that a defect in *nef* could lead to a non-progressive phenotype, and could greatly impact viral replication [4]. Additional studies in a cohort of LTNPs showed similar findings [5,6]. The majority of patients possess intact, functional *nef*, while a single patient was observed to have a significant portion of defect *nef* alleles. In this patient, *nef* protein was dysfunctional and could not downregulate CD4 [5]. A more recent case study has also implicated deficiencies in *nef* as causal to the EC phenotype. In this study, a patient was infected for 20 years with a virus that contained a large deletion in *nef* and regions in the U3 LTR [6]. These studies highlight the consequences of *nef* deletion, but also suggest that defects in this gene alone cannot explain elite control or long-term non-progression. They also suggest that progressive evolution can continue in some patients infected with viruses containing *nef* deletions. These findings support studies in the SIV model, and reinforce the role of *nef* in the pathogenesis of HIV [4–6].

There have been reports of defects in *rev, gag-pol and vif* isolated from LTNPs, indicating that viruses harboring *nef* mutations are not solely responsible for poor viral replication in LTNPs [7–9]. In one case study, while sequence analysis of *env* from a LTNP did not reveal any large deletions, a functional assay revealed a replication deficiency was observed compared to HIV-1$_{NL4-3}$ control virus. It was shown that this defect could actually be explained by mutations in a *rev* activating domain [7]. Another study isolated virus from eight LTNPs, and *gag* and *pol* sequences were extensively characterized. While no large deletions or insertions were seen in any of the patients, it was noted that premature stop codons in *gag* and *pol* were observed in some patients. Thus, similar to other studies, some LTNPs were found to harbor genetic defects while others had no signs of unusual viral sequence [8]. A recent case study documented a unique mother-to-child transmission study in which both individuals developed a non-progressive disease course. HIV-1 isolates from both patients were found to be replication deficient, and a unique 2-amino-acid insertion in *vif* was shown to be the cause of the attenuated viral phenotype [9].

Viral defects could be present in the infecting virus, or they could be directly related to a host response which forces viral attenuation. In one study it was argued and demonstrated that ECs and LTNPs were infected with HIV-1 isolates which had rare or unusual polymorphisms in key genes, thus allowing their replication to be controlled more readily by the immune system in these patients. Replication-competent virus was isolated from eight LTNPs, and the virus subjected to full genome sequence analysis. Unusual or difficult to revert polymorphisms were identified in each of these patients, which suggests an inherent defect in infecting viruses in LTNPs [10]. It is worth noting that while HAART-treated, chronic progressors offer the best comparison in studies looking at the mechanism of elite control, they are clearly an imperfect control. In all cases, control patients have already been affected irrevocably by robust HIV-1 replication in acute and chronic infection. Thus, virus isolated from these patients also reflects this robust replication and evolution before the initiation of HAART treatment could have optimized viral fitness.

While it is clear that infection with a defective or attenuated virus may increase the likelihood of developing an EC phenotype, there is ample evidence that defective virus alone cannot predict the clinical outcome of infection. In the aforementioned Syndey Blood Bank cohort, longitudinal studies have shown that, despite being infected from a single source, the cohort is comprised of both slow progressors eventually requiring HAART treatment, and some ECs with undetectable viral loads [11]. Interestingly, viral isolates from these patients have shown progressive loss of *nef*/LTR sequence even as viral loads increased in a subset of the cohort [11]. While infection with defective *nef* initially led to the LTNP phenotype, some patients still developed progressive disease. Thus, in patients with dramatically deficient viral strains, with deletion of entire genes, HIV-1 still has the potential to mutate and evolve to increase the fitness of the virus, or to escape the host immune response. Additionally, in many of these early studies many of the LTNPs studied did not have any known viral defects as determined by sequences analysis [4,5]. Overall, these data indicate that infection with defective virus cannot be the exclusive explanation for the dramatic control of viral replication seen in LTNPs and ECs.

EVIDENCE OF REPLICATION-COMPETENT VIRUS

Key studies have since suggested that replication competent virus, without gross defects, could be isolated from ECs and LTNPs. In a study of 95 EC patients, HIV-1 clones were amplified from CD4+ T cells in 94 percent of the population, and plasma viral clones were amplified from 78 percent. No large defects were observed in sequencing analysis, and comparative phylogenetic analysis showed EC sequences were clustered with sequence from chronic progressors. No length polymorphisms were observed, and individual codon polymorphisms were shown to have no correlation with elite control. While this work was not performed on replication-competent virus, it suggested that large deletions were not present in viral isolates from ECs [12]. Actual replication-competent virus was isolated from a small cohort of ECs, utilizing a sensitive, limiting dilution co-culture assay originally used to culture virus from patients on HAART therapy [13,14]. In this method individual viruses were amplified and expanded over a period of 2 weeks, and thus only viruses with robust replicative capabilities were isolated [14]. Replication-competent virus was cultured from 4 out of 10 subjects, and in-depth genotypic and phenotypic assays were utilized to search for attenuating mutations. No large deletions, stop codons or insertions were observed when the isolates were subjected to full genome sequencing. Overall, replication levels of viral isolates from these ECs were seen to be equal to both CCR5-tropic and X4R5-tropic standard reference strains. This work indicated, for the first time, that ECs were infected with replication-competent viruses, suggesting that host factors played a large role in the control of viral replication. Other studies have supported the hypothesis that ECs are infected with replication-competent virus. In one such study, stimulation of EC CD4 T cells resulted in detection of Gag within cells [15]. Other work demonstrated that replication-competent virus could be isolated from CD4 T cells of EC after stimulation with either PHA and IL-2, or IL-7. *Vpr* and *vpu* from all recovered isolates were sequenced, and showed no evidence of insertions or deletions that could explain the clinical outcome of infection. All viral isolates had full-length *nef* [16]. Similarly, in an additional study viral outgrowth from ECs' CD4 T cells occurred rarely, but robust replication was observed, indicating replication-competent virus. In 14 ECs studied, virus was detected *in vitro* for only 3 patients after activation of EC CD4 T cells. Interestingly, in this study viral outgrowth was more frequent in HAART-treated patients and in patients with progressive disease [17].

Unique case studies have enabled a greater understanding of how viral factors relate to control of HIV-1 replication. In one study, virologic break-through was observed in an HLA-B*57-positive EC. While this patient had the attenuating M184V drug resistance mutation in RT that eventually reverted, the replication capacity of viral isolates before and after breakthrough was similar, and full genome sequence analysis suggested that escape mutations in HLA B*5701 Gag epitopes led to a loss of control. This indicates that escape from host-mediated immunologic factors played a bigger role in the loss of control than did changes in viral fitness [18].

ELITE CONTROLLERS HAVE A LOW FREQUENCY OF LATENTLY INFECTED CD4+ T CELLS

Resting CD4 T cells have been identified as the primary reservoir of HIV-1 infection in patients on HAART. These latently infected memory cells are long-lived, and represent a barrier to the eradication of HIV-1 with current treatment strategies [19]. Briefly, latency is established early in infection, when active CD4 T cells are infected and then revert to a resting state. As well as being long-lived, these cells are quiescent and indistinguishable from non-infected, resting CD4 T cells. Interestingly, LTNPs and ECs have a reduced number of latently infected CD4 T cells with integrated provirus. Studies have shown that ECs have very low frequencies of CD4+ T cells that contain HIV DNA [20], and infrequent recovery of replication-competent HIV from EC latent reservoir has been observed [13,17]. In one study the median frequency of replication-competent virus in ECs was found to be 0.2 IUPM in the latent reservoir in resting CD4 T cells, a 1.5-log lower average value than in patients on HAART therapy [13]. ECs have been shown to have a blunted peak viremia during acute infection [21,22], and it is reasonable to assume that reduced replication would result in a reduced seeding of the latent reservoir. The mechanisms for this blunted peak viremia are currently unclear, but this rapid control of viral replication suggests that innate immune effectors may play some role.

ELITE CONTROLLERS HAVE PLASMA LEVELS OF VIREMIA THAT ARE SIMILAR TO PATIENTS ON HAART

To further the understanding of latency in ECs, multiple studies utilized ultrasensitive viral load assays to analyze residual viremia in these subjects. This distinction is what was originally used to clinically define an EC. ECs were originally seen to have viral loads below the limit of detection by standard clinical assays, meaning residual viremia of below 50 copies/ml. While ECs are defined as having "undetectable" viral loads by standard clinical assays, the development of ultrasensitive assays has allowed a deeper understanding of viral replication in these patients. Multiple studies have shown that ECs actually maintain extremely low levels of residual viremia ($<$ 50 copies/ml). The implications of this low-level viral production and its impact on the infected individual are currently poorly understood. All current studies to date have shown that the majority of ECs maintain extremely low levels of residual viremia that are approximately equal to the levels of viremia seen in HAART-treated patients [23–26]. This is in contrast to the latent reservoir in these patients, which is much smaller than that seen in patients on HAART. In a large cohort study analyzing viral load in ECs, 70 percent of ECs had some detectable low-level viremia, with a median value of two copies/ml [24]. This viremia was seen to fluctuate over time, as has been seen in other studies [24,25]. The source of this viremia is currently unknown, but could either be a result of random release from the latent reservoir or represent ongoing viral replication. Identifying the nature and source of this low-level circulating virus is important in understanding the nature of elite control and evolution of virus in ECs.

EVIDENCE OF VIRAL EVOLUTION IN ELITE CONTROLLERS

The relationship between immune pressure and residual viremia, specifically viral evolution within ECs, can provide insights into the nature of host control of replication, potentially forming the basis for an HIV-1 vaccine. Central to this understanding is answering whether ECs have ongoing rounds of infection, how their viruses respond to immune pressure, and what effect escape mutations have on viral fitness. Here we will focus on those viral factors important to this relationship, while immune parameters will be discussed elsewhere.

Initial evidence showed discordance between *gag* plasma viral sequences and sequences from archived provirus in resting CD4 T cells from HLA-B*57-positive ECs. Utilizing a sensitive RT-PCR assay, near full-length *gag* was amplified and sequenced from both proviral and plasma virons. This allows both an in-depth look at evolution in *gag* epitopes, and a comparison between proviral and plasma virons (Figure 9.1). This work showed evidence of low-level viremia present in ECs, and discordance between those virons seen in the plasma and those in provirus. All plasma viral clones amplified had mutations in HLA-B*57-restricted epitopes, indicating that evolution was occurring in these epitopes in response to selective pressure from cytotoxic T lymphocytes (CTLs). In contrast, almost all proviral clones were wild-type, indicating that patients were not infected with viruses containing escape mutations. Interestingly, even though mutations were present in these *gag*-restricted epitopes, there was no virologic breakthrough. Since a lower frequency of escape mutants was seen in proviral clones, it was argued that plasma virus was not reseeding the latent reservoir to a significant degree [27]. Utilizing the same sensitive RT-PCR based assay, full-length *nef* sequences were analyzed phylogenetically. A similar discordance between plasma and proviral sequences was seen. Some but not all of the mutations seen in *nef* were seen to be escape mutations from host CTL response. These data provide further evidence of ongoing replication in ECs. Like the previous study, the development of escape mutations in *nef* was not associated with virologic breakthrough [28]. Potentially, mutations which mediate escape from the host immune response result in a reduced viral fitness which could prevent robust replication.

Recent studies have provided evidence of viral evolution in chronic infection in ECs. In a 5-year longitudinal study of HLA-B*57- and/or HLA-B*27-positive ECs, clonal *gag* sequences were amplified from resting CD4+ T cells and plasma. Phylogenetic analysis showed clear evidence of evolution in the plasma viruses, but not in the proviral sequence amplified from resting CD4+ T cells. Furthermore, the proviral clones clustered together and were ancestral to the plasma clones, suggesting that virus in this compartment represented isolates that had been archived in the latent reservoir. As described above, the plasma virus has evidence of evolution in response to selective pressure from HIV-specific CTLs. After this initial evolution occurs, there is continued low-level ongoing replication, as demonstrated by the accumulation of synonymous mutations in *gag* in plasma virus over time [29]. A companion study similarly analyzed temporal evolution in plasma *nef* in the same patient population in chronic infection, and similar results were obtained. One again, proviral clones were found to be ancestral to plasma clones and evolution occurred in plasma virus over time, as evidenced by the accumulation of non synonymous mutations [30]. Overall, both studies suggest that low-level ongoing replication is occurring in ECs, but there is little reseeding of the latent reservoir in these patients, as seen by the discordance in plasma and proviral sequences [29,30] (Figure 9.2).

Another study has demonstrated evidence of evolution in *pro-RT* and *env* in ECs. Twenty-one HIV-1 ECs were enrolled, and all had low-level viremia as documented by the single copy assay. Clonal isolates of *pro-RT* and *env* were sequenced for 18 out of 21 patients, and analyzed by phylogenetic analysis. Evidence for ongoing replication was confirmed in the majority of ECs in this study, due to increasing viral diversity over time. Evolution was observed in patients both with and without protective HLA allele types [31]. Taken together, these results suggest that after initial escape from host immune responses, possibly in acute infection, ongoing replication continues, but there is little evidence of non-synonymous mutations as equilibrium between immune evasion and viral fitness is achieved [25,30]. This may explain why there is reduced env diversity in EC proviral and plasma isolates compared to isolates from HAART patients and chronic progressors [32].

ATTENUATED PLASMA VIRUS; CAUSE OR EFFECT OF ELITE CONTROL?

Other studies have shown that gag, pol and env isolated from the plasma of ECs have reduced replication capacity when compared to virus from patients with progressive disease [33,34]. In one such study, recombinant viruses were engineered which contained RT and integrase sequences from 58 elite controllers and also from 50 progressors. The replicative fitness of recombinant EC pseudotyped viruses was seen to be reduced compared to recombinant virus containing pol genes from patients with progressive disease and to the wild-type HIV-1$_{NL4-3}$ reference strain [33]. A similar study looking at Gag fitness was recently performed. In this study plasma *gag-protease* clones from 54 ECs and 41 progressive patients were inserted into HIV-1$_{NL4-3}$ backbone, and

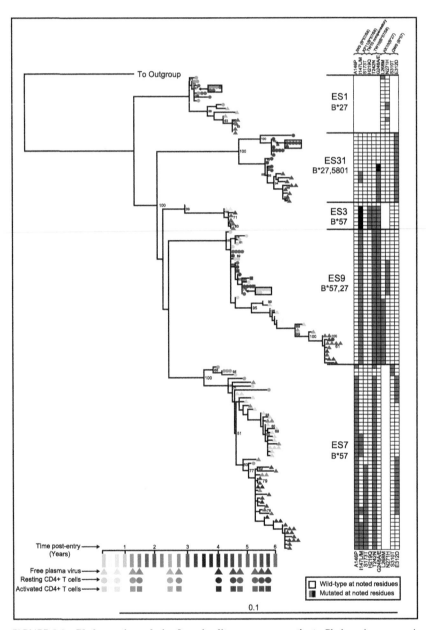

FIGURE 9.2   Phylogenetic analysis of *gag* in elite suppressor patients. Phylogenies were estimated by using a classical approach, functioning under a maximum-likelihood (ML) optimality criterion. All sequences are clonal, and APOBEC-mediated hypermutated sequences were removed from analysis. Bootstrap values of 50 and higher are displayed. Protective HLA B alleles are noted beneath the patient number. Patients are not related in any way, but are placed on the same tree for display purposes. Colors indicate time, with the scale below in years. Triangles represent clonal

replicative fitness was compared. It was seen that clones from ECs were less fit than those from progressive patients. Additionally, mutations in epitopes restricted by protective HLA alleles were correlated with viral fitness. These data suggest attenuation in plasma viral isolates from ECs, but it is unclear whether this attenuation explains clinical outcome, or whether it is a result of the strong CTL response in ECs [34]. Another study looking at early HIV-1 infection showed that plasma gag-protease clones from patients who had viral loads of < 2,000 copies/ml were less fit and more likely to have drug resistance and escape mutations than clones from patients with progressive disease [35]. Finally, plasma *env* clones from ECs were found to be less efficient at entry into a cell line than plasma *env* clones from patients with progressive disease [36]. It is important to note that in each of these studies only individual genes were isolated and inserted into a reference backbone strain; thus only the fitness of individual genes could be assayed, as opposed to the overall fitness of infecting viruses in ECs. It should also be noted that plasma clones from ECs have been subjected to selective pressure and have evolved significantly, as previously described. Thus, plasma clones are probably not representative of the virus ECs were infected with, and the observed attenuated phenotype may therefore very well be an effect rather than the cause of elite control.

This is best highlighted by the *gag* gene in HLA-B*57-positive ECs. Gag T242N, a well-studied CTL escape mutation in an epitope restricted by HLA-B*57, is associated with a significant fitness cost. Reversion to wild-type virus occurs when virus with this mutation is transmitted to HLA-B*57-negative patients. As described earlier, T242N and other similar mutants are found in virtually every plasma clone amplified from ECs, but are rare in proviral clones. It thus appears likely that ECs were infected with wild-type virus which does not contain these attenuating escape mutations. It should also be noted that studies that have sequence provirus from ECs have not reported a high incidence of drug resistance mutations [12,13], so viral attenuation caused by these mutations is likely not a common cause of elite control.

Furthermore, as discussed above, the rate of viral evolution is significantly lower in ECs than in patients with progressive disease. In chronic infection synonymous mutations predominate in ECs, whereas non-synonymous mutations are seen in patients with progressive disease [37]. It thus follows that virus evolves over time towards increased fitness in patients with progressive disease, which could explain why these patients are more likely to have compensatory mutations [37] that restore the fitness of T242N mutants. Similarly, it has been shown that *env* in patients with progressive disease evolves to a state where it is

---

plasma sequences, squares represent proviral sequences from HLA-DR+ CD4+ T cells, and circles represent clonal proviral sequences from HLA-DR− CD4+ T cells. To the right, escape mutations in HLA-B*57- and -B*27-restricted epitopes are denoted in black or gray and aligned with the appropriate symbol on the tree. Escape mutations are listed above the grid, with the epitopes in which the mutations occurred listed above the mutations. *Reproduced from O'Connell et al., 2010 [29]* (J.Virol., 4, 7018–7028, 2010), with permission. Copyright ©American Society for Microbiology.

more efficient at viral entry than clones present in primary infection [38]. Cross-sectional studies that compare virus from chronic infection in ECs to patients with progressive disease would thus be comparing virus that has undergone limited evolution, to virus that has evolved over many years of uncontrolled replication. In fact, in one study it was shown that virus isolated from both HLA-B*57-positive LTNPs and chronic progressors (CPs) in primary infection had poor replication capacity. Virus from CPs, however, became progressively more fit over time, whereas virus from LTNPS did not [39]. This strongly suggests that the diminished fitness seen in many studies may be an effect rather than a cause of elite control, and the amount of viral evolution that occurs has a major impact on viral fitness.

CLUES FROM TRANSMISSION PAIRS

Due to the difficult nature of working with human subjects, where ideal experimental situations are often not possible, it is hard to discern the mechanism of viral control. It is probable that host, viral and environmental factors, in complex association, all play some role in control. However, true causality is hard to define, and difficult to discern experimentally. By exploiting unique clinical situations, researchers have been able to glean important evidence regarding the nature of elite control. Situations where progressive patients transmit virus to patients capable of elite control offer insightful snapshots into the mechanism of host control. These aptly named transmission pairs reduce confounding factors and answer the question: if the infecting virus is the same, or extremely similar, how do ECs suppress viral replication when other patients cannot?

The first documented transmission pair was confirmed by phylogenetics and by sequence analysis [40]. Rare polymorphisms were present in both the transmitter's and the recipient's virus, present in less than 1 percent of clade B isolated in the Los Alamos HIV Sequence Database, indicating the close similarity between the viruses. However, it was seen that viral isolates from the EC were attenuated when compared to the progressive patient's virus. Both patients were HLA-B*57 positive, and contained the Gag T242N mutation which has been shown to infer a reduction in viral fitness [41]. However, only the progressor had compensatory mutations which restored viral fitness, thus potentially explaining the viral attenuation seen in the EC's viral isolates. Furthermore, a novel escape mutation in the immunodominant Gag KK 10 HLA-B*27-restricted epitope was also shown to affect viral fitness in the EC, who was also HLA-B*27 positive. Given these data, it was suggested that ECs control viral isolates both by a potent CTL response which limits viral evolution, and through the maintenance of viral isolates with attenuating escape mutations. Through both of these mechanisms, it was hypothesized that the EC in this transmission pair was able to control a viral isolate that was pathogenic enough to cause progressive disease in the other patient. Therefore, in this study the EC virus's lower replication capacity was the result of elite control, and not the cause [40].

Unpublished data show evidence of a second transmission pair, where an LTNP, with detectable viral loads, transmitted virus to an individual able to maintain elite control. Virus isolated from each patient has been shown to have attenuated replication kinetics, but the cause of viral deficiency is currently unknown. While attenuating virus is clearly the root cause of control, individual host factors are still playing some role in the differing clinical outcome of infection [42]. In contrast to both of these transmission pairs, there is evidence for transmission pairs where viral strains infecting each patient are equally fit, and replicate as well as laboratory reference strains. Even in these cases, the EC is able to control the replication of the fully pathogenic virus while their partner progresses (unpublished data). The mechanism of host control is currently unknown in these pairs, but in one case the EC was HLA-B*57 positive, suggesting a role for CD8+ T cell mediated control of viral replication. Thus, looking at these three case studies we see clear evidence of CTL-induced viral attenuation, as well as host-mediated suppression of viral replication in the absence of attenuation. Additionally, a transmission pair where both patients were infected with a defective virus argues that viral deficiencies can still play some role in the EC phenotype. Thus, a clear picture of a balance of host and viral factors is clearly demonstrated, in which the individual contributions of these factors dictate clinical progression. Studies of other transmission pairs are crucial to elucidate new information on the nature of elite control.

Studies of transmission pairs provide a picture of the varying nature, and possibly different mechanisms, of host control of viral replication. While infection with attenuating virus clearly can increase the probability of being able to control replication to some degree, it has become evident that many ECs are infected with replication-competent virus. In fact, some ECs have been shown to have virus which is able to cause progressive disease in other individuals. Initially seen in small cohort studies, this hypothesis has since been confirmed in a large number of patients. It is clear that ECs maintain low levels of viral replication, and limited evolution characterized by synonymous mutations is observed in plasma viral isolates. Further research will be needed to determine whether virus seen in the plasma is from the latent reservoir of resting CD4 T cells or from some other novel reservoir. It is therefore appropriate to view elite control as a tentative balance between viral replication and host control. Thus, varying viral and host factors can tip the balance in either direction. The remarkable degree to which ECs are able to suppress viral replication provides hope for a therapeutic HIV-1 vaccine aimed at tipping this balance in favor of immune control.

CLINICAL IMPLICATIONS

The fact that some ECs harbor fully replication-competent virus suggests that a therapeutic vaccine may be a feasible goal if we fully understand which host factors are responsible for the control of viral replication.

CONCLUSIONS

While some ECs have defective virus, others have fully replication-competent virus that is controlled by host factors. There is compartmentalization of virus in these patients, with provirus typically containing wild-type ancestral viral clones that may have been archived during primary infection, whereas plasma virus has been subjected to selective pressure from CD8+T cells and contains escape mutations. Low-level evolution consisting of the accumulation of synonymous mutations continues in plasma virus but not provirus during chronic infection as an equilibrium between viral fitness and immunologic escape is achieved.

Main Points

1. Some ECs may be infected with defective or attenuated HIV-1 isolates.
2. Many ECs appear to harbor fully replication-competent HIV-1 isolates in their latent reservoir.
3. The latent reservoir in ECs is much smaller than that found in patients with progressive disease on HAART, whereas the amount of residual plasma viremia is similar in the two groups of patients.
4. Attenuated plasma viral clones may be an effect rather than the cause of elite control.

REFERENCES

[1] Ockulicz J, Lambotte O. Epidemiology and clinical characteristics of elite controllers. Curr Opin HIV AIDS 2011, in press.
[2] Deacon NJ, Tsykin A, Solomon A, Smith K, Ludford-Menting M, Hooker D, et al. Genomic structure of an attenuated quasi species of HIV-1 from a blood transfusion donor and recipients. Science 1995;270:891−988.
[3] Kestler III HW, Ringler DJ, Mori K, Panicali DL, Sehgal PK, Daniel MD, et al. Importance of the *nef* gene for maintenance of high virus loads and for development of AIDS. Cell 1991;65:651−62.
[4] Calugi G, Montella F, Favalli C, Benedetto A. Entire genome of a strain of human immunodeficiency virus type 1 with a deletion of nef that was recovered 20 years after primary infection: Large pool of proviruses with deletions of env. J Virol 2006;80:11892−6.
[5] Mariani R, Kirchhoff F, Greenough TC, Sullivan JL, Desrosiers RC, Skowronski J. High frequency of defective *nef* alleles in a long-term survivor with nonprogressive human immunodeficiency virus type 1 infection. J Virol 1996;70:7752−64.
[6] Kirchhoff F, Greenough TC, Brettler DB, Sullivan JL, Desrosiers RC. Brief report: Absence of intact nef sequences in a long-term survivor with nonprogressive HIV-1 infection. N Engl J Med 1995;332:228−32.
[7] Iversen AK, Shpaer EG, Rodrigo AG, Hirsch MS, Walker BD, Sheppard HW, et al. Persistence of attenuated rev genes in a human immunodeficiency virus type 1-infected asymptomatic individual. J Virol 69:5743−53.

[8] Huang Y, Zhang L, Ho DD. Characterization of gag and pol sequences from long-term survivors of human immunodeficiency virus type 1 infection. Virology 1998;240:36−49.

[9] Alexander L, Aquino-DeJesus MJ, Chan M, Andiman WA. Inhibition of human immuno-deficiency virus type 1 (HIV-1) replication by a two-amino-acid insertion in HIV-1 Vif from a nonprogressing mother and child. J Virol 2002;76:10533−9.

[10] Alexander L, Weiskopf E, Greenough TC, Gaddis NC, Auerbach MR, Malim MH, et al. Unusual polymorphisms in human immunodeficiency virus type 1 associated with nonpro-gressive infection. J Virol 2000;74:4361−76.

[11] Churchill MJ, Rhodes DI, Learmont JC, Sullivan JS, Wesselingh SL, Cooke IR, et al. Longitudinal analysis of human immunodeficiency virus type 1 nef/long terminal repeat sequences in a cohort of long-term survivors infected from a single source. J Virol 2006;80:1047−52.

[12] Miura T, Brockman MA, Brumme CJ, Brumme ZL, Carlson JM, Pereyra F, et al. Genetic characterization of human immunodeficiency virus type 1 in elite controllers: Lack of gross genetic defects or common amino acid changes. J Virol 2008;82: 8422−30.

[13] Blankson JN, Bailey JR, Thayil S, Yang HC, Lassen K, Lai J, et al. Isolation and charac-terization of replication-competent human immunodeficiency virus type 1 from a subset of elite suppressors. J Virol 2007;81:2508−18.

[14] Siliciano JD, Siliciano RF. Enhanced culture assay for detection and quantitation of latently infected, resting CD4+ T-cells carrying replication-competent virus in HIV-1-infected individuals. Methods Mol Biol 2005;304:3−15.

[15] Migueles SA, Laborico AC, Imamichi H, Shupert WL, Royce C, McLaughlin M, et al. The differential ability of HLA B*5701+ long-term nonprogressors and progressors to restrict human immunodeficiency virus replication is not caused by loss of recognition of autologous viral gag sequences. J Virol 2003;77:6889−98.

[16] Lamine A, Caumont-Sarcos A, Chaix ML, Saez-Cirion A, Rouzioux C, Delfraissy JF, et al. Replication-competent HIV strains infect HIV controllers despite undetectable viremia (ANRS EP36 study). AIDS 2007;21:1043−5.

[17] Julg B, Pereyra F, Buzón MJ, Piechocka-Trocha A, Clark MJ, Baker BM, et al. Infrequent recovery of HIV from but robust exogenous infection of activated CD4(+) T cells in HIV elite controllers. Clin Infect Dis 2010;51:233−8.

[18] Bailey JR, Zhang H, Wegweiser BW, Yang HC, Herrera L, Ahonkhai A, et al. Evolution of HIV-1 in an HLA-B*57-positive patient during virologic escape. J Infect Dis 2007;196:50−5.

[19] Finzi D, Hermankova M, Pierson T, Carruth LM, Buck C, Chaisson RE, et al. Identification of a reservoir for HIV-1 in patients on highly active antiretroviral therapy. Science 1997;278:1295−300.

[20] Lambotte O, Boufassa F, Madec Y, Nguyen A, Goujard C, Meyer L, et al. SEROCO-HEMOCO Study Group, HIV controllers: A homogeneous group of HIV-1-infected patients with spontaneous control of viral replication. Clin Infect Dis 2005;41:1053−6.

[21] Goujard C, Chaix ML, Lambotte O, Deveau C, Sinet M, Guergnon J, et al. Agence Nationale de Recherche sur le Sida PRIMO Study Group., Spontaneous control of viral replication during primary HIV infection: When is "HIV controller" status established? Clin Infect Dis 2009;49:982−6.

[22] Altfeld M, Addo MM, Rosenberg ES, Hecht FM, Lee PK, Vogel M, et al. Influence of HLA-B57 on clinical presentation and viral control during acute HIV-1 infection. AIDS 2003;17:2581−91.

[23] Hatano H, Delwart EL, Norris PJ, Lee TH, Dunn-Williams J, Hunt PW, et al. Evidence for persistent low-level viremia in individuals who control human immunodeficiency virus in the absence of antiretroviral therapy. J Virol 2009;83:329−35.

[24] Pereyra F, Palmer S, Miura T, Block BL, Wiegand A, Rothchild AC, et al. Persistent low-level viremia in HIV-1 elite controllers and relationship to immunologic parameters. J Infect Dis 2009;200:984−90.

[25] Dinoso JB, Kim SY, Siliciano RF, Blankson JN. A comparison of viral loads between HIV-1-infected elite suppressors and individuals who receive suppressive highly active antiretroviral therapy. Clin Infect Dis 2008;47:102−4.

[26] Migueles SA, Osborne CM, Royce C, Compton AA, Joshi RP, Weeks KA, et al. Lytic granule loading of CD8+ T cells is required for HIV-infected cell elimination associated with immune control. Immunity 2008;29:1009−21.

[27] Bailey JR, Williams TM, Siliciano RF, Blankson JN. Maintenance of viral suppression in HIV-1-infected HLA-B*57+ elite suppressors despite CTL escape mutations. J Exp Med 2006;203:1357−69.

[28] Bailey JR, Brennan TP, O'Connell KA, Siliciano RF, Blankson JN. Evidence of CD8+ T-cell-mediated selective pressure on human immunodeficiency virus type 1 nef in HLA-B*57+ elite suppressors. J Virol 2009;83:88−97.

[29] O'Connell KA, Brennan TP, Bailey JR, Ray SC, Siliciano RF, Blankson JN. Control of HIV-1 in elite suppressors despite ongoing replication and evolution in plasma virus. J Virol 2010;84:7018−28.

[30] Salgado M, Brennan TP, O'Connell KA, Bailey JR, Ray SC, Siliciano RF, et al. Evolution of the HIV-1 nef gene in HLA-B*57 positive elite suppressors. Retrovirology 2010;7:94.

[31] Mens H, Kearney M, Wiegand A, Shao W, Schønning K, Gerstoft J, et al. HIV-1 continues to replicate and evolve in patients with natural control of HIV infection. J Virol 2010;84:12971−81.

[32] Bailey JR, Lassen KG, Yang HC, Quinn TC, Ray SC, Blankson JN, et al. Neutralizing antibodies do not mediate suppression of human immunodeficiency virus type 1 in elite suppressors or selection of plasma virus variants in patients on highly active antiretroviral therapy. J Virol 2006;80:4758−70.

[33] Brumme ZL, Li C, Miura T, Sela J, Rosato PC, Brumme CJ, et al. Reduced replication capacity of NL4-3 recombinant viruses encoding reverse transcriptase-integrase sequences from HIV-1 elite controllers. J Acquir Immune Defic Syndr 2011;56:100−8.

[34] Miura T, Brockman MA, Brumme ZL, Brumme CJ, Pereyra F, Trocha A, et al. HLA-associated alterations in replication capacity of chimeric NL4-3 viruses carrying gag-protease from elite controllers of human immunodeficiency virus type 1. J Virol 2009;83:140−9.

[35] Miura T, Brumme ZL, Brockman MA, Rosato P, Sela J, Brumme CJ, et al. Impaired replication capacity of acute/early viruses in persons who become HIV controllers. J Virol 2010;84:7581−91.

[36] Lassen KG, Lobritz MA, Bailey JR, Johnston S, Nguyen S, Lee B, et al. Elite suppressor-derived HIV-1 envelope glycoproteins exhibit reduced entry efficiency and kinetics. PLoS Pathog 2009;5:e1000377.

[37] Schneidewind A, Brockman MA, Yang R, Adam RI, Li B, Le Gall S, et al. Escape from the dominant HLA-B27-restricted cytotoxic T-lymphocyte response in Gag is associated with a dramatic reduction in human immunodeficiency virus type 1 replication. J Virol 2007;81:12382−93.

[38] Etemad B, Fellows A, Kwambana B, Kamat A, Feng Y, Lee S, et al. Human immunodeficiency virus type 1 V1-to-V5 envelope variants from the chronic phase of infection use CCR5 and fuse more efficiently than those from early after infection. J Virol 2009;83:9694—708.

[39] Navis M, Schellens I, van Baarle D, Borghans J, van Swieten P, Miedema F, et al. Viral replication capacity as a correlate of HLA B57/B5801-associated nonprogressive HIV-1 infection. J Immunol 2007;179:3133—43.

[40] Bailey JR, O'Connell K, Yang HC, Han Y, Xu J, Jilek B, et al. Transmission of human immunodeficiency virus type 1 from a patient who developed AIDS to an elite suppressor. J Virol 2008;82:7395—410.

[41] Martinez-Picado J, Prado JG, Fry EE, Pfafferott K, Leslie A, Chetty S, et al. Fitness cost of escape mutations in p24 Gag in association with control of human immunodeficiency virus type 1. J Virol 2006;80:3617—23.

[42] Buckheit RW III, Sexauer S, Cofrancesco Jr J, Apuzzo LG, Margolick JB, Siliciano RF, Blankson JN. Transmission of human immunodeficiency type 1 from a long-term non-progressor to an elite suppressor. Conference on Retroviruses and Opportunistic Infections. Abstract, 2011, in press.

Chapter 10

Immune Responses Associated to Viral Control

Florencia Pereyra and Bruce D. Walker

Ragon Institute of MGH, MIT & Harvard, Massachusetts General Hospital—East Campus, Charlestown, Massachusetts, USA

Chapter Outline

INTRODUCTION

Although enormous knowledge has been created by the study of HIV-infected persons, and the key role of viral load [1,2] and CD4 counts [3] in disease progression has been defined, the precise immune responses that govern outcome have remained largely elusive. Nowhere is this more a puzzle than among those who remain well without treatment despite having been infected, in some cases for more than three decades [4]. In this chapter, we will review what is known (Table 10.1) and the critical gaps in knowledge and interpretation related to adaptive and innate immune responses in HIV controllers.

For the purposes of this review, we will consider HIV controllers by a simple albeit limited definition that involves only viral load, considering HIV controllers to be those who have maintained viral loads of less than 2,000 copies/ml for at least a year of observation [5]. The use of this functional definition is based on population studies that demonstrate a marked decrease in the likelihood of not

Models of Protection Against HIV/SIV. DOI: 10.1016/B978-0-12-387715-4.00010-1

TABLE 10.1   Immune responses associated with durable viral control

Immune correlate	Type of response	Reference
Targeting of conserved group-specific antigen (*Gag*) epitopes	CD8+ T cell	5, 17, 18
Expression of central/effector memory phenotype	CD8+ T cell	31
Cell proliferation upon stimulation	CD8+ T cell CD4+ T cell	49, 51, 56
Polyfunctionality (*defined by secretion of multiple cytokines*)	CD8+ T cell	41
Killing capacity, perforin and granzyme	CD8+ T cell	34, 46, 47, 53, 54
Inhibition of HIV replication (*in vitro*)	CD8+ T cell	18
Targeting of vulnerable areas of the HIV proteome (*where mutations have a high fitness cost*)	CD8+ T cell	24, 39, 40
Maintenance and enhanced effective CD8 T cell responses	CD4+ T helper cells CD4+ IL-21+ cells	61, 75
Cytolyis	CD4+ T cells	72
Cytotoxicity	KIR3DL1[pos] NK cells and Bw04 ligand	98
Inhibition of HIV replication (*in vitro*)	KIR3DS1[pos] NK cells and Bw04 ligand	95, 96
Antibody-dependent cellular cytotoxicity	NK cells via Fc receptor and ADCC inducing Ab	86, 102
Autologous Ab neutralization	B cells and NAb	87

only transmission but also disease progression [6,7]. Indeed, the recent HPTN trial results further support viral load as a critical parameter in transmission, with a 96 percent reduction in transmission among those on antiretroviral therapy in a randomized trial of discordant couples (http://www.hptn.org/web%20documents/PressReleases/HPTN052PressReleaseFINAL5_12_118am.pdf).

In this review, we will also attempt to define the current state of knowledge as to the actual mechanisms by which each of these immune responses may be playing a role, and the immune dysregulation that impairs effective functioning.

CD8 T CELL IMMUNE RESPONSES

Of the many adaptive immune responses generated in viral infections, and the extensive interplay among them, the overwhelming majority of data suggest that HIV-specific CD8 T cells play the major role in modulating viral load. Historically, the strongest association has been between specific HLA class I alleles and disease progression [8]. Although this suggests a role for the most proximate interacting ligand, namely virus-specific CD8 T cells, the association alone could also be due to the impact of class I on cells of the innate immune system [9,10]. However, a recent genome-wide association study, coupled to inferred sequencing of the HLA class I alleles, shows that the major genetic determinants of viral control involve amino acids lining the HLA-B peptide binding groove, together with a single-nucleotide polymorphism (SNP) that is associated with HLA-C expression levels [11,12] (see Chapter 12). This study, the result of a collaborative international effort involving hundreds of investigators and laboratories, extends prior studies of genetic association with viral load [13,14] by showing that the physicochemical properties of viral peptide binding in the class I binding groove account for the signal that had previously been linked to certain protective (B*27, B*57 and others) and risk (B*35, B*07 and other) alleles, and shows that the same amino acid positions, depending on their composition, account for both protective and risk associations with viral load. It is important to note, however, that some persons who control HIV replication without the need for antiviral therapy do so without the presence of any detectable CTL responses [15], underscoring the fact that this response, at least as measured by IFN-γ Elispot, is not a requirement for spontaneous control. Moreover, to the extent that they are important, the challenge at this time is to define the functional correlates of CD8 T cells. As more studies are conducted on persons with controlled *versus* progressive infection, those parameters are beginning to be defined, but suffice it to say that we still lack an immunologic measurement that is highly predictive of viral load.

Immunodominance

There are now numerous studies that show an association between targeting of Gag by HIV-specific CD8 T cells and viral control, and a similar association has been observed in HIV controllers [5,16–19]. More specifically, the depletion of Gag specific CD8 T cell responses strongly affects the suppressive activity of these cells on *in vitro* assays [20].

The most conclusive evidence that specific epitopes targeted by the CTL response matters comes from the study of persons expressing HLA B*27, in whom targeting of a single B*27-restricted 10-amino-acid epitope in Gag termed KK10 is associated with lower viral load, and escape from this response is associated with higher viral load and disease progression [21], remarkably suggesting that even a single specificity can be sufficient for immune control.

It may not only be targeting of Gag that is important, but also the relative targeting of this protein compared to others. Preferential targeting of Gag is seen in HIV controllers [5], and other studies have shown that broader Env-specific responses are associated with higher viral loads [17]. However, attempts to link specific epitopic responses to viral control on a population level have thus far not revealed a clear association [22,23]. Also, targeting of specific regions that are critical to virus viability may be a key factor in prolonged immune control [24].

Comprehensive studies of targeting have all relied on the use of IFN-γ Elispot assay as a read-out, but this assay has multiple limitations. Whereas it may be the preferred way to define what is immunogenic, it does not address T cell function [25−27], reflect critical steps in antigen processing [28] or represent physiologic expression of peptide epitopes on the cell surface, and it can only be an approximation of responses to autologous virus since in almost all cases reference strains of HIV are used, rather than peptide representing autologous virus [29,30]. Indeed, IFN-γ is the last cytokine to be lost on the way to T cell exhaustion.

Animal models suggest that patterns of immunodominance, as well as maintenance of HIV specific effector memory T cells responses [31], may impact AIDS virus control, but defining what is important has been difficult. Indeed, comprehensive analysis of immunodominance in elite controllers has revealed no significant differences in persons of a given HLA type who control viremia or progress to disease [32,33]. It is important to note that the true breadth of responses to HIV in HIV controllers remains unknown, since all assays to date have relied on targeting of a reference strain of virus. Indeed, studies suggest that the breadth of responses may be much greater than initially indicated, as targeting of autologous virus is associated with up to 30 percent increases in targeted epitopes in the limited studies reported thus far [29,30]. Also, although some studies have used *in vitro* stimulation and expansion to measure CD8 T cell function [34], comprehensive examination of the true memory cell populations in elite controllers has not been performed. Moreover, studies have shown that dendritic cells have unique antigen-presenting properties in HIV controllers, and allow for a highly-efficient generation of memory-like T cell responses, while simultaneously secreting diminished amounts of pro-inflammatory cytokines. These extraordinary functional characteristics appear to be mediated and maintained by a selective upregulation of two immunoregulatory receptors from the leukocyte immunoglobulin-like receptor family [35], and they underscore the potential role that memory T cell responses play in HIV control.

Finally, a major way in which immunodominance may impact CD8 T cell mediated control is through the induction of fitness-impairing mutations. In fact, in studies comparing cell-associated provirus and plasma viral sequences of HIV controllers, powerful immune selection pressure in B*57 Gag restricted epitopes and Nef sequences has been demonstrated, some of these being associated with novel responses targeting the plasma viral variants [36,37] (see Chapter 9). Just as partial drug selection pressure can lead to viral mutations and resistance, so can partial immune selection pressure lead to mutations that allow for escape from detection of these responses, but at the same time can impair viral fitness, thus conferring an overall advantage [38–40]. Thus any analysis of immune selection pressure also needs to assess the impact on viral replication capacity and induction of immune responses against epitopes with escape mutations.

Magnitude

The magnitude of HIV responses, as measured by overlapping peptides spanning the entire viral proteome, is similar in persons with chronic progressive disease and in persons with controlled infection [23]. Moreover, despite a strong association between Gag targeting and viral load, the absolute magnitude of Gag responses in HIV controllers is actually lower than in persons with progressive infection [5], likely because the IFN-γ Elispot assay used measures effector memory rather than central memory cells, and the former are stimulated to expand in the presence of ongoing antigenemia [5]. Since these studies measure effector cell responses, which are driven by antigen exposure, rather than central memory cells, they may be expected to be lower in persons who control HIV spontaneously, as has been reported [5]. Interestingly, in studies that measured HLA-restricted epitope-specific Gag immune responses, the magnitude of the responses was higher in HIV controllers than in viremic patients [20]. The extent to which responses restricted by protective HLA alleles contribute to this difference is not known.

Although the observed discrepancy suggests that the use of overlapping peptides underestimates the true magnitude of the Gag response, other qualitative differences in immune responses might not be differentiated based on IFN-γ production.

Polyfunctionality

The ability of cells to secrete multiple cytokines has become an area of intense interest, with polyfunctionality defined as the ability to simultaneously secrete multiple cytokines. Betts and colleagues assessed antigen-specific secretion of five different cytokines, including IFN-γ, TNF-α, MIP-1 β, CD107a and IL-2, and found that HIV controllers consistently maintained more highly functional responses compared to progressors, and that T cell responses with the highest functionality correlated with control of viremia [41]. These and other studies [42] suggest that the quality of responses is important rather than just the presence of responses [43], although what is the cause and what is the consequence of controlled viral load remains to be determined. Differentiation status may also affect control, given that fully differentiated CD8 T cell responses are enriched in controllers [44], although within a given individual the maturation status is quite heterogeneous, suggesting epitope-specific influences on CD8+ T cell function.

Perforin, Granzyme and Cell Killing

HIV-specific CD8 T cells are thought to exert antiviral control by one of at least two mechanisms: direct cell killing [45] and the release of antiviral cytokines [46]. Studies of T cell responses in elite controllers have shown that the ability to directly upregulate perforin upon exposure to antigen is a correlate of control [47]. More recent studies have indicated that the ability to upregulate perforin may be related to the T-box transcription factor T-bet, which is involved in CD8 T cell effector function and differentiation [48]. HIV-specific CD8 T cells in elite controllers express higher levels of T-bet, and these levels correlate positively with levels of perforin and granzyme B [48]. Other studies indicate that loading of lytic granules following antigen encounter is more effective in CD8 T cells from controllers [34,49]. Since a major antiviral mechanism of CD8 T cells is lysis of infected cells, these studies suggest that direct cell killing may be an important function of these cells. Indeed, *in vitro* studies have shown that HIV-specific CTL can not only lyze infected cells before progeny virions are produced [45] but also select for immune escape mutations *in vitro* [46], suggesting potent antiviral function.

Proliferation

Upon encounter with infected cells, CD8 T cells must necessarily rapidly expand to contain the infection by eliminating infected cells and by activation-induced release of antiviral cytokines. Numerous studies have now shown that the ability of HIV-specific CD8 T cells to expand following recognition of infected target cells is associated with lower viral load [49−52], and may in part be linked to preservation of T helper cell function in these persons [50]. These studies suggest that functional attributes of these cells are important, and are consistent with the observation that upregulation of PD-1, a negative immunoregulatory molecule, on HIV-specific CD8 T cells is associated with higher viral loads [25−27]. Proliferative capacity may also be linked to specificity, in that freshly isolated PBMCs from persons with strong Gag-specific antiviral activity (see below) are better able to proliferate [19].

Inhibition of Viral Replication

As alluded to above, direct killing of infected cells may be critical to their antiviral function. Attempts to model this *in vitro* have shown that recognition of infected cells by CTL leads to two antiviral functions: direct cell killing, which can occur before progeny virions are produced, as well as release of antiviral cytokines [45,46]. In the *in vitro* situation cell killing seems to be the most important effector function, but the relative contribution of these two mechanisms *in vivo* remains to be defined. Indeed, in the three-dimensional space *in vivo* it may be that bathing the surrounding environment with antiviral cytokines is more effective than serial killing by CTLs to limit virus replication, and these cytokines would be operative against virions that had already been released from infected cells.

Examination of antiviral function *in vivo* has been reported in HIV elite controllers, both in freshly isolated PBMCs and at the single epitope-specific level. In elegant studies using freshly isolated PBMCs from HIV controllers, Sáez-Cirión and colleagues showed high frequencies of HIV-specific CD8 T cells, which expressed HLA DR but not the activation marker CD38 and effectively suppressed viral replication *in vitro*, without the need for *in vitro* stimulation [53]. These results indicate that cells with immediate effector function are present in elite controllers, and the mechanism of inhibition is consistent with killing of infected CD4 T cells. In studies of *in vitro* expanded HIV epitope-specific CTL responses, Chen and colleagues showed marked differences in antiviral function in a similar *in vitro* inhibition assay, using production of p24 antigen over time in infected CD4 cells as a read-out [54]. These studies indicate that the responses directed at Gag have greater antiviral efficacy than those directed against Env, and this could not be linked to avidity of responses [55]. Additional studies using this type of assay have shown that persons with broad Gag-specific responses have greater inhibitory activity in freshly isolated PBMCs than do those with narrow responses, and these were associated with lower viral loads *in vivo*, greater proliferative capacity, and increased polyfunctionality [19]. However, there are clearly HIV controllers who appear to lack this inhibitory activity, suggesting that other mechanisms of control may also be contributing *in vivo* [20].

CD4 T CELL IMMUNE RESPONSES

One of the major hallmarks of HIV infection is the lack of virus-specific CD4 T cells in persons with chronic infection—something that was noted very early in the epidemic. Indeed, it was through the study of elite controllers that the ability of HIV to induce strong virus-specific CD4 T cell responses, as measured by proliferation in response to HIV antigens, was first detected [56]. The fact that strong responses can be detected in persons with controlled HIV infection provides some level of evidence that these cells cannot be all bad—and that concerns that strong HIV-specific CD4 T cell responses may provide more fuel for the fire [57,58] may not be warranted. Indeed, these responses have been essential for effective antiviral T cell and B cell responses in all of the model systems in which they have been studied, so it is reasonable to think that these are an important component of effective immune control in HIV-infected persons as well [59]. In an animal model of chronic viral infection, the outcome in terms of control or progressive disease appears to depend on the rapidity of development of these responses [60]. Also, the maintenance of effective CD8 T cell responses, which are clearly linked to immune control of HIV as noted above, requires the presence of virus-specific T helper cell responses [61].

There have been a number of studies of HIV-specific CD4 T cells in HIV controllers, but the scope of these studies has been far more limited than in similar studies of HIV-specific CD8 T cell responses. Important to note is the finding that CD4 T cell responses, as measured by IFN-γ secretion, can be detected in both progressive and controlled infection [62], but the functionality of these cells, such as the ability to secrete IL-2 and proliferate upon stimulation, is enhanced in controllers [56,63−65]. Such responses have also been detected in transfusion-related HIV control in humans [64]; furthermore, strong responses have been seen in macaque elite controllers infected with SIV [66]. In addition, HIV controllers have a preserved CD4 T central memory cell compartment and immune activation that appears to be restricted to the CD4 T effector memory compartment [65]; these memory T cells show high avidity for Gag antigens and are capable of maintaining robust responses despite low-level viremia [67]. In addition, controllers have been shown to have higher levels of polyfunctional CD4 T cell responses in the gut mucosa [68], and future studies should place an emphasis on tissue-specific responses. The lack of function seen in HIV-specific CD4 T cells from progressors compared to controllers may well relate to induction of T cell exhaustion, associated with upregulation of negative immunoregulatory molecules such as PD-1, TIM-3 and CTLA-4, in the face of ongoing viremia [25,69,70].

Although HIV-specific CD4 T cell responses are predominantly targeted against Gag and Nef, there are only limited data regarding the precise viral epitopes targeted [71,72]. Some studies indicate that CD4 T cells can be directly cytolytic [72], but whether these exert sufficient selection pressure to lead to immune escape remains unclear [73]. *In vivo* reduction in CD4 T cells does not affect viral load in macaques [74], raising questions regarding the requirement for help once effective CD8 T cells have been induced. Exactly what HIV-specific CD4 T cells provide in terms of help may relate to the production of the interleukin 21 (IL-21). Exposure to HIV antigens leads to the specific triggering of IL-21 production by CD4 T cells in HIV controllers, whereas this capacity is lost in persons with progressive disease [75,76]. In addition, IL-21 production by CD4 T cells leads to increased perforin production by HIV-specific CD8 T cells even in the later stages of disease, and these CD8 T cells possess enhanced ability to inhibit virus replication. HIV-specific CD4 T cells have also been detected in exposed uninfected persons, but whether this implies a role in protection remains unclear [77] (see Chapter 7). Clearly, there is a future need for more emphasis on dissecting the effector role of HIV-specific CD4 cells in natural control of HIV.

HUMORAL IMMUNE RESPONSES

The role of humoral immune responses in HIV controllers has been investigated in numerous studies, but clear involvement in maintaining a low viral set-point is less clear. Early studies suggested that broad neutralizing antibodies are seen in persons with long-term non-progressing HIV infection [78—81], but when viral load testing became available and more sensitive assays for viral load were introduced it became clear that this was not always the case [82]. More recent data have instead shown a direct association between plasma virus load and HIV neutralizing and non-neutralizing antibody levels [83,84], suggesting that a low antigen burden may affect the generation and maintenance of potent humoral responses in this population.

An important component of the humoral immune response to HIV is that of neutralization of viral particles. By binding to *env* proteins and preventing viral entry, neutralizing antibodies (NAbs) have the potential to reduce the pool of cells that become latently infected—a crucial step towards HIV eradication. In HIV controllers, studies have shown significantly lower levels of heterologous neutralization compared to individuals with low-level and high viremia [5,85,86] and little in the way of NAb titers against contemporaneous plasma viruses [85]. Together these data suggest that despite the maintenance of broad cross-neutralizing antibodies during the chronic phases of HIV infection, continuous generation of escape variants limits the efficacy of these Abs in suppressing viral replication. More recent detailed studies looking at longitudinal autologous neutralization in controllers have found that despite having low or undetectable virus load, there is considerable *env* evolution over relatively short periods of time [87]. More so, there is neutralization activity against individual contemporaneous viral variants, and a positive correlation between virus load and autologous neutralizing antibodies (ANAbs) [87].

Among HIV controllers with broadly neutralizing antibody activity, it has been demonstrated that their serum neutralizing activity is the result of multiple responses with neutralizing activity directed against several *env* epitopes [88].

Together these data suggest a model in which there is continuous selection and turnover of strong ANAbs, but the extent to which these actually contribute to the durable control of HIV replication remains to be better defined. Although anecdotal, a single case of an elite controller treated with rituximab, a B-cell depleting therapeutic monoclonal antibody, is reported to have maintained elite control of his virus [89], suggesting against a dominant role of NAb in at least some elite controllers.

In addition to NAbs, other potentially protective antibodies have gained interest as correlates of protection in HIV controllers; they can inhibit viral replication in macrophages and dendritic cells via interactions with Fc receptors [90] and can effectively recruit innate immune effectors. Antibody-dependent cell-mediated cytotoxicity (ADCC) has been associated with lower viral set-points in animal models challenged with SIV [91], as well as implicated in the modest protection provided by the RV144 vaccine trial. In contrast to NAbs, ADCC-inducing antibodies appear to block autologous contemporaneous virus in longitudinal studies of acute infection cohorts [92]. In HIV controllers ADCC activity appears to be higher compared to individuals with progressive disease [86], and it has been demonstrated that non-neutralizing binding Abs are involved in the effective recruitment of NK cells and monocytes to mediate a stronger ADCC effect. Furthermore, gp120-binding titers appear to correlate with the level of ADCC inducing antibodies, but not with their serum neutralizing activity [93].

NATURAL KILLER CELLS

Natural killer (NK) cells have a central role in the early immune responses against several viral infections. They express, on their surface, numerous inhibitory and activating receptors that modulate the elimination of infected targets via direct cytotoxicity or induction of antibody-dependent cellular cytotoxicity (ADCC).

The strongest evidence supporting a role for NK cells in control of HIV infection comes from large population-based genetic studies which have demonstrated that members of the killer cell immunoglobulin-like receptors (KIRs) are associated with slower disease progression. Specifically, allotypes encoded by the KIR3DL1 gene in combination with its ligands, HLA-B alleles of the Bw4-80I group, have been associated with protection against HIV disease progression, opportunistic infections and plasma HIV-RNA [9,10]. Interestingly, some of the class I HLA alleles that are associated with HIV control, namely HLA-B*57/27/58/51, are of the Bw4-80I subtype, suggesting that their mechanisms of protection might be mediated, at least in part, via interactions with NK cells. These associations have been demonstrated with the common activating allotype KIR3DS1, as well as several inhibitory allotypes.

Functional studies have demonstrated that the inhibitory capacity of NK cells of specific KIR3DL1 allotypes is closely linked to the amount of these molecules that is expressed on the NK cell population of an individual. Similarly, KIR3DS1/L1-positive NK cells exhibit enhanced IFN-γ production and functionality in the presence of their putative ligands; this effect is apparent in the context of protective HLA alleles that are over-represented in HIV controllers [94]. The mechanism by which co-expression of these protective KIR and class I molecules confers protection varies according to the KIR receptor. Individuals with the KIR3DS1/Bw4-80I genotype have enhanced IFN-γ production, cytotoxicity and HIV-suppression capacity [95,96]. For the inhibitory KIR3DL1 variants, it has been proposed that inhibitory signals during development result in the development of more functionally competent NK cells—a process called "licensing" [97,98].

An SNP located 35 kb upstream from HLA-C has been associated with differential viral set-points and spontaneous HIV control [11,13]; this SNP was subsequently associated with higher expression of HLA-C alleles on the surface of cells [99] and, given that HLA-C serves as the dominant ligand for KIR2D alleles and is not downregulated upon infection by HIV like HLA-A and -B are, it is possible that higher expression may render NK cells more effective. More recently, in comprehensive studies looking at MicroRNAs, it has been demonstrated that the interaction between miR-148a and its polymorphic binding site in the 3'UTR of HLA-C, rather than the −35-kb SNP, is the most likely causal explanation for variable levels of HLA-C expression. As demonstrated by comparing the specific 3'UTR variants in large cohorts of HIV controllers and progressors, the effect is independent of individual HLA-A, -B, or -C alleles. These data indicate diversity in the HLA-C locus beyond the peptide-binding region of the gene, and suggest that multiple mechanisms might explain the different HLA correlates of protection; they likely include the type of peptides they bind and their level of expression [12].

In HIV controllers and long-term non-progressors, extensive phenotyping and functional characterization has shown high frequency of IFN-γ secreting NK cells and high cytolytic activity, as measured by their ability to kill highly susceptible infected targets [100]. Whether this preserved NK cell functionality and "non-exhausted" phenotype is a cause or consequence of HIV control has not been definitively answered.

Despite having high NK-cell cytokine secretion and degranulation, in some studies HIV controllers exhibit low capacity for direct cytolyis of infected autologous CD4 T cells [100], presumably due to lower expression of NKp44, a natural cytotoxicity receptor. Moreover, in HIV controllers, *in vitro* studies have shown that CD8 T cells inhibit viral replication to a greater extent than NK cells, suggesting that NK-cell mediated reduction of viral replication may not be a dominant mechanism of spontaneous HIV control [101].

In addition to direct cytotoxicity, NK cells are involved in the clearance of infected cells through the induction of antibody-dependent cell cytotoxicity. This process occurs via activation of an Fc-receptor on innate immune cells—a mechanism that has been shown to correlate with slower disease progression [102] and spontaneous HIV control [86], as described earlier in this chapter.

CONCLUSIONS

Although HIV controllers represent only a small proportion of the overall HIV-infected population, they, given their unique ability to remain healthy and maintain very low levels of viral replication, represent an excellent model to understand natural immunity against HIV-1.

The enrichment of certain class I HLA alleles in cohorts of HIV controllers, as well as the footprints that these alleles leave on the HIV virus, have indirectly linked effective immune responses to HIV-1-specific cytotoxic T lymphocytes (CTLs). In addition, the mapping of all classical HLA allele associations to specific amino acids located within the peptide binding groove of the HLA molecule has underscored the critical causal role that the viral peptide−MHC complex and, indirectly, CTLs play in spontaneous HIV control [11].

However, as we have highlighted in this chapter, emerging data support a complex model that involves other components of the immune system (Figure 10.1). Moreover, several studies have described substantial variation and marked heterogeneity underlying HIV controllers' immune responses.

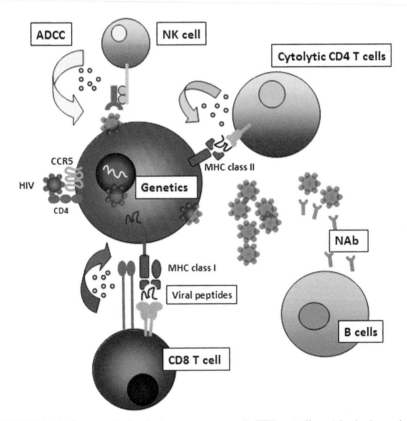

FIGURE 10.1   Innate and adaptive immune responses in HIV controllers. Adaptive immunity is mediated by cytotoxic CD8 T cells via recognition of HIV peptides presented by class I HLA molecules, neutralizing antibodies (NAb) against HIV *env* and cytolytic CD4 T cells via recognition of HIV peptides presented by class II HLA molecules. Innate immunity is mediated by natural killer (NK) cells via FC-receptor recognition of antibody-coated cells.

This variation suggest that within controllers there might be two subpopulations of individuals: those with an inflammatory immune profile that is characterized by high levels of HIV-1-specific immune responses, expression of pro-inflammatory transcriptional gene profiles and higher levels of HIV-1 reservoirs; and an alternative subgroup with a more quiescent immune system, possibly with intrinsic resistance to HIV-1 infection, immune activation signatures that are indistinguishable from HIV-1 uninfected persons, and minimally detectable levels of persistent HIV-1 reservoirs [20,103,104].

The past decade has seen great advances in the quest to find correlates of protection in HIV controllers, facilitated largely by the establishment of large clinical cohorts along with specimen repositories. Despite this, critical questions underlying the mechanism of HIV control remain unanswered: What are the biologic and functional mechanisms that explain the observed genetic associations? What represents an effective T cell response, and what is the contribution of T cell memory to immune control? What is the relationship between low-level viral replication, effective immune responses and the viral reservoirs in blood and tissue compartments? What are the critical areas of the virus that the immune system targets to achieve durable immune control? What is the role of innate immunity in durable HIV control? What are the strongest predictors of HIV control?

Additional studies will be needed to better characterize this population, and to bring the field a step closer to a much-needed therapeutic or preventive HIV vaccine.

REFERENCES

[1] Mellors JW, Rinaldo Jr CR, Gupta P, White RM, Todd JA, Kingsley LA. Prognosis in HIV-1 infection predicted by the quantity of virus in plasma. Science 1996;272:1167−70.

[2] Lyles RH, Munoz A, Yamashita TE, Bazmi H, Detels R, Rinaldo CR, et al. Natural history of human immunodeficiency virus type 1 viremia after seroconversion and proximal to AIDS in a large cohort of homosexual men. Multicenter AIDS Cohort Study. J Infect Dis 2000;181:872−80.

[3] Rodriguez B, Sethi AK, Cheruvu VK, Mackay W, Bosch RJ, Kitahata M, et al. Predictive value of plasma HIV RNA level on rate of CD4 T-cell decline in untreated HIV infection. J Am Med Assoc 2006;296:1498−506.

[4] Deeks SG, Walker BD. Human immunodeficiency virus controllers: Mechanisms of durable virus control in the absence of antiretroviral therapy. Immunity 2007;27:406−16.

[5] Pereyra F, Addo MM, Kaufmann DE, Liu Y, Miura T, Rathod A, et al. Genetic and immunologic heterogeneity among persons who control HIV infection in the absence of therapy. J Infect Dis 2008;197:563−71.

[6] Wawer MJ, Gray RH, Sewankambo NK, Serwadda D, Li X, Laeyendecker O, et al. Rates of HIV-1 transmission per coital act, by stage of HIV-1 infection, in Rakai, Uganda. J Infect Dis 2005;191:1403−9.

[7] Quinn TC, Wawer MJ, Sewankambo N, Serwadda D, Li C, Wabwire-Mangen F, et al. Viral load and heterosexual transmission of human immunodeficiency virus type 1. Rakai Project Study Group. N Engl J Med 2000;342:921−9.

[8] Kaslow RA, Carrington M, Apple R, Park L, Munoz A, Saah AJ, et al. Influence of combinations of human major histocompatibility complex genes on the course of HIV-1 infection. Nat Med 1996;2:405−11.

[9] Martin MP, Gao X, Lee JH, Nelson GW, Detels R, Goedert JJ, et al. Epistatic interaction between KIR3DS1 and HLA-B delays the progression to AIDS. Nat Genet 2002;31:429−34.

[10] Martin MP, Qi Y, Gao X, Yamada E, Martin JN, Pereyra F, et al. Innate partnership of HLA-B and KIR3DL1 subtypes against HIV-1. Nat Genet 2007;39:733−40.

[11] Pereyra F, Jia X, McLaren PJ, Telenti A, de Bakker PI, Walker BD, et al. The major genetic determinants of HIV-1 control affect HLA class I peptide presentation. Science 2010;330:1551−7.

[12] Kulkarni S, Savan R, Qi Y, Gao X, Yuki Y, Bass SE, et al. Differential microRNA regulation of HLA-C expression and its association with HIV control. Nature 2011;472:495−8.

[13] Fellay J, Shianna KV, Ge D, Colombo S, Ledergerber B, Weale M, et al. A whole-genome association study of major determinants for host control of HIV-1. Science 2007;317:944−7.

[14] Limou S, Le Clerc S, Coulonges C, Carpentier W, Dina C, Delaneau O, et al. Genomewide Association Study of an AIDS, nonprogression cohort emphasizes the role played by HLA genes (ANRS Genomewide Association Study 02). J Infect Dis 2009;199:419−26.

[15] Emu B, Sinclair E, Hatano H, Ferre A, Shacklett B, Martin JN, et al. HLA class I-restricted T-cell responses may contribute to the control of human immunodeficiency virus infection, but such responses are not always necessary for long-term virus control. J Virol 2008;82:5398−407.

[16] Edwards BH, Bansal A, Sabbaj S, Bakari J, Mulligan MJ, Goepfert PA. Magnitude of functional CD8+ T-cell responses to the gag protein of human immunodeficiency virus type 1 correlates inversely with viral load in plasma. J Virol 2002;76:2298−305.

[17] Kiepiela P, Ngumbela K, Thobakgale C, Ramduth D, Honeyborne I, Moodley E, et al. CD8+ T-cell responses to different HIV proteins have discordant associations with viral load. Nat Med 2007;13:46−53.

[18] Zuniga R, Lucchetti A, Galvan P, Sanchez S, Sanchez C, Hernandez A, et al. Relative dominance of Gag p24-specific cytotoxic T lymphocytes is associated with human immunodeficiency virus control. J Virol 2006;80:3122−5.

[19] Julg B, Williams KL, Reddy S, Bishop K, Qi Y, Carrington M, et al. Enhanced anti-HIV functional activity associated with Gag-specific CD8 T-cell responses. J Virol 2010; 84:5540−9.

[20] Sáez-Cirión A, Sinet M, Shin SY, Urrutia A, Versmisse P, Lacabaratz C, et al. Heterogeneity in HIV suppression by CD8 T cells from HIV controllers: Association with Gag-specific CD8 T cell responses. J Immunol 2009;182:7828−37.

[21] Goulder PJ, Brander C, Tang Y, Tremblay C, Colbert RA, Addo MM, et al. Evolution and transmission of stable CTL escape mutations in HIV infection. Nature 2001;412:334−8.

[22] Betts MR, Ambrozak DR, Douek DC, Bonhoeffer S, Brenchley JM, Casazza JP, et al. Analysis of total human immunodeficiency virus (HIV)-specific CD4(+) and CD8(+) T-cell responses: Relationship to viral load in untreated HIV infection. J Virol 2001;75:11983−91.

[23] Addo MM, Yu XG, Rathod A, Cohen D, Eldridge RL, Strick D, et al. Comprehensive epitope analysis of human immunodeficiency virus type 1 (HIV-1)-specific T-cell responses directed against the entire expressed HIV-1 genome demonstrate broadly directed responses, but no correlation to viral load. J Virol 2003;77:2081−92.

[24] Dahirel V, Shekhar K, Pereyra F, Miura T, Artyomov N, Talsania S, et al. Coordinate linkage of HIV evolution reveals regions of immunologic vulnerability. Proc Natl Acad Sci USA, submitted 2011.

[25] Day CL, Kaufmann DE, Kiepiela P, Brown JA, Moodley ES, Reddy S, et al. PD-1 expression on HIV-specific T cells is associated with T-cell exhaustion and disease progression. Nature 2006;443:350−4.

[26] Petrovas C, Casazza JP, Brenchley JM, Price DA, Gostick E, Adams WC, et al. PD-1 is a regulator of virus-specific CD8+ T cell survival in HIV infection. J Exp Med 2006;203:2281−92.

[27] Trautmann L, Janbazian L, Chomont N, Said EA, Gimmig S, Bessette B, et al. Upregulation of PD-1 expression on HIV-specific CD8+ T cells leads to reversible immune dysfunction. Nat Med 2006;12:1198−202.

[28] Le Gall S, Stamegna P, Walker BD. Portable flanking sequences modulate CTL epitope processing. J Clin Invest 2007;117:3563−75.

[29] Goonetilleke N, Liu MKP, Salazar-Gonzalez JF, Ferrari G, Giorgi E, Ganusov VV, et al. The first T cell response to transmitted/founder virus contributes to the control of acute viremia in HIV-1 infection. J Exp Med 2009;206:1253−72.

[30] Altfeld M, Addo MM, Shankarappa R, Lee PK, Allen TM, Yu XG, et al. Enhanced detection of human immunodeficiency virus type 1-specific T-cell responses to highly variable regions by using peptides based on autologous virus sequences. J Virol 2003;77:7330−40.

[31] Hansen SG, Vieville C, Whizin N, Coyne-Johnson L, Siess DC, Drummond DD, et al. Effector memory T cell responses are associated with protection of rhesus monkeys from mucosal simian immunodeficiency virus challenge. Nat Med 2009;15:293−9.

[32] Maness NJ, Yant LJ, Chung C, Loffredo JT, Friedrich TC, Piaskowski SM, et al. Comprehensive immunological evaluation reveals surprisingly few differences between elite controller and progressor Mamu-B*17-positive simian immunodeficiency virus-infected rhesus macaques. J Virol 2008;82:5245−54.

[33] Migueles SA, Laborico AC, Imamichi H, Shupert WL, Royce C, McLaughlin M, et al. The differential ability of HLA B*5701+ long-term nonprogressors and progressors to restrict human immunodeficiency virus replication is not caused by loss of recognition of autologous viral gag sequences. J Virol 2003;77:6889−98.

[34] Migueles SA, Osborne CM, Royce C, Compton AA, Joshi RP, Weeks KA, et al. Lytic granule loading of CD8+ T cells is required for HIV-infected cell elimination associated with immune control. Immunity 2008;29:1009−21.

[35] Huang J, Burke PS, Cung TD, Pereyra F, Toth I, Walker BD, et al. Leukocyte immunoglobulin-like receptors maintain unique antigen-presenting properties of circulating myeloid dendritic cells in HIV-1 elite controllers. J Virol 2010;84:9463−71.

[36] Bailey JR, Williams TM, Siliciano RF, Blankson JN. Maintenance of viral suppression in HIV-1-infected HLA-B*57+ elite suppressors despite CTL escape mutations. J Exp Med 2006;203:1357−69.

[37] Bailey JR, Brennan TP, O'Connell KA, Siliciano RF, Blankson JN. Evidence of CD8+ T-cell-mediated selective pressure on human immunodeficiency virus type 1 nef in HLA-B*57+ elite suppressors. J Virol 2009;83:88−97.

[38] Lassen KG, Lobritz MA, Bailey JR, Johnston S, Nguyen S, Lee B, et al. Elite suppressor-derived HIV-1 envelope glycoproteins exhibit reduced entry efficiency and kinetics. PLoS Pathog 2009;5:e1000377.

[39] Miura T, Brockman MA, Brumme ZL, Brumme CJ, Pereyra F, Trocha A, et al. HLA-associated alterations in replication capacity of chimeric NL4-3 viruses carrying gag-protease from elite controllers of human immunodeficiency virus type 1. J Virol 2009;83:140−9.

[40] Martinez-Picado J, Prado JG, Fry EE, Pfafferott K, Leslie A, Chetty S, et al. Fitness cost of escape mutations in p24 Gag in association with control of human immunodeficiency virus type 1. J Virol 2006;80:3617−23.

[41] Betts MR, Nason MC, West SM, De Rosa SC, Migueles SA, Abraham J, et al. HIV non-progressors preferentially maintain highly functional HIV-specific CD8+ T cells. Blood 2006;107:4781–9.

[42] Quigley M, Pereyra F, Nilsson B, Porichis F, Fonseca C, Eichbaum Q, et al. Transcriptional analysis of HIV-specific CD8+ T cells shows that PD-1 inhibits T cell function by upregulating BATF. Nat Med 2010;16:1147–51.

[43] Almeida JR, Price DA, Papagno L, Arkoub ZA, Sauce D, Bornstein E, et al. Superior control of HIV-1 replication by CD8+ T cells is reflected by their avidity, polyfunctionality, and clonal turnover. J Exp Med 2007;204:2473–85.

[44] Addo MM, Draenert R, Rathod A, Verrill CL, Davis BT, Gandhi RT, et al. Fully differentiated HIV-1 specific CD8+ T effector cells are more frequently detectable in controlled than in progressive HIV-1 infection. PLoS One 2007;2:e321.

[45] Yang OO, Kalams SA, Rosenzweig M, Trocha A, Jones N, Koziel M, et al. Efficient lysis of human immunodeficiency virus type 1-infected cells by cytotoxic T lymphocytes. J Virol 1996;70:5799–806.

[46] Yang OO, Kalams SA, Trocha A, Cao H, Luster A, Johnson RP, et al. Suppression of human immunodeficiency virus type 1 replication by CD8+ cells: Evidence for HLA class I-restricted triggering of cytolytic and noncytolytic mechanisms. J Virol 1997;71:3120–8.

[47] Hersperger AR, Pereyra F, Nason M, Demers K, Sheth P, Shin LY, et al. Perforin expression directly *ex vivo* by HIV-specific CD8 T-cells is a correlate of HIV elite control. PLoS Pathog 2010;6:e1000917.

[48] Hersperger AR, Martin JN, Shin LY, Sheth PM, Kovacs CM, Cosma GL, et al. Increased HIV-specific CD8+ T-cell cytotoxic potential in HIV elite controllers is associated with T-bet expression. Blood 2011;117:3799–808.

[49] Migueles SA, Laborico AC, Shupert WL, Sabbaghian MS, Rabin R, Hallahan CW, et al. HIV-specific CD8+ T cell proliferation is coupled to perforin expression and is maintained in nonprogressors. Nat Immunol 2002;3:1061–8.

[50] Lichterfeld M, Kaufmann DE, Yu XG, Mui SK, Addo MM, Johnston MN, et al. Loss of HIV-1-specific CD8+ T cell proliferation after acute HIV-1 infection and restoration by vaccine-induced HIV-1-specific CD4+ T cells. J Exp Med 2004;200:701–12.

[51] Day CL, Kiepiela P, Leslie AJ, van der Stok M, Nair K, Ismail N, et al. Proliferative capacity of epitope-specific CD8 T-cell responses is inversely related to viral load in chronic human immunodeficiency virus type 1 infection. J Virol 2007;81:434–8.

[52] Horton H, Frank I, Baydo R, Jalbert E, Penn J, Wilson S, et al. Preservation of T cell proliferation restricted by protective HLA alleles is critical for immune control of HIV-1 infection. J Immunol 2006;177:7406–15.

[53] Sáez-Cirión A, Lacabaratz C, Lambotte O, Versmisse P, Urrutia A, Boufassa F, et al. HIV controllers exhibit potent CD8 T cell capacity to suppress HIV infection *ex vivo* and peculiar cytotoxic T lymphocyte activation phenotype. Proc Natl Acad Sci 2007;104:6776–81.

[54] Chen H, Piechocka-Trocha A, Miura T, Brockman MA, Julg BD, Baker BM, et al. Differential neutralization of human immunodeficiency virus (HIV) replication in autologous CD4 T cells by HIV-specific cytotoxic T lymphocytes. J Virol 2009;83:3138–49.

[55] Almeida JR, Sauce D, Price DA, Papagno L, Shin SY, Moris A, et al. Antigen sensitivity is a major determinant of CD8+ T-cell polyfunctionality and HIV-suppressive activity. Blood 2009;113:6351–60.

[56] Rosenberg ES, Billingsley JM, Caliendo AM, Boswell SL, Sax PE, Kalams SA, et al. Vigorous HIV-1-specific CD4+ T cell responses associated with control of viremia. Science 1997;278:1447–50.

[57] Douek DC, Brenchley JM, Betts MR, Ambrozak DR, Hill BJ, Okamoto Y, et al. HIV preferentially infects HIV-specific CD4+ T cells. Nature 2002;417:95−8.

[58] Staprans SI, Barry AP, Silvestri G, Safrit JT, Kozyr N, Sumpter B, et al. Enhanced SIV replication and accelerated progression to AIDS in macaques primed to mount a CD4 T cell response to the SIV envelope protein. Proc Natl Acad Sci USA 2004;101:13026−31.

[59] Virgin HW, Walker BD. Immunology and the elusive AIDS vaccine. Nature 2010;464:224−31.

[60] Pike R, Filby A, Ploquin MJ-Y, Eksmond U, Marques R, Antunes I, et al. Race between retroviral spread and CD4+ T-cell response determines the outcome of acute Friend virus infection. J Virol 2009;83:11211−22.

[61] Zajac AJ, Blattman JN, Murali-Krishna K, Sourdive DJ, Suresh M, Altman JD, et al. Viral immune evasion due to persistence of activated T cells without effector function. J Exp Med 1998;188:2205−13.

[62] Pitcher CJ, Quittner C, Peterson DM, Connors M, Koup RA, Maino VC, et al. HIV-1-specific CD4+ T cells are detectable in most individuals with active HIV-1 infection, but decline with prolonged viral suppression. Nat Med 1999;5:518−25.

[63] McNeil AC, Shupert WL, Iyasere CA, Hallahan CW, Mican JA, Davey Jr RT, et al. High-level HIV-1 viremia suppresses viral antigen-specific CD4(+) T cell proliferation. Proc Natl Acad Sci USA 2001;98:13878−83.

[64] Dyer WB, Zaunders JJ, Yuan FF, Wang B, Learmont JC, Geczy AF, et al. Mechanisms of HIV non-progression; robust and sustained CD4+ T-cell proliferative responses to p24 antigen correlate with control of viraemia and lack of disease progression after long-term transfusion-acquired HIV-1 infection. Retrovirology 2008;5:112.

[65] Potter SJ, Lacabaratz C, Lambotte O, Perez-Patrigeon S, Vingert B, Sinet M, et al. Preserved central memory and activated effector memory CD4+ T-cell subsets in human immunodeficiency virus controllers: An ANRS EP36 study. J Virol 2007;81:13904−15.

[66] Giraldo-Vela JP, Rudersdorf R, Chung C, Qi Y, Wallace LT, Bimber B, et al. The major histocompatibility complex class II alleles Mamu-DRB1*1003 and -DRB1*0306 are enriched in a cohort of simian immunodeficiency virus-infected rhesus macaque elite controllers. J Virol 2008;82:859−70.

[67] Vingert B, Perez-Patrigeon S, Jeannin P, Lambotte O, Boufassa F, Lemaitre F, et al. HIV controller CD4+ T cells respond to minimal amounts of Gag antigen due to high TCR avidity. PLoS Pathog 2010;6:e1000780.

[68] Ferre AL, Hunt PW, McConnell DH, Morris MM, Garcia JC, Pollard RB, et al. HIV controllers with HLA-DRB1*13 and HLA-DQB1*06 alleles have strong, polyfunctional mucosal CD4+ T-cell responses. J Virol 2010;84:11020−9.

[69] Kaufmann DE, Kavanagh DG, Pereyra F, Zaunders JJ, Mackey EW, Miura T, et al. Upregulation of CTLA-4 by HIV-specific CD4+ T cells correlates with disease progression and defines a reversible immune dysfunction. Nat Immunol 2007;8:1246−54.

[70] Kassu A, Marcus RA, D'Souza MB, Kelly-McKnight EA, Golden-Mason L, Akkina R, et al. Regulation of virus-specific CD4+ T cell function by multiple costimulatory receptors during chronic HIV infection. J Immunol 2010;185:3007−18.

[71] Kaufmann DE, Bailey PM, Sidney J, Wagner B, Norris PJ, Johnston MN, et al. Comprehensive analysis of human immunodeficiency virus type 1-specific CD4 responses reveals marked immunodominance of gag and nef and the presence of broadly recognized peptides. J Virol 2004;78:4463−77.

[72] Norris PJ, Moffett HF, Brander C, Allen TM, O'Sullivan KM, Cosimi LA, et al. Fine specificity and cross-clade reactivity of HIV type 1 Gag-specific CD4+ T cells. AIDS Res Hum Retroviruses 2004;20:315−25.

[73] Rychert J, Saindon S, Placek S, Daskalakis D, Rosenberg E. Sequence variation occurs in CD4 epitopes during early HIV infection. J Acquir Immune Defic Syndr 2007; 46:261−7.

[74] Mudd PA, Ericsen AJ, Price AA, Wilson NA, Reimann KA, Watkins DI. Reduction of CD4+ T cells *in vivo* does not affect virus load in macaque elite controllers. J Virol 2011. in press.

[75] Chevalier MF, Julg B, Pyo A, Flanders M, Ranasinghe S, Soghoian DZ, et al. HIV-1-specific interleukin-21+ CD4+ T cell responses contribute to durable viral control through the modulation of HIV-specific CD8+ T cell function. J Virol 2011;85:733−41.

[76] Williams LD, Bansal A, Sabbaj S, Heath SL, Song W, Tang J, et al. Interleukin-21-producing HIV-1-specific CD8 T cells are preferentially seen in elite controllers. J Virol 2011;85:2316−24.

[77] Ritchie AJ, Campion SL, Kopycinski J, Moodie Z, Wang ZM, Pandya K, et al. Differences in HIV-specific T cell responses between HIV-exposed and -unexposed HIV-seronegative individuals. J Virol 2011;85:3507−16.

[78] Cao Y, Qin L, Zhang L, Safrit J, Ho DD. Virologic and immunologic characterization of long-term survivors of human immunodeficiency virus type 1 infection. N Engl J Med 1995;332:201−8.

[79] Montefiori DC, Pantaleo G, Fink LM, Zhou JT, Zhou JY, Bilska M, et al. Neutralizing and infection-enhancing antibody responses to human immunodeficiency virus type 1 in long-term nonprogressors. J Infect Dis 1996;173:60−7.

[80] Pantaleo G, Menzo S, Vaccarezza M, Graziosi C, Cohen OJ, Demarest JF, et al. Studies in subjects with long-term nonprogressive human immunodeficiency virus infection. N Engl J Med 1995;332:209−16.

[81] Pilgrim AK, Pantaleo G, Cohen OJ, Fink LM, Zhou JY, Zhou JT, et al. Neutralizing antibody responses to human immunodeficiency virus type 1 in primary infection and long-term-nonprogressive infection. J Infect Dis 1997;176:924−32.

[82] Harrer T, Harrer E, Kalams SA, Elbeik T, Staprans SI, Feinberg MB, et al. Strong cytotoxic T cell and weak neutralizing antibody responses in a subset of persons with stable non-progressing HIV type 1 infection. AIDS Res Hum Retroviruses 1996;12:585−92.

[83] Hatano H, Delwart EL, Norris PJ, Lee TH, Dunn-Williams J, Hunt PW, et al. Evidence for persistent low-level viremia in individuals who control human immunodeficiency virus in the absence of antiretroviral therapy. J Virol 2009;83:329−35.

[84] Pereyra F, Palmer S, Miura T, Block BL, Wiegand A, Rothchild AC, et al. Persistent low-level viremia in HIV-1 elite controllers and relationship to immunologic parameters. J Infect Dis 2009;200:984−90.

[85] Bailey JR, Lassen KG, Yang HC, Quinn TC, Ray SC, Blankson JN, et al. Neutralizing antibodies do not mediate suppression of human immunodeficiency virus type 1 in elite suppressors or selection of plasma virus variants in patients on highly active antiretroviral therapy. J Virol 2006;80:4758−70.

[86] Lambotte O, Ferrari G, Moog C, Yates NL, Liao HX, Parks RJ, et al. Heterogeneous neutralizing antibody and antibody-dependent cell cytotoxicity responses in HIV-1 elite controllers. AIDS 2009;23:897−906.

[87] Mahalanabis M, Jayaraman P, Miura T, Pereyra F, Chester EM, Richardson B, et al. Continuous viral escape and selection by autologous neutralizing antibodies in drug-naive human immunodeficiency virus controllers. J Virol 2009;83:662−72.

[88] Scheid JF, Mouquet H, Feldhahn N, Seaman MS, Velinzon K, Pietzsch J, et al. Broad diversity of neutralizing antibodies isolated from memory B cells in HIV-infected individuals. Nature 2009;458:636−40.

[89] Gaillard S, Dinoso JB, Marsh JA, Dezern AE, O'Connell KA, Spivak AM, et al. Sustained elite suppression of replication competent HIV-1 in a patient treated with rituximab based chemotherapy. J Clin Virol 2011. in press.

[90] Hessell AJ, Hangartner L, Hunter M, Havenith CE, Beurskens FJ, Bakker JM, et al. Fc receptor but not complement binding is important in antibody protection against HIV. Nature 2007;449:101−4.

[91] Gomez-Roman VR, Patterson LJ, Venzon D, Liewehr D, Aldrich K, Florese R, et al. Vaccine-elicited antibodies mediate antibody-dependent cellular cytotoxicity correlated with significantly reduced acute viremia in rhesus macaques challenged with SIVmac251. J Immunol 2005;174:2185−9.

[92] Behzad Etemad A-SD, Axten K, Rosenberg E, Alter G, Sagar M. Antibody-dependent cellular cytotoxicity response differs from neutralizing antibodies against autologous virus. 18th Conference on Retrovirus and Opportunistic Infections. Boston: MA; 2011.

[93] Dugast A, Barkume C, Ruberman C, Alter G. Elite controllers elicit HIV-specific antibodies that in the absence of neutralizing activity can efficiently mediate ADCC. 18th Conference of Retrovirus and Opportunistic Infections. Boston: MA; 2011.

[94] Long BR, Ndhlovu LC, Oksenberg JR, Lanier LL, Hecht FM, Nixon DF, et al. Conferral of enhanced natural killer cell function by KIR3DS1 in early human immunodeficiency virus type 1 infection. J Virol 2008;82:4785−92.

[95] Alter G, Martin MP, Teigen N, Carr WH, Suscovich TJ, Schneidewind A, et al. Differential natural killer cell-mediated inhibition of HIV-1 replication based on distinct KIR/HLA subtypes. J Exp Med 2007;204:3027−36.

[96] Alter G, Rihn S, Walter K, Nolting A, Martin M, Rosenberg ES, et al. HLA class I subtype-dependent expansion of KIR3DS1+ and KIR3DL1+ NK cells during acute human immunodeficiency virus type 1 infection. J Virol 2009;83:6798−805.

[97] Kim S, Poursine-Laurent J, Truscott SM, Lybarger L, Song YJ, Yang L, et al. Licensing of natural killer cells by host major histocompatibility complex class I molecules. Nature 2005;436:709−13.

[98] Kim S, Sunwoo JB, Yang L, Choi T, Song YJ, French AR, et al. HLA alleles determine differences in human natural killer cell responsiveness and potency. Proc Natl Acad Sci USA 2008;105:3053−8.

[99] Thomas R, Apps R, Qi Y, Gao X, Male V, O'HUigin C, et al. HLA-C cell surface expression and control of HIV/AIDS correlate with a variant upstream of HLA-C. Nat Genet 2009;41:1290−4.

[100] Vieillard V, Fausther-Bovendo H, Samri A, Debre P. Specific phenotypic and functional features of natural killer cells from HIV-infected long-term nonprogressors and HIV controllers. J Acquir Immune Defic Syndr 53:564−73.

[101] O'Connell KA, Han Y, Williams TM, Siliciano RF, Blankson JN. Role of natural killer cells in a cohort of elite suppressors: Low frequency of the protective KIR3DS1 allele and limited inhibition of human immunodeficiency virus type 1 replication in vitro. J Virol 2009;83:5028−34.

[102] Baum LL, Cassutt KJ, Knigge K, Khattri R, Margolick J, Rinaldo C, et al. HIV-1 gp120-specific antibody-dependent cell-mediated cytotoxicity correlates with rate of disease progression. J Immunol 1996;157:2168−73.

[103] Vigneault F, Woods M, Buzon M, Li C, Pereyra F, Crosby SD, et al. Transcriptional profiling of CD4 T cells identifies distinct subgroups of HIV-1 elite controllers. J Virol 2010;85:3015−9.

[104] Chen H, Li C, Huang J, Cung T, Seiss K, Beamon J, et al. CD4+ T cells from elite controllers resist HIV-1 infection by selective upregulation of p21. J Clin Invest 2011;121:1549−60.

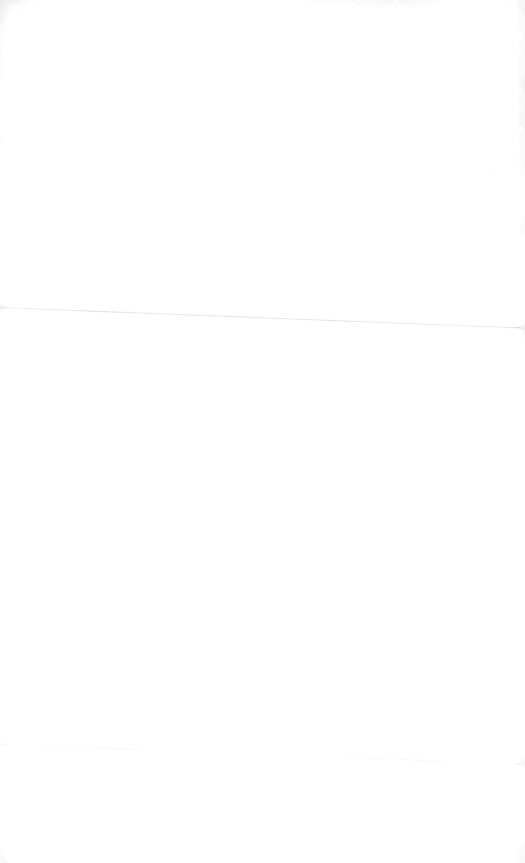

Chapter 11

Immune Mechanisms of Viral Control in HIV-2 Infection

Eirini Moysi, Thushan de Silva and Sarah Rowland-Jones

Nuffield Department of Medicine, Weatherall Institute of Molecular Medicine, John Radcliffe Hospital, Oxford, UK

Chapter Outlines

INTRODUCTION

Origins of HIV-2 Infection

The first cases of HIV-2 infection were recognized in 1985, when Senegalese patients were noted to have antibodies that were more cross-reactive against simian immunodeficiency virus (SIV) than against HIV-1 [1]. The virus responsible was isolated the following year from the blood of two West African AIDS patients, from Guinea-Bissau and the Cape Verde islands [2]. Shortly afterwards, the structure and sequence of HIV-2 was characterized and shown to be remarkably similar to HIV-1 [3,4].

Models of Protection Against HIV/SIV. DOI: 10.1016/B978-0-12-387715-4.00011-3

We now know HIV-2 infection to be a zoonosis in which SIV from a West African monkey species, the sooty mangabey (*Cercocebus torquatus atys*), is thought to have entered the human population on at least eight separate occasions. This has given rise to eight distinct HIV-2 groups, of which only groups A and B have continued to spread amongst humans; the other clades appear only to have led to single-person infections (reviewed in [5,6]). These groups tend to be found in different parts of West Africa (group A predominating in Senegal, the Gambia and Guinea-Bissau, with group B more commonly found in Côte d'Ivoire and Ghana); there are no reported epidemiological data to suggest that they are associated with different clinical outcomes (reviewed in [7]). The entry date of the HIV-2 subtype A ancestor into humans is estimated to be 1940 ± 16 years, approximately a decade after the introduction of HIV-1 into the human population [8]. Although it is not known exactly how humans became infected with SIVsmm, the most plausible route is through the bush-meat trade: in one study, 7 of 12 sooty mangabey bush-meat samples being sold in West African markets were infected with SIV [9].

Epidemiology of HIV-2 Infection

HIV-2 infection is largely confined to West Africa, coinciding with the distribution of the sooty mangabey in the 1940s—1950s, but has strong epidemiological linkages with Portugal and former Portuguese colonies: within Europe, the largest number of cases is in Portugal [10], and HIV-2 infection has also been described in Mozambique, Angola, India and Brazil [11—13]. The country with the highest recorded prevalence of HIV-2 is Guinea-Bissau: a community survey in 1989 in the capital, Bissau, documented a seroprevalence of 8 percent in adults and up to 20 percent in individuals over 40 years of age [14]. The prevalence was highest amongst women in the 45—60 years age-group, leading to speculation that older women may be more susceptible to infection (possibly due to hormonal changes affecting the vaginal mucosa) [15]. Guinea-Bissau is a former Portuguese colony that had a protracted war of independence in the 1960s, which coincides with the rapid spread of HIV-2 infection for reasons that are not entirely clear but are assumed to relate to social instability during the war and subsequent movement of Portuguese military forces [8,16]. At its height the overall prevalence of HIV-2 infection was estimated at around 1 million people [17], but currently there are few reliable incidence or prevalence data available, compounded by the fact that not all countries perform specific HIV-2 testing in their HIV surveillance programs.

In recent years, HIV-2 prevalence has shown signs of decline in some countries in West Africa [18—20]. However, a recent report from Japan describes, for the first time, a circulating recombinant form (CRF) of HIV-2, CRF01_AB, detected in three subjects, two African (from Nigeria and Ghana) and one Japanese, all of whom showed evidence of advanced disease [21]. The sequence is very similar to a recombinant form first found in Côte d'Ivoire [22], but the full extent of the distribution of this CRF is not known. Another new form of HIV-2 (a circulating form of clade F) has been reported in Sierra Leone [23]. There is a strong case for studies to determine how widespread the CRF and other HIV-2 clades have become in West Africa, and whether these are associated with increased likelihood of disease progression, as this could herald the development of a new epidemic of HIV-2 infection.

NATURAL HISTORY AND CLINICAL FEATURES OF HIV-2 INFECTION

The original isolation of HIV-2 infection from two AIDS patients clearly indicated that this virus is able to cause severe immunodeficiency: the clinical picture of AIDS caused by HIV-2 appears to be indistinguishable from that due to HIV-1 infection [24,25], although both presentation with and death from AIDS tend to occur at a higher CD4+ count than for HIV-1 in the same clinical setting [26], and, curiously, Kaposi's sarcoma is significantly rarer in African patients with HIV-2 infection [27].

However, further studies showed that, despite approximately 30—60 percent sequence identity at the amino acid level between HIV-1 and HIV-2, HIV-2 infection does not lead to significant immunodeficiency or disease for most infected adults [17,28,29]. This is particularly striking for older HIV-2-infected adults, in whom the mortality rates are no different from uninfected people [30], in stark contrast to HIV-1 infection, where age at infection is a powerful co-factor for accelerated disease progression [31]. Similarly, although vertical HIV-2 transmission is rare [32], HIV-2-infected children are much less likely to develop disease progression than HIV-1 vertically-infected children [33], and may survive well into adulthood without clinical complications of infection [34].

Although the proviral load is similar between HIV-1- and HIV-2-infected people at the same stage of infection [35,36], the plasma viral load is significantly lower in most people with HIV-2 infection [37,38]. Viral "controllers", who maintain a plasma viral load below detection for many years, show survival curves that are the same as in the uninfected population: moreover, in contrast to HIV-1 infection, the "controller" clinical phenotype can be maintained for a decade or more without any signs of disease [39].

In HIV-2-infected patients with a detectable viral load (even with loads that would be considered modest in HIV-1 infection) disease progression can develop [38], and the rates of CD4 decline and progression to disease for a given level of plasma viral load are very similar between HIV-1 and HIV-2 [40,41]. Progressors with HIV-2 infection are in the minority (an estimated 15—20 percent of the Caió community HIV-2 cohort in Guinea-Bissau), developing a syndrome characterized by high levels of plasma virus and CD4+ T cell decline [42], leading to a clinical picture indistinguishable from AIDS caused by HIV-1 [26]. The Caió community cohort is based in a string of rural settlements in the Cacheu region of Guinea-Bissau, and is one of the very few community cohorts of HIV-2 infection.

This provides the advantage of assessing the large group of HIV-2-infected non-progressors who would not normally require medical attention, as well as the benefits of long-term follow-up for over two decades, so provides a reasonable estimate of the relative proportion of HIV-2-infected long-term non-progressors (LTNPs) from the HIV-2-infected community as a whole. However, because of the length of time between full community serosurveys, it is possible that newly HIV-2-infected individuals with very rapid disease progression may have been missed, and the proportion of LTNPs would therefore be an over-estimate. Moreover, the Caió cohort derives from a distinct ethnic group, the Manjako, who because of their animist beliefs and practices have not mixed to any significant extent with the other ethnic groups in the region. As described later in this chapter, the human leukocyte antigen (HLA) and killer cell immunoglobulin-like receptor (KIR) distribution of the Manjago in Caió show significant differences from those reported in Gambian and Senegalese populations, suggesting that this ethnic group is genetically quite distinct from those in neighboring countries. It is therefore quite possible that observations about the natural history of HIV-2 infection in Caió may not necessarily apply to other ethnic groups with different genetic backgrounds, particularly as they may also be infected with different HIV-2 strains.

With these caveats in mind, it is worth noting that long-term follow-up of the French ANRS CO5 HIV-2 cohort has recently been reported [43] and describes a much lower proportion of LTNPs than we have observed in Caió. Using a definition of a LTNP as an HIV-2-infected individual who has been infected for at least 8 years and has maintained a CD4 count of > 500 cells/µl, only 6.1 percent of the cohort (of 749 subjects) could be described as LTNPs. Viral controllers, subjects who have maintained plasma viral load at or below 500 copies/ml for 10 years or more (all but one of whom had viral load < 100 copies/ml), accounted for 9.1 percent of the cohort; whilst most LTNPs (81 percent) were controllers, only 55 percent of the controllers were LTNPs. These data differ from our observations in Caió, where viral control strongly predicts normal survival and is seen in a much larger proportion of the HIV-2-infected cohort (37 percent had an undetectable viral load at study entry) [39]. It is important to remember that a clinical cohort would inevitably tend to select patients who have symptomatic disease and therefore over-estimate the proportion of progressors, but it may also be the case that the natural history of HIV-2 infection differs according to host genetic and viral factors that are distinct in different cohorts.

Drug therapy for HIV-2 infection is more challenging than for HIV-1, as the virus is intrinsically resistant to two classes of antiretroviral drugs (non-nucleoside reverse transcriptase inhibitors and fusion inhibitors) and there are no randomized clinical trial data to guide therapy (reviewed in [44]).

In keeping with the low plasma viral load of most HIV-2-infected subjects, the likelihood of transmission is much lower for HIV-2 than for HIV-1. Vertical transmission from HIV-2-infected breastfeeding mothers in the absence of antiretroviral therapy (ART) is less than 4 percent, compared to up to 24.4 percent for HIV-1 in the same population [32]; mothers who transmitted had high plasma viral loads. Although the sexual transmission efficiency of HIV-2 has not been estimated, the lesser shedding of HIV-2 in semen [45] and in the female genital tract [46] makes it likely that this is also significantly lower than for HIV-1.

Primary HIV-2 infection has only rarely been observed: in one case report, a European woman presented with fever, rash and lymphadenopathy 3 weeks after presumed exposure and was subsequently shown to be HIV-2 positive [47]. However, observations of recently-infected subjects in a cohort in Guinea-Bissau showed profoundly lower levels of set-point viremia (median level 2,500 copies/ml) than seen in HIV-1 infection [48].

Thus, HIV-2 presents the intriguing picture of a human retrovirus that has many similarities to HIV-1 but with which most infected people behave as LTNPs, although in many cases the virus is capable of causing profound immunodeficiency and death. The discrepancy between the plasma and proviral load in most HIV-2-infected patients is compatible with enhanced immune control of viral replication, or defective HIV-2 replicative capacity, or a combination of both these mechanisms. Elucidating the reasons for the relatively attenuated course of HIV-2 infection, and identifying the key differences between progressors and non-progressors with HIV-2 infection, could shed light on the mechanisms of HIV-1 pathogenesis and lead to a better understanding of protective immunity to HIV infection.

IMMUNE ACTIVATION AND HIV-2 PATHOGENESIS

Chronic immune activation is believed to be central to the pathogenesis of HIV-1 infection [49], and may in part be driven by translocation of bacterial products (such as lipopolysaccharide, LPS) from the gut across a damaged mucosal barrier [50]. In contrast, the natural host of HIV-2, the sooty mangabey, tolerates very high levels of replicating SIVsmm without developing chronic immune activation [51]. In a key study on immune activation in HIV-2 infection, levels were shown to be lower in HIV-2- than HIV-1-infected subjects studied in Portugal who were matched according to CD4 count, but elevated levels of immune activation were seen in HIV-2-infected patients in relation to plasma viral load [52]. In the Caió community cohort in Guinea-Bissau, the level of circulating beta-2 microglobulin, a soluble marker of immune activation, predicted clinical outcome as well as (and in some cases better than) plasma viral load [53]. We also observed a linear relationship between various markers of immune activation and plasma viral load in the Caió cohort [54]; however, some subjects with undetectable viral load also showed a significant degree of systemic immune activation. As an important study had highlighted the link between the ability of the *nef* gene of different retroviruses to downregulate the CD3 protein linked to the T cell receptor, thereby reducing unwanted non-specific immune activation [55], we explored the relationship between HIV-2 *nef* gene variation and immune activation in the Caió cohort. We found that the ability of individual nef proteins from different donors to downregulate CD3 correlated with the level of immune activation, as predicted by Schindler and colleagues [55], but this did not necessarily predict clinical status [56], presumably because of the many individuals with undetectable viral load and elevated immune activation [54]. The relationship between mucosal integrity and disease progression has not been studied to date in HIV-2 infection, but it has recently been shown that immune activation levels correlate well with circulating LPS [57].

VIROLOGICAL ASPECTS OF HIV-2 PATHOGENESIS

It is worth noting that much of the reported data about the behavior and characteristics of HIV-2 *in vitro* has been derived from isolates collected from individuals with high viral loads, usually with evidence of disease progression; indeed, the "prototype" HIV-2 strain LAV-2/HIV-2 ROD was isolated from a Cape Verdean patient with AIDS in 1985 [2]. It has been technically demanding to generate viral isolates and sequence data from HIV-2-infected people with plasma viral loads below detection, but more recent studies have provided some information about virus isolated and sequenced from non-progressors [58,59].

Is HIV-2 merely an "attenuated" form of HIV? Although some HIV-2 isolates are less cytopathic *in vitro* [60], systematic studies in a lymphoid histoculture model showed no overall differences in cytopathicity between HIV-1 and HIV-2 and suggested that coreceptor usage determines the cytopathic effect of both viruses [61]. Generally HIV-2 uses similar coreceptors to HIV-1, but some isolates are able to use additional coreceptors, potentially extending the range of susceptible cells, although the *in vivo* relevance of this broader repertoire is not clear. Overall, HIV-2 isolates are less fit than HIV-1 group M viruses when compared by competition between viral strains in tissue culture [62], although some HIV-2 isolates replicate very efficiently; moreover, it is not clear how well these kind of studies reflect *in vivo* viral fitness in the infected person. However, the replication kinetics of isolates from aviremic HIV-2 non-progressors are slower than in HIV-2 progressor isolates and virus from HIV-1 LTNPs [63]. The accumulation of viral mRNA is lower for HIV-2 than HIV-1, suggesting that there is tighter transcriptional control of the HIV-2 provirus [64]. Interestingly, the HIV-2 long terminal repeat (LTR) is different from that in HIV-1 [65], with only a single NF-κB binding site, which could contribute to differential mRNA expression; thus the LTR is less readily activated by CD3 activation [66]. However, a recent study comparing untreated HIV-2 and HIV-1 patients matched for the degree of CD4 T cell depletion showed similar levels of gag mRNA in both groups, suggesting that significant viral transcription occurs in HIV-2 patients despite the lower viremia [67].

In addition, the rate of viral replication between HIV-1 and HIV-2 patients at CD4+ T cell counts below 200 cells/μl is the same [68], further demonstrating HIV-2's pathogenic potential.

Are there viral sequence characteristics that distinguish HIV-2 from progressors and controllers? The first study to examine viral sequence variation between HIV-2-infected subjects with distinct clinical outcomes looked at proviral sequence in *gag, pol, LTR* and *env (V3)* in 131 subjects in the Caió community cohort in Guinea-Bissau [69]. The authors used a novel phylogenetic approach to compare the association between viral genotype and clinical outcome with other parameters (such as age and gender). All the sequences were from clade A HIV-2, and a phylogenetic analysis showed a degree of correlation between survival and viral genotype using a joint alignment of *LTR, gag* and *pol* sequences, but this was no longer significant when these genes were examined separately, and neither was there a correlation between genotype and either CD4 count or proviral load. A subsequent study in the same cohort looking at gag p26 sequences predominantly from viral RNA identified distinct viral sequence motifs within the capsid that were linked with the progression group [59]; the most striking associations were with three separate amino acid positions in the capsid, which were more likely to be prolines in aviremic individuals. The first of these amino acids has been shown to be a determinant of susceptibility to the host restriction factor TRIM5α [70], and modeling of the other residues suggested that they may contribute to capsid stability [59]. This raises the question of whether more virulent forms of HIV-2 are circulating that lead to more progressive disease; however, phylogenetic analysis of *gag* and *env* sequences showed that the HIV-2 progressor disease phenotype is not exclusive to certain viral lineages and sequences from progressors and non-progressors often cluster together ([59], and T. de Silva, personal communication). Also relevant to this question are studies of clinical outcome in the rare cases of vertical HIV-2 transmission. In one such study, despite high viral load and progressive disease in their mothers only one of four infected children also showed progressive disease [33], making it less likely that particularly virulent strains of HIV-2 lead to both disease progression and transmission. It is possible, therefore, that viral motifs identified as being more common in HIV-2 non-progressors are the result of adaptive interactions between the virus and host immune responses.

Little is known about the rate of evolution of HIV-2. One study of the HIV-2 envelope in 8 Senegalese patients studied over 10 years showed slower rates of diversification than are reported for HIV-1 [71]. However, when advanced HIV-2 and HIV-1 patients, matched for CD4 counts, are compared, then a faster rate of evolution can be seen for some HIV-2 genes, notably the envelope glycoprotein gp125, compared to HIV-1 [72]. To date no full viral genome studies have been reported for HIV-2, and there is a strong case for performing more extensive HIV-2 sequence analysis in order to address adequately the relationship between viral characteristics and clinical outcome in HIV-2 infection.

HOST GENETICS AND CLINICAL OUTCOME IN HIV-2 INFECTION

Few studies have been performed to examine host genetic influences on clinical outcome in HIV-2 infection. A small study in Senegalese sex workers suggested that HLA-B35 is linked with an increased risk of disease progression [73]. HLA-B35 has also been linked with rapid disease progression in HIV-1 infection [74], but this applies only to the subtypes of HLA-B35 that present peptides with a "PX" motif [75]. Interestingly, most people with HLA-B35 in the Senegambia region have the B*3501 subtype (L. M. Yindom, personal communication), which presents peptides containing the "PY" motif and is not linked with rapid HIV-1 disease progression [75]. A larger study in the Caió community HIV-2 cohort recently examined HLA class I and KIR gene polymorphisms, which have both been shown to have a substantial impact on the clinical course of HIV-1 infection [74,76]. In contrast to HIV-1, in which some of the strongest effects come from class I HLA molecules associated with viral control (HLA-B27, 57 and 51) [77], the major association with HIV-2 disease outcome was with HLA-B*1503, which was linked with low CD4 count and raised viral load [78]. Furthermore, whilst there are few data implicating class I HLA with susceptibility to HIV-1 infection, HLA-B*08 was significantly associated with HIV-2 susceptibility in Caió. No significant individual KIR gene associations were seen with HIV-2 disease progression, but the data suggested that the compound genotypes 2DS2:HLA-C1/x and/or 2DL2:HLA-C1/x (where x could be C1 or C2) might protect against HIV-2 acquisition. The Caió community consists largely of an animist ethnic group, the Manjago, whose HLA and KIR repertoire are distinct in several regards from those of other ethnic groups in the sub-region [78], so it will be important to examine immunogenetic associations in other HIV-2 cohorts, which may be different from Caió.

There are no published reports of other genetic associations with HIV-2 outcome, but it will be interesting to study the potential role of polymorphisms in host restriction factors, such as TRIM5α. This host cellular protein restricts HIV-2 more efficiently than HIV-1 [79], and polymorphisms in rhesus macaque TRIM5α, particularly in the SPRY domain, have a significant impact on the outcome of experimental SIV infection, in terms of both viral load set-point and clinical course [80].

IMMUNE CONTROL IN HIV-2 INFECTION

Initial studies of immune response in HIV-2 infection tended to compare parameters between HIV-1 and HIV-2 infection, rather than between the distinct HIV-2 progression groups. In contrast to HIV-1 infection, HIV-2 infection elicits a potent neutralizing antibody (nAb) response and strong HIV-2 specific cellular (both CD4+ and CD8+) responses in most subjects [81], which sometimes show cross-reactivity against HIV-1 antigens [82−85].

The high titers of nAb in most people with HIV-2 infection are intriguing [86], especially given the importance of this response in HIV vaccine strategies and the rarity of broadly neutralizing responses in HIV-1 infection. Nevertheless, no association has been seen between the breadth or magnitude of heterologous nAbs and lower viral load in HIV-2 infection [87]. More recent data suggest that neither autologous nor heterologous nAb, even in high titers, are associated with undetectable viral load and lack of disease progression (T. de Silva, personal communication). The only longitudinal study of HIV-2 neutralizing antibodies to date showed little evidence of neutralization escape over time, and, in contrast to HIV-1, patient sera from baseline were able to neutralize autologous virus isolated many years later [88]. The potential lack of neutralization escape in chronic HIV-2 infection in the face of high autologous nAbs is intriguing and is in stark contrast to HIV-1 infection, where rapid escape occurs from an early stage and is a major obstacle to defining protective humoral immune responses. It is possible that this characteristic in HIV-2 infection is due to factors such as the persistence of proviral sequences, the lower replication rate of most HIV-2 isolates relative to HIV-1, or greater functional constraints on HIV-2 envelope evolution [62,89].

When HIV-specific CD8+ T cell responses were compared between HIV-1- and HIV-2-infected subjects matched for disease stage, no significant differences were found in frequency, magnitude or phenotype [90−92], although more detailed studies demonstrated greater polyfunctionality in HIV-2-specific CD4 and CD8 T cells than seen in HIV-1 infection [93,94]. CD8+ T cell polyfunctionality was demonstrated by the observation that over 60 percent of responding cells produced the cytokines IFN-γ, TNF-α, MIP-1β and CD107a upon stimulation with the cognate antigen; other studies have shown that HIV-2-specific T cells are potent producers of the CC chemokines that are associated with suppression of viral replication [95]. Studies of the T cell response to overlapping peptides representing the entire HIV-2 proteome show that the response focuses on a narrow set of viral epitopes in HIV-2 infection. Recognition of T cell epitopes follows a hierarchical pattern: gag is the most recognized region, followed by epitopes in env and pol, and, in marked contrast to HIV-1 infection, responses to nef are rare, being seen in less than 10 percent of subjects [96]. This pattern of T cell responses to some extent resembles those detected early in acute HIV-1 infection (although in acute HIV-1 infection nef is the most commonly recognized target [97]), as well as those developed early in elite controllers, which are then lost during the course of infection [98]. However, when HIV-2-infected donors with undetectable plasma viral load are compared with viremic subjects, there are substantial differences in the magnitude and specificity of the virus-specific T cell response. An early study showed an inverse relationship between HIV-2-specific cytotoxic lymphocyte (CTL) activity and proviral load [99]. More recently, individuals with viral control were shown to have significantly higher T cell responses to peptides spanning the HIV-2 proteome, and to target the gag protein more frequently than subjects with elevated viral load [96]. In particular, responses directed towards highly conserved regions of gag were strongly associated with unde-tectable viral load; these responses can be very large in magnitude, even in donors who have maintained viral load below detection for a decade or more [100]. HIV-2 *gag* encodes a number of viral proteins, notably the matrix (p17), capsid (p26), nucleocapsid (p7) and vpr binding p6 proteins [101], which share a 58.0−59.4 percent sequence identity with the corresponding HIV-1 products (increasing up to 95 percent for more distant HIV-1 isolates [65]).

Lower plasma viral load in HIV-1 infection is also associated with T cell responses to three or more epitopes in gag [102,103], and viral controllers exhibit strong gag-specific responses that are associated with potent *in vitro* viral suppressive ability [104]. However, in contrast to HIV-2 infection, the overall magnitude of the HIV-1-specific CD4+ and CD8+ T cell response shows no association with viral load [105,106] and is not increased in viral controllers [107].

Therefore, there is good evidence to suggest that the control of viral repli-cation in HIV-2 infection is due, at least in part, to robust CD8+ T cell responses, particularly directed towards conserved regions of the viral antigen gag.

CHARACTERISTICS OF HIV-SPECIFIC CD8+ T-CELLS ASSOCIATED WITH VIRAL CONTROL

In addition to high-magnitude responses targeting conserved regions of gag, are there also qualitative features of the HIV-2-specific T cell response that are linked with viral control? In addition to generalized polyfunctionality, CD8+ T cells from HIV-2 non-progressors also secrete IL-2 and IL-4 [100], but there are no reports to date of a distinct functional phenotype that differentiates CTLs from progressors and non-progressors with HIV-2 infection.

HIV-1-specific CD8+ T cells characteristically display an unusual inter-mediate differentiation phenotype (CD28− CD27+ CDRA− CCR7−) [108], even in subjects with delayed disease progression or ART-induced viral control [107,109], and it has been suggested that this is related to impaired function [110,111]. Interestingly some reports suggest that the HIV-specific T cells from viral controllers, whilst heterogeneous, show in general a more advanced differentiation phenotype (being more likely to be CD27− [112] or CD45RA+/CCR7− [5]) than those seen in progressors; however, in another study HIV-specific T cells that had downregulated CD27− were shown to accumulate with advanced disease, elevated immune activation and increased viral load [113], leading to speculation that HIV-1 pathogenesis may in part reflect more rapid "aging" of the immune system [114]. Relating the differentiation phenotype of virus-specific T cells to function and clinical status is therefore a complex issue where clear consensus has not yet been reached.

We sought to investigate the phenotype of HIV-2-specific T cells using peptide−HLA tetrameric complexes ("tetramers"), and found in initial studies that this was broadly similar to that seen in HIV-1 infection [92]. However, we noted that in some donors HIV-2-specific CD8+ T cells showed an early-differentiated phenotype (CD28+ CD27+), and further studies in the Caió cohort showed that the proportion of early-differentiated tetramer-staining cells positively associated with higher CD4 counts and showed an inverse relationship with levels of immune activation [100].

It is striking that large populations of antigen-specific CD8+ T cells (up to 10.5 percent of CD8+ T cells) can be detected in people who have been infected with HIV-2 for over a decade and have an undetectable viral load [100]; moreover, these cells strongly express PD-1, which in HIV-1 infection has been clearly associated with higher viral loads and impaired function [115, 116]. It is possible that these expanded populations may show enhanced proliferative capacity because of preserved CD4+ T cell help in HIV-2 infection [93].

We recently examined functional aspects of the HIV-2-specific T cell response in 60 members of the Caió cohort, comparing subjects with an undetectable viral load (controllers), with those with a viral load above 100 copies/ml (viremic). Of the controllers, 85 percent had been infected with HIV-2 for at least 14 years; the average age of participants in both groups was 62 years (T. de Silva, personal communication). In these studies, a significantly higher CD8+T cell IFN-γ response to pooled HIV-2 gag peptides was observed in controllers than in viremic individuals, in keeping with our previous observations [96]. A significantly higher proportion of the CD8+ T cell response in controllers was made up of IFN-γ-producing and TNF-α-producing cells, whereas the converse was true for CD107a secretion. There was a significant inverse correlation between the proportion and magnitude of IFN-γ + TNF-α + CD107a + CD8 + T cells responding to gag peptides and plasma viral load. The median fluorescence intensity (MFI) for IFN-γ and TNF-α in these CD8+ T cells secreting multiple soluble factors simultaneously was also higher than in the monofunctional CD8+ T cells dominating the progressor responses, indicating that the production of antiviral factors on a per cell basis was also significantly higher for CD8+ T cells in HIV-2 controllers. Taken together, these data suggest that both the magnitude and the quality of the gag-specific CD8+ T cell response are greater in HIV-2 elite controllers (T. de Silva, personal communication).

The most striking finding in HIV-2 infection that could contribute significantly to viral control is the persistence of virus-specific CD8+ T cells of exceptional functional avidity in asymptomatic HIV-2 patients [100]. Functional avidity is a measure of cellular sensitivity to antigen, and reflects the amount of peptide that is needed for 50 percent maximal CTL activity (EC_{50}). In the case of HLA-B35-restricted CTL clones generated from HIV-2-infected non-progressors in the Caió cohort, this lies within the uppermost limits of all natural functional avidities reported to date (Figure 11.1). CD8+ T cells of high functional avidity, as measured by IFN-γ, MIP-1β, CD107a/b expression and

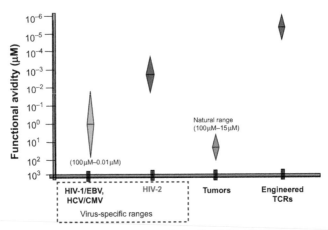

FIGURE 11.1 Comparison of HIV-2 specific CD8+ T-cell functional avidities with natural and engineered avidities reported to date.

tetramer dissociation, also appear during early HIV-1 infection. However, in most cases they do not persist but rather become deleted or replaced by less avid CTLs that were previously subdominant as high-level antigenemia establishes, presumably because of increased levels of activation in higher-avidity T cells [98]. High-avidity CD8+ T cells are believed to contribute significantly to the control of viral replication in HIV-1 infection [117], and are associated with increased polyfunctionality in CTLs from viral controllers [118]. High avidity CD8+ T cells are also linked with the control of chronic viral infections in mice, monkeys and humans [119]; for instance, adoptive transfers of highly avid CTL lines into SCID mice result in the clearance of the infecting recombinant vaccinia strains within 3 days from challenge [120]. A considerable body of evidence regarding the role of highly avid CD8+ T cells in retroviral infection also comes from non-human primate vaccination studies. Macaques vaccinated mucosally with a prime-boost vaccinia/SHIV strategy (NYVAC/SHIV) and challenged with SHIV-Ku2 develop highly avid CTLs in the colon, mesenteric lymph nodes and mucosa which appeared to delay the development of peak viremia at the early stages of infection [121]. Such high-avidity CTLs have been found to persist for at least 6 months post-vaccination [43], but have also been associated with a higher rate of viral escape in epitopes from proteins such as nef, vpr and tat in acute SIV infection, with no profound effect on viral fitness [122]. Interestingly, in contrast to the frequently observed CTL-driven escape mutations in HIV-1 infection, to date there are no published data describing similar CTL escape in HIV-2-infected individuals.

Similar findings have been reported in humans in a number of settings. In hepatitis C virus (HCV) infection, patients who have effective viral clearance harbor HCV-specific CD8+ T cells of higher avidity than chronically infected patients [123], and studies of human cytomegalovirus (CMV) infection suggest an oligoclonal narrowing of the CD8+ responses in cases of viral reactivation and/or chronic inflammation that is dominated by cell clonotypes which display higher avidity for their antigens [124]. Finally, studies in mouse models of influenza infection also support the notion that distinct Vβ clonotypes, rather than cellular subsets with more polyfunctional profiles, account for the observed higher avidity [125]. It has thus been proposed that high-avidity clones may have a kinetic advantage over less avid clonotypes that could emerge from the ability of such clonotypes to sense their cognate epitopes early in infection, when antigenemia is still quite low [98]. In the context of HIV-2 infection, this may permit the persistence of large populations of virus-specific T cells even when the viral load is below detection.

High functional avidity has also been associated with increased cross-reactivity in HIV-1 infection [126]. When a natural TCR recovered from an HIV-1 long-term non-progressor targeting the gag epitope SLYNTVATL (SL9) was mutated to increase avidity, its ability to control different viral isolates and escape variants also increased [127]. Similarly, in a study by Bennett and colleagues, the engineering of TCRs of higher avidity through CDR3 amino-acid swapping broadened the antiviral recognition for some TCR mutants [128]. However, whether or not the higher avidity in HIV-2 infection also correlates with higher cross-recognition is not yet clear. Cross-reactive responses against the corresponding HIV-1 epitope have been previously described in HIV-2 infection in patients expressing the HLA-B*35 and HLA*58 alleles that target gag epitopes [83,85], but, interestingly, not for the very dominant HLA-B*53-restricted [81] or B*2703-restricted [129] responses to HIV-2 gag. One study has suggested that whilst HIV-2-infected patients mount strong CD8+ T cell responses to gag, cross-reactivity against corresponding HIV-1 epitopes is less commonly seen in HIV-2 than cross-reactive responses to HIV-2 gag in HIV-1 infection: the extent of cross-reactivity correlates inversely with CD4+ count [126]. HIV-1/2 cross-reactive responses have previously been thought to emerge from a broader TCR usage [130] rather than from the action of highly avid cross-reactive CTL clonotypes, but more detailed studies are needed to confirm this hypothesis.

How these avid clonotypes can persist over time in HIV-2 infection is not yet clear. Immune activation in HIV-2 infection is more pronounced in viremic individuals, where activation markers such as HLA-DR, CD38, and Fas (CD95) are highly upregulated [67] and show a linear relationship with viral load [54]; therefore, one plausible explanation could be that there is less clonal turnover in aviremic patients because of the lower degree of immune activation. Findings from HIV-1 infection also render this hypothesis plausible. For instance, even though avidity differences do not appear to translate into differences in functionality between different clonotypes in HIV-1 infection, they do associate with different cellular differentiation phenotypes, whereby highly avid clonotypes are more likely to display a profile of replicative senescence (CD27-CD45RO-CD57+) [131]. It has also been proposed that the maintenance of clonotypic patterns in HIV-1 infection is associated with low-level set-point HIV-1 viremia [98], whereas high doses of antigen may induce the apoptotic death of highly avid CTLs [120,132].

Hence, as for HIV-1 infection, the decline of highly avid, dominant clonotypes could reflect the replicative senescence of CD8+ T cells at the clonal level [117] in the face of continuing antigen exposure in HIV-2+ progressors, whereas clonotypes that display a higher functional avidity can survive in the context of low viremia and immune activation which they serve to promote in non-progressors.

As in other models of viral control, it is difficult to disentangle cause and effect between low viral replication and superior immune responses. Whilst the case for immune control in non-progression with HIV-2 infection is stronger than that for HIV-1 infection, formal proof could come from studies in which non-progressor-like responses are induced in viremic subjects by therapeutic vaccination or T cell receptor transfer strategies, to determine if this would lead to control of viral replication. This would provide a valuable "proof of concept" of the potential for cellular immune control of human HIV infection, as well as having potential utility as an adjunct to ART in HIV-2-infected progressors, which poses particular challenges for the clinician.

CONCLUSIONS

Although comparative studies of HIV-1- and HIV-2-infected individuals have yielded several features of host immunity that are selectively preserved, superior or distinct in natural HIV-2 infection, currently the most compelling evidence suggests a role for T cell immunity in defining the HIV-2 controller phenotype. Thus, viral control in HIV-2 infection is associated with several distinct features—a high-magnitude cellular immune response directed towards conserved Gag epitopes, an earlier-differentiated CD8+ T cell phenotype with increased polyfunctionality and exceptionally high functional avidity, supported by polyfunctional virus-specific CD4+ T cells, against a background of substantially less extensive immune activation than is seen in HIV-1 infection. Recent sequence data have also revealed key motifs in the HIV-2 capsid associated with undetectable plasma viremia, although the mechanisms for their selection or their role in viral control are yet to be fully investigated. Emerging as one of the most striking differences from HIV-1 infection is the slower evolution and possible lower frequency of adaptive immune escape in asymptomatic HIV-2-infected individuals. It is tempting to speculate that these features may be the direct result of a highly avid and polyfunctional HIV-2-specific cellular immune response that controls viremia to such an extent that HIV-2 is unable to successfully replicate, persist and adapt in its host—hallmarks of HIV-1 that define the fundamental obstacles in designing an HIV-1 vaccine. However, the question arises as to whether these findings, which have been largely derived from the Caió village community cohort, are specific to the Manjago ethnic group—which our immunogenetic studies suggests is quite distinct from other groups in the sub-region—or if they can be generalized to people of other ethnicities and/or infected with different HIV-2 strains. Further studies are needed to confirm or extend these observations in different clinical settings, which would help to determine whether or not HIV-2 infection does indeed represent a robust model of host immune control in the majority of cases.

REFERENCES

[1] Barin F, M'Boup S, Denis F, Kanki P, Allan JS, Lee TH, et al. Serological evidence for virus related to simian T-lymphotropic retrovirus III in residents of West Africa. Lancet 1985;2:1387−9.

[2] Clavel F, Guetard D, Brun-Vezinet F, Chamaret S, Rey MA, Santos-Ferreira MO, et al. Isolation of a new human retrovirus from West African patients with AIDS. Science 1986;233:343−6.

[3] Clavel F, Guyader M, Guetard D, Salle M, Montagnier L, Alizon M. Molecular cloning and polymorphism of the human immune deficiency virus type 2. Nature 1986;324:691−5.

[4] Guyader M, Emerman M, Sonigo P, Clavel F, Montagnier L, Alizon M. Genome organisation and transactivation of the human immunodeficiency virus type 2. Nature 1987;326:662−9.

[5] Addo MM, Draenert R, Rathod A, Verrill CL, Davis BT, Gandhi RT, et al. Fully differentiated HIV-1 specific CD8+ T effector cells are more frequently detectable in controlled than in progressive HIV-1 infection. PLoS ONE 2007;2:e321.

[6] Damond F, Apetrei C, Robertson DL, Souquiere S, Lepretre A, Matheron S, et al. Variability of human immunodeficiency virus type 2 (HIV-2) infecting patients living in France. Virology 2001;280:19−30.

[7] Hodges-Mameletzis I, De Bree G, Rowland-Jones SL. An underestimated lentivirus model: What can HIV-2 research contribute to the development of an effective HIV-1 vaccine? Exp Rev Anti-Infect Ther 2011;9:195−206.

[8] Lemey P, Pybus OG, Wang B, Saksena NK, Salemi M, Vandamme AM. Tracing the origin and history of the HIV-2 epidemic. Proc Natl Acad Sci USA 2003;100:6588−92.

[9] Apetrei C, Metzger MJ, Richardson D, Ling B, Telfer PT, Reed P, et al. Detection and partial characterization of simian immunodeficiency virus SIVsm strains from bush meat samples from rural Sierra Leone. J Virol 2005;79:2631−6.

[10] Valadas E, Franca L, Sousa S, Antunes F. 20 years of HIV-2 infection in Portugal: Trends and changes in epidemiology. Clin Infect Dis 2009;48:1166−7.

[11] Schim van der Loeff MF, Aaby P. Towards a better understanding of the epidemiology of HIV-2. AIDS 1999;13(Suppl A):S69−84.

[12] Cortes E, Detels R, Aboulafia D, Li XL, Moudgil T, Alam M, et al. HIV-1, HIV-2, and HTLV-I infection in high-risk groups in Brazil. N Engl J Med 1989;320:953−8.

[13] Kannangai R, Ramalingam S, Vijayakumar TS, Prabu K, Jesudason MV, Sridharan G. HIV-2 sub-epidemic not gathering speed: Experience from a tertiary care center in South India. J Acquir Immune Defic Syndr 2003;32:573−5.

[14] Poulsen AG, Kvinesdal B, Aaby P, Molbak K, Frederiksen K, Dias F, et al. Prevalence of and mortality from human immunodeficiency virus type 2 in Bissau, West Africa. Lancet 1989;1:827−31.

[15] Aaby P, Ariyoshi K, Buckner M, Jensen H, Berry N, Wilkins A, et al. Age of wife as a major determinant of male-to-female transmission of HIV-2 infection: A community study from rural West Africa. AIDS 1996;10:1585−90.

[16] Poulsen AG, Aaby P, Jensen H, Dias F. Risk factors for HIV-2 seropositivity among older people in Guinea-Bissau. A search for the early history of HIV-2 infection. Scand J Infect Dis 2000;32:169−75.

[17] Marlink R, Kanki P, Thior I, Travers K, Eisen G, Siby T, et al. Reduced rate of disease development after HIV-2 infection as compared to HIV-1. Science 1994;265:1587−90.

[18] Hamel DJ, Sankale JL, Eisen G, Meloni ST, Mullins C, Gueye-Ndiaye A, et al. Twenty years of prospective molecular epidemiology in Senegal: Changes in HIV diversity. AIDS Res Hum Retrovir 2007;23:1189−96.

[19] da Silva ZJ, Oliveira I, Andersen A, Dias F, Rodrigues A, et al. Changes in prevalence and incidence of HIV-1, HIV-2 and dual infections in urban areas of Bissau, Guinea-Bissau: Is HIV-2 disappearing? AIDS 2008;22:1195−202.

[20] Van Tienen C, van der Loeff MS, Zaman SM, Vincent T, Sarge-Njie R, Peterson I, et al. Two distinct epidemics: The rise of HIV-1 and decline of HIV-2 infection between 1990 and 2007 in rural Guinea-Bissau. J Acquir Immune Defic Syndr 2010;53:640−7.

[21] Ibe S, Yokomaku Y, Shiino T, Tanaka R, Hattori J, Fujisaki S, et al. HIV-2 CRF01_AB: First circulating recombinant form of HIV-2. J Acquir Immune Defic Syndr 2010;54:241−7.

[22] Gao F, Yue L, Robertson DL, Hill SC, Hui H, Biggar RJ, et al. Genetic diversity of human immunodeficiency virus type 2: Evidence for distinct sequence subtypes with differences in virus biology. J Virol 1994;68:7433−47.

[23] Smith SM, Christian D, de Lame V, Shah U, Austin L, Gautam R, et al. Isolation of a new HIV-2 group in the US. Retrovirology 2008;5:103.

[24] Clavel F, Mansinho K, Chamaret S, Guetard D, Favier V, Nina J, et al. Human immuno-deficiency virus type 2 infection associated with AIDS in West Africa. N Engl J Med 1987;316:1180−5.

[25] Brun-Vezinet F, Rey MA, Katlama C, Girard PM, Roulot D, Yeni P, et al. Lymphadenop-athy-associated virus type 2 in AIDS and AIDS-related complex. Clinical and virological features in four patients. Lancet 1987;1:128−32.

[26] Martinez-Steele E, Awasana AA, Corrah T, Sabally S, van der Sande M, Jaye A, et al. Is HIV-2- induced AIDS different from HIV-1-associated AIDS? Data from a West African clinic. AIDS 2007;21:317−24.

[27] Ariyoshi K, Schim van der Loeff M, Cook P, Whitby D, Corrah T, Jaffar S, et al. Kaposi's sarcoma in the Gambia, West Africa is less frequent in human immunodeficiency virus type 2 than in human immunodeficiency virus type 1 infection despite a high prevalence of human herpesvirus 8. J Hum Virol 1998;1:193−9.

[28] Marlink RG, Ricard D, M'Boup S, Kanki PJ, Romet-Lemonne JL, N'Doye I, et al. Clinical, hematologic, and immunologic cross-sectional evaluation of individuals exposed to human immunodeficiency virus type-2 (HIV-2). AIDS Res Hum Retroviruses 1988;4:137−48.

[29] Poulsen AG, Aaby P, Larsen O, Jensen H, Naucler A, Lisse IM, et al. 9-year HIV-2-asso-ciated mortality in an urban community in Bissau, W. Africa. Lancet 1997;349:911−4.

[30] Poulsen AG, Aaby P, Larsen O, Jensen H, Naucler A, Lisse IM, et al. 9-year HIV-2-associated mortality in an urban community in Bissau, West Africa. Lancet 1997;349: 911−4.

[31] Darby SC, Ewart DW, Giangrande PL, Spooner RJ, Rizza CR. Importance of age at infection with HIV-1 for survival and development of AIDS in UK haemophilia population. UK Haemophilia Centre Directors' Organisation. Lancet 1996;347:1573−9.

[32] O'Donovan D, Ariyoshi K, Milligan P, Ota M, Yamuah L, Sarge-Njie R, et al. Maternal plasma viral RNA levels determine marked differences in mother-to-child transmission rates of HIV-1 and HIV-2 in The Gambia. MRC/Gambia Government/University College London Medical School Working Group on Mother–Child Transmission of HIV. AIDS 2000;14:441–8.

[33] Ota MO, O'Donovan D, Alabi AS, Milligan P, Yamuah LK, N'Gom PT, et al. Maternal HIV-1 and HIV-2 infection and child survival in The Gambia. AIDS 2000;14:435–9.

[34] Barroso H, Araujo F, Gomes MH, Mota-Miranda A, Taveira N. Phylogenetic demonstration of two cases of perinatal human immunodeficiency virus type 2 infection diagnosed in adulthood. AIDS Res Hum Retrovir 2004;20:1373–6.

[35] Ariyoshi K, Berry N, Wilkins A, Ricard D, Aaby P, Naucler A, et al. A community-based study of human immunodeficiency virus type 2 provirus load in rural village in West Africa. J Infect Dis 1996;173:245–8.

[36] Popper SJ, Sarr AD, Gueye-Ndiaye A, Mboup S, Essex ME, Kanki PJ. Low plasma human immunodeficiency virus type 2 viral load is independent of proviral load: Low virus production *in vivo*. J Virol 2000;74:1554–7.

[37] Popper SJ, Sarr AD, Travers KU, Gueye-Ndiaye A, Mboup S, Essex ME, et al. Lower human immunodeficiency virus (HIV) type 2 viral load reflects the difference in pathogenicity of HIV-1 and HIV-2. J Infect Dis 1999;180:1116–21.

[38] Berry N, Jaffar S, Van Der Loeff MS, Ariyoshi K, Harding E, N'Gom PT, et al. Low level viremia and high CD4% predict normal survival in a cohort of HIV type-2-infected villagers. AIDS Res Hum Retrovir 2002;18:1167–73.

[39] van der Loeff MF, Larke N, Kaye S, Berry N, Ariyoshi K, Alabi A, et al. Undetectable plasma viral load predicts normal survival in HIV-2-infected people in a West African village. Retrovirology 2010;7:46.

[40] Gottlieb GS, Sow PS, Hawes SE, Ndoye I, Redman M, Coll-Seck AM, et al. Equal plasma viral loads predict a similar rate of CD4+ T cell decline in human immunodeficiency virus (HIV) type 1- and HIV-2-infected individuals from Senegal, West Africa. J Infect Dis 2002;185:905–14.

[41] Hansmann A, Schim van der Loeff MF, Kaye S, Awasana AA, Sarge-Njie R, O'Donovan D, et al. Baseline plasma viral load and CD4 cell percentage predict survival in HIV-1- and HIV-2-infected women in a community-based cohort in The Gambia. J Acquir Immune Defic Syndr 2005;38:335–41.

[42] Ariyoshi K, Jaffar S, Alabi AS, Berry N, van der Loeff MS, Sabally S, et al. Plasma RNA viral load predicts the rate of CD4 T cell decline and death in HIV-2-infected patients in West Africa. AIDS 2000;14:339–44.

[43] Thiebaut R, Matheron S, Taieb A, Brun-Vezinet F, Chene G, Autran B. Long-term nonprogressors and elite controllers in the ANRS CO5 HIV-2 cohort. AIDS 2011;25:865–7.

[44] Peterson K, de Silva T, Rowland-Jones SL, Jallow S. Antiretroviral therapy for HIV-2 infection: Recommendations for management in low-resource settings. AIDS Res Treatment 2011. in press.

[45] Gottlieb GS, Hawes SE, Agne HD, Stern JE, Critchlow CW, Kiviat NB, et al. Lower levels of HIV RNA in semen in HIV-2 compared with HIV-1 infection: Implications for differences in transmission. AIDS 2006;20:895–900.

[46] Hawes SE, Sow PS, Stern JE, Critchlow CW, Gottlieb GS, Kiviat NB. Lower levels of HIV-2 than HIV-1 in the female genital tract: Correlates and longitudinal assessment of viral shedding. AIDS 2008;22:2517–25.

[47] Besnier JM, Barin F, Baillou A, Liard F, Choutet P, Goudeau A. Symptomatic HIV-2 primary infection. Lancet 1990;335:798.

[48] Andersson S, Norrgren H, da Silva Z, Biague A, Bamba S, Kwok S, et al. Plasma viral load in HIV-1 and HIV-2 singly and dually infected individuals in Guinea-Bissau, West Africa: Significantly lower plasma virus set point in HIV-2 infection than in HIV-1 infection. Arch Intern Med 2000;160:3286−93.

[49] Grossman Z, Meier-Schellersheim M, Sousa AE, Victorino RM, Paul WE. CD4+ T-cell depletion in HIV infection: Are we closer to understanding the cause? Nat Med 2002;8:319−23.

[50] Brenchley JM, Price DA, Schacker TW, Asher TE, Silvestri G, Rao S, et al. Microbial translocation is a cause of systemic immune activation in chronic HIV infection. Nat Med 2006;12:1365−71.

[51] Silvestri G, Sodora DL, Koup RA, Paiardini M, O'Neil SP, McClure HM, et al. Nonpathogenic SIV infection of sooty mangabeys is characterized by limited bystander immunopathology despite chronic high-level viremia. Immunity 2003;18:441−52.

[52] Sousa AE, Carneiro J, Meier-Schellersheim M, Grossman Z, Victorino RM. CD4 T cell depletion is linked directly to immune activation in the pathogenesis of HIV-1 and HIV-2 but only indirectly to the viral load. J Immunol 2002;169:3400−6.

[53] Jaffar S, Van der Loeff MS, Eugen-Olsen J, Vincent T, Sarje-Njie R, Ngom P, et al. Immunological predictors of survival in HIV type 2-infected rural villagers in Guinea-Bissau. AIDS Res Hum Retrovir 2005;21:560−4.

[54] Leligdowicz A, Feldmann J, Jaye A, Cotten M, Dong T, McMichael A, et al. Direct relationship between virus load and systemic immune activation in HIV-2 infection. J Infect Dis 2010;201:114−22.

[55] Schindler M, Munch J, Kutsch O, Li H, Santiago ML, Bibollet-Ruche F, et al. Nef-mediated suppression of T cell activation was lost in a lentiviral lineage that gave rise to HIV-1. Cell 2006;125:1055−67.

[56] Feldmann J, Leligdowicz A, Jaye A, Dong T, Whittle H, Rowland-Jones SL. Down-regulation of the T-cell receptor by human immunodeficiency virus type 2 Nef does not protect against disease progression. J Virol 2009;83:12968−72.

[57] Nowroozalizadeh S, Mansson F, da Silva Z, Repits J, Dabo B, Pereira C, et al. Microbial translocation correlates with the severity of both HIV-1 and HIV-2 infections. J Infect Dis 2010;201:1150−4.

[58] Blaak H, Boers PH, Schutten M, Van Der Enden ME, Osterhaus AD. HIV-2-infected individuals with undetectable plasma viremia carry replication-competent virus in peripheral blood lymphocytes. J Acquir Immune Defic Syndr 2004;36:777−82.

[59] Onyango CO, Leligdowicz A, Yokoyama M, Sato H, Song H, Nakayama EE, et al. HIV-2 capsids distinguish high and low virus load patients in a West African community cohort. Vaccine 2010;28(Suppl 2):B60−7.

[60] Kong LI, Lee SW, Kappes JC, Parkin JS, Decker D, Hoxie JA, et al. West African HIV-2-related human retrovirus with attenuated cytopathicity. Science 1988;240:1525−9.

[61] Schramm B, Penn ML, Palacios EH, Grant RM, Kirchhoff F, Goldsmith MA. Cytopathicity of human immunodeficiency virus type 2 (HIV-2) in human lymphoid tissue is coreceptor dependent and comparable to that of HIV-1. J Virol 2000;74:9594−600.

[62] Arien KK, Abraha A, Quinones-Mateu ME, Kestens L, Vanham G, Arts EJ. The replicative fitness of primary human immunodeficiency virus type 1 (HIV-1) group M, HIV-1 group O, and HIV-2 isolates. J Virol 2005;79:8979−90.

[63] Blaak H, van der Ende ME, Boers PH, Schuitemaker H, Osterhaus AD. *In vitro* replication capacity of HIV-2 variants from long-term aviremic individuals. Virology 2006;353: 144−54.

[64] MacNeil A, Sarr AD, Sankale JL, Meloni ST, Mboup S, Kanki P. Direct evidence of lower viral replication rates *in vivo* in human immunodeficiency virus type 2 (HIV-2) infection than in HIV-1 infection. J Virol 2007;81:5325−30.

[65] Guyader M, Emerman M, Sonigo P, Clavel F, Montagnier L, Alizon M. Genome organization and transactivation of the human immunodeficiency virus type 2. Nature 1987;326:662−9.

[66] Markovitz DM, Hannibal M, Perez VL, Gauntt C, Folks TM, Nabel GJ. Differential regulation of human immunodeficiency viruses (HIVs): A specific regulatory element in HIV-2 responds to stimulation of the T-cell antigen receptor. Proc Natl Acad Sci USA 1990;87:9098−102.

[67] Soares RS, Tendeiro R, Foxall RB, Baptista AP, Cavaleiro R, Gomes P, et al. Cell-associated viral burden provides evidence of ongoing viral replication in aviremic HIV-2-infected patients. J Virol 2011;85:2429−38.

[68] Simon F, Matheron S, Tamalet C, Loussert-Ajaka I, Bartczak S, Pepin JM, et al. Cellular and plasma viral load in patients infected with HIV-2. AIDS 1993;7:1411−7.

[69] Grassly NC, Xiang Z, Ariyoshi K, Aaby P, Jensen H, Schim van der Loeff M, et al. Mortality among human immunodeficiency virus type 2-positive villagers in rural Guinea-Bissau is correlated with viral genotype. J Virol 1998;72:7895−9.

[70] Song H, Nakayama EE, Yokoyama M, Sato H, Levy JA, Shioda T. A single amino acid of the human immunodeficiency virus type 2 capsid affects its replication in the presence of cynomolgus monkey and human TRIM5alphas. J Virol 2007;81:7280−5.

[71] MacNeil A, Sankale JL, Meloni ST, Sarr AD, Mboup S, Kanki P. Long-term intrapatient viral evolution during HIV-2 infection. J Infect Dis 2007;195:726−33.

[72] Skar H, Borrego P, Wallstrom TC, Mild M, Marcelino JM, Barroso H, et al. HIV-2 genetic evolution in patients with advanced disease is faster than that in matched HIV-1 patients. J Virol 2010;84:7412−5.

[73] Diouf K, Sarr AD, Eisen G, Popper S, Mboup S, Kanki P. Associations between MHC class I and susceptibility to HIV-2 disease progression. J Hum Virol 2002;5:1−7.

[74] Carrington M, Nelson GW, Martin MP, Kissner T, Vlahov D, Goedert JJ, et al. HLA and HIV-1: Heterozygote advantage and B*35-Cw*04 disadvantage. Science 1999;283: 1748−52.

[75] Gao X, Nelson GW, Karacki P, Martin MP, Phair J, Kaslow R, et al. Effect of a single amino acid change in MHC class I molecules on the rate of progression to AIDS. N Engl J Med 2001;344:1668−75.

[76] Martin MP, Gao X, Lee JH, Nelson GW, Detels R, Goedert JJ, et al. Epistatic interaction between KIR3DS1 and HLA-B delays the progression to AIDS. Nat Genet 2002; 31:429.

[77] Pereyra F, Jia X, McLaren PJ, Telenti A, de Bakker PI, et al. The major genetic determinants of HIV-1 control affect HLA class I peptide presentation. Science 2010;330:1551−7.

[78] Yindom LM, Leligdowicz A, Martin MP, Gao X, Qi Y, Zaman SM, et al. Influence of HLA class I and HLA-KIR compound genotypes on HIV-2 infection and markers of disease progression in a Manjako community in West Africa. J Virol 2010;84:8202−8.

[79] Ylinen LM, Keckesova Z, Wilson SJ, Ranasinghe S, Towers GJ. Differential restriction of human immunodeficiency virus type 2 and simian immunodeficiency virus SIVmac by TRIM5alpha alleles. J Virol 2005;79:11580−7.

[80] Lim SY, Rogers T, Chan T, Whitney JB, Kim J, Sodroski J, et al. TRIM5alpha modulates immunodeficiency virus control in rhesus monkeys. PLoS Pathog 2010;6:e1000738.

[81] Gotch F, McAdam SN, Allsopp CE, Gallimore A, Elvin J, Kieny MP, et al. Cytotoxic T cells in HIV2-seropositive Gambians. Identification of a virus-specific MHC-restricted peptide epitope. J Immunol 1993;151:3361−9.

[82] Weiss RA, Clapham PR, Weber JN, Whitby D, Tedder RS, O'Connor T, et al. HIV-2 antisera cross-neutralize HIV-1. AIDS 1988;2:95−100.

[83] Rowland-Jones SL, Sutton J, Ariyoshi K, Dong T, Gotch FM, McAdam S, et al. HIV-specific cytotoxic T cells in HIV-exposed but uninfected Gambian women. Nat Med 1995;1:59−64.

[84] Pinto LA, Covas MJ, Victorino RM. T-helper cross reactivity to viral recombinant proteins in HIV-2-infected patients [letter] [published erratum appears in AIDS (1993) 7(11), following 1541]. AIDS 1993;7:1389−91.

[85] Bertoletti A, Cham F, McAdam S, Rostron T, Rowland-Jones S, Sabally S, et al. Cytotoxic T cells from human immunodeficiency virus type 2-infected patients frequently cross-react with different human immunodeficiency virus type 1 clades. J Virol 1998;72:2439−48.

[86] Bjorling E, Scarlatti G, von GA, Albert J, Biberfeld G, Chiodi F, et al. Autologous neutralizing antibodies prevail in HIV-2 but not in HIV-1 infection. Virology 1993;193:528−30.

[87] Rodriguez SK, Sarr AD, MacNeil A, Thakore-Meloni S, Gueye-Ndiaye A, Traore I, et al. Comparison of heterologous neutralizing antibody responses of human immuno-deficiency virus type 1 (HIV-1)- and HIV-2-infected Senegalese patients: Distinct patterns of breadth and magnitude distinguish HIV-1 and HIV-2 infections. J Virol 2007;81:5331−8.

[88] Shi Y, Brandin E, Vincic E, Jansson M, Blaxhult A, Gyllensten K, et al. Evolution of human immunodeficiency virus type 2 coreceptor usage, autologous neutralization, envelope sequence and glycosylation. J Gen Virol 2005;86:3385−96.

[89] Barroso H, Taveira N. Evidence for negative selective pressure in HIV-2 evolution *in vivo*. Infect Genet Evol 2005;5:239−46.

[90] Jaye A, Sarge-Njie R, van der Loeff MS, Todd J, Alabi A, Sabally S, et al. No differences in cellular immune responses between asymptomatic HIV type 1- and type 2-infected Gambian patients. J Infect Dis 2004;189:498−505.

[91] Zheng NN, Kiviat NB, Sow PS, Hawes SE, Wilson A, Diallo-Agne H, et al. Comparison of human immunodeficiency virus (HIV)-specific T-cell responses in HIV-1- and HIV-2-infected individuals in Senegal. J Virol 2004;78:13934−42.

[92] Gillespie GM, Pinheiro S, Sayeid-Al-Jamee M, Alabi A, Kaye S, Sabally S, et al. CD8(+) T cell responses to human immunodeficiency viruses type 2 (HIV-2) and type 1 (HIV-1) gag proteins are distinguishable by magnitude and breadth but not cellular phenotype. Eur J Immunol 2005;35:1445−53.

[93] Duvall MG, Jaye A, Dong T, Brenchley JM, Alabi AS, Jeffries DJ, et al. Maintenance of HIV-specific CD4+ T cell help distinguishes HIV-2 from HIV-1 infection. J Immunol 2006;176:6973−81.

[94] Duvall MG, Precopio ML, Ambrozak DA, Jaye A, McMichael AJ, Whittle HC, et al. Polyfunctional T cell responses are a hallmark of HIV-2 infection. Eur J Immunol 2008;38:350−63.

[95] Ahmed RK, Norrgren H, da Silva Z, Blaxhult A, Fredriksson EL, Biberfeld G, et al. Antigen-specific beta-chemokine production and CD8 T-cell noncytotoxic antiviral activity in HIV-2-infected individuals. Scand J Immunol 2005;61:63−71.

[96] Leligdowicz A, Yindom LM, Onyango C, Sarge-Njie R, Alabi A, Cotten M, et al. Robust Gag-specific T cell responses characterize viremia control in HIV-2 infection. J Clin Invest 2007;117:3067−74.

[97] Lichterfeld M, Yu XG, Cohen D, Addo MM, Malenfant J, Perkins B, et al. HIV-1 Nef is preferentially recognized by CD8 T cells in primary HIV-1 infection despite a relatively high degree of genetic diversity. AIDS 2004;18:1383−92.

[98] Lichterfeld M, Yu XG, Mui SK, Williams KL, Trocha A, Brockman MA, et al. Selective depletion of high-avidity human immunodeficiency virus type 1 (HIV-1)-specific CD8+ T cells after early HIV-1 infection. J Virol 2007;81:4199−214.

[99] Ariyoshi K, Cham F, Berry N, Jaffar S, Sabally S, Corrah T, et al. HIV-2-specific cytotoxic T-lymphocyte activity is inversely related to proviral load. AIDS 1995;9:555−9.

[100] Leligdowicz A, Onyango C, Yindom LM, Peng Y, Cotten M, Jaye A, et al. Highly avid, oligoclonal, early-differentiated antigen-specific CD8+ T cells in chronic HIV-2 infection. Eur J Immunol 2010;40:1963−72.

[101] Gottlinger HG. The HIV-1 assembly machine. AIDS 2001;15(Suppl 5):S13−20.

[102] Kiepiela P, Ngumbela K, Thobakgale C, Ramduth D, Honeyborne I, Moodley E, et al. CD8+ T-cell responses to different HIV proteins have discordant associations with viral load. Nat Med 2007;13:46−53.

[103] Edwards BH, Bansal A, Sabbaj S, Bakari J, Mulligan MJ, Goepfert PA. Magnitude of functional CD8+ T-cell responses to the gag protein of human immunodeficiency virus type 1 correlates inversely with viral load in plasma. J Virol 2002;76:2298−305.

[104] Saez-Cirion A, Sinet M, Shin SY, Urrutia A, Versmisse P, Lacabaratz C, et al. Heterogeneity in HIV suppression by CD8 T cells from HIV controllers: Association with Gag-specific CD8 T cell responses. J Immunol 2009;182:7828−37.

[105] Betts MR, Ambrozak DR, Douek DC, Bonhoeffer S, Brenchley JM, Casazza JP, et al. Analysis of total human immunodeficiency virus (HIV)-specific CD4(+) and CD8(+) T-cell responses: Relationship to viral load in untreated HIV infection. J Virol 2001;75:11983−91.

[106] Addo MM, Yu XG, Rathod A, Cohen D, Eldridge RL, Strick D, et al. Comprehensive epitope analysis of human immunodeficiency virus type 1 (HIV-1)-specific T-cell responses directed against the entire expressed HIV-1 genome demonstrate broadly directed responses, but no correlation to viral load. J Virol 2003;77:2081−92.

[107] Papagno L, Appay V, Sutton J, Rostron T, Gillespie GM, Ogg GS, et al. Comparison between HIV- and CMV-specific T cell responses in long-term HIV infected donors. Clin Exp Immunol 2002;130:509−17.

[108] Appay V, Dunbar PR, Callan M, Klenerman P, Gillespie GM, Papagno L, et al. Memory CD8+ T cells vary in differentiation phenotype in different persistent virus infections. Nat Med 2002;8:379−85.

[109] Appay V, Hansasuta P, Sutton J, Schrier RD, Wong JK, Furtado M, et al. Persistent HIV-1-specific cellular responses despite prolonged therapeutic viral suppression. AIDS 2002;16:161−70.

[110] Champagne P, Ogg GS, King AS, Knabenhans C, Ellefsen K, Nobile M, et al. Skewed maturation of memory HIV-specific CD8 T lymphocytes. Nature 2001;410:106−11.

[111] van Baarle D, Kostense S, van Oers MH, Hamann D, Miedema F. Failing immune control as a result of impaired CD8+ T-cell maturation: CD27 might provide a clue. Trends Immunol 2002;23:586−91.

[112] Saez-Cirion A, Lacabaratz C, Lambotte O, Versmisse P, Urrutia A, Boufassa F, et al. HIV controllers exhibit potent CD8 T cell capacity to suppress HIV infection *ex vivo* and peculiar cytotoxic T lymphocyte activation phenotype. Proc Natl Acad Sci USA 2007;104:6776−81.

[113] Papagno L, Spina CA, Marchant A, Salio M, Rufer N, Little S, et al. Immune activation and CD8(+) T-cell differentiation towards senescence in HIV-1 infection. PLoS Biol 2004;2:E20.

[114] Appay V, Rowland-Jones SL. Premature ageing of the immune system: The cause of AIDS? Trends Immunol 2002;23:580–5.

[115] Day CL, Kaufmann DE, Kiepiela P, Brown JA, Moodley ES, Reddy S, et al. PD-1 expression on HIV-specific T cells is associated with T-cell exhaustion and disease progression. Nature 2006;443:350–4.

[116] Trautmann L, Janbazian L, Chomont N, Said EA, Gimmig S, Bessette B, et al. Upregulation of PD-1 expression on HIV-specific CD8+ T cells leads to reversible immune dysfunction. Nat Med 2006;12:1198–202.

[117] Almeida JR, Price DA, Papagno L, Arkoub ZA, Sauce D, Bornstein E, et al. Superior control of HIV-1 replication by CD8+ T cells is reflected by their avidity, polyfunctionality, and clonal turnover. J Exp Med 2007;204:2473–85.

[118] Almeida JR, Sauce D, Price DA, Papagno L, Shin SY, Moris A, et al. Antigen sensitivity is a major determinant of CD8+ T-cell polyfunctionality and HIV-suppressive activity. Blood 2009;113:6351–60.

[119] Chakrabarti LA, Simon V. Immune mechanisms of HIV control. Curr Opin Immunol 2010;22:488–96.

[120] Alexander-Miller MA, Leggatt GR, Berzofsky JA. Selective expansion of high- or low-avidity cytotoxic T lymphocytes and efficacy for adoptive immunotherapy. Proc Natl Acad Sci USA 1996;93:4102–7.

[121] Belyakov IM, Kuznetsov VA, Kelsall B, Klinman D, Moniuszko M, Lemon M, et al. Impact of vaccine-induced mucosal high-avidity CD8+ CTLs in delay of AIDS viral dissemination from mucosa. Blood 2006;107:3258–64.

[122] O'Connor DH, Allen TM, Vogel TU, Jing P, DeSouza IP, Dodds E, et al. Acute phase cytotoxic T lymphocyte escape is a hallmark of simian immunodeficiency virus infection. Nat Med 2002;8:493–9.

[123] Neveu B, Debeaupuis E, Echasserieau K, le Moullac-Vaidye B, Gassin M, Jegou L, et al. Selection of high-avidity CD8 T cells correlates with control of hepatitis C virus infection. Hepatology 2008;48:713–22.

[124] Trautmann L, Rimbert M, Echasserieau K, Saulquin X, Neveu B, Dechanet J, et al. Selection of T cell clones expressing high-affinity public TCRs within human cytomegalovirus-specific CD8 T cell responses. J Immunol 2005;175:6123–32.

[125] Moffat JM, Handel A, Doherty PC, Turner SJ, Thomas PG, La Gruta NL. Influenza epitope-specific CD8+ T cell avidity, but not cytokine polyfunctionality, can be determined by TCRbeta clonotype. J Immunol 2010;185:6850–6.

[126] Jennes W, Camara M, Dieye T, Mboup S, Kestens L. Higher homologous and lower cross-reactive Gag-specific T-cell responses in human immunodeficiency virus type 2 (HIV-2) than in HIV-1 infection. J Virol 2008;82:8619–28.

[127] Varela-Rohena A, Molloy PE, Dunn SM, Li Y, Suhoski MM, Carroll RG, et al. Control of HIV-1 immune escape by CD8 T cells expressing enhanced T-cell receptor. Nat Med 2008;14:1390–5.

[128] Bennett MS, Joseph A, Ng HL, Goldstein H, Yang OO. Fine-tuning of T-cell receptor avidity to increase HIV epitope variant recognition by cytotoxic T lymphocytes. AIDS 2010;24:2619–28.

[129] Rowland-Jones S, Colbert RA, Dong T, McAdam S, Brown M, Ariyoshi K, et al. Distinct recognition of closely-related HIV-1 and HIV-2 cytotoxic T-cell epitopes presented by HLA-B*2703 and B*2705 [letter]. AIDS 1998;12:1391–3.

[130] Lopes AR, Jaye A, Dorrell L, Sabally S, Alabi A, Jones NA, et al. Greater CD8+ TCR heterogeneity and functional flexibility in HIV-2 compared to HIV-1 infection. J Immunol 2003;171:307−16.

[131] Price DA, Brenchley JM, Ruff LE, Betts MR, Hill BJ, Roederer M, et al. Avidity for antigen shapes clonal dominance in CD8+ T cell populations specific for persistent DNA viruses. J Exp Med 2005;202:1349−61.

[132] Dong T, Moran E, Vinh Chau N, Simmons C, Luhn K, Peng Y, et al. High pro-inflammatory cytokine secretion and loss of high avidity cross-reactive cytotoxic T-cells during the course of secondary dengue virus infection. PLoS ONE 2007;2:e1192.

Genetic Basis of Protection Against HIV

Genetic Associations with Resistance to HIV-1 Infection, Viral Control and Protection Against Disease

Jacques Fellay [1,2] and Amalio Telenti [2]

[1] *Global Health Institute, School of Life Sciences, Federal Institute of Technology—EPFL, Lausanne, Switzerland,* [2] *Institute of Medical Microbiology, University Hospital, University of Lausanne, Lausanne, Switzerland*

INTRODUCTION

The recent progress in genomics [1,2] opens multiple possibilities in HIV research. The field of genomics allows high-throughput investigation of DNA variation, epigenetic modification and RNA regulation, and, of particular relevance for the field of HIV/SIV and research in animal models, the possibility of comparative studies across species. Genetic and genomic research has gone through periods of doubt due to the difficulties in validating results from candidate gene studies, and to the anticipation and impatience generated by the first tools for genome-wide investigation (i.e., genome-wide association studies (GWAS), RNA expression analyses, and siRNA screens). Progress is, however,

Models of Protection Against HIV/SIV. DOI: 10.1016/B978-0-12-387715-4.00012-5

more solid than occasionally perceived, and great advances in technology will continue to generate information on the genetic basis of susceptibility to HIV-1 infection and disease. The next series of tools for exome and whole genome sequencing, deep sequencing analysis of the transcriptome and spliceosome, analysis of epigenetic modification, and new-generation gene silencing and gain-of-function screens should be applied to best materials, and validated with the best functional assays. This chapter will review the state of this field and identify opportunities in research and in vaccine development.

GENETICS OF RESISTANCE AGAINST HIV INFECTION

One of the most remarkable host genetic influences on an infectious disease, homozygosity for a 32-bp deletion in the CCR5 gene (CCR5-Δ32) confers strong resistance against HIV-1 infection [3−5]. The CCR5 molecule, acting as a retroviral coreceptor on the surface of CD4+ T lymphocytes, is required for infection by macrophage-tropic (or R5) viruses, which are responsible for the vast majority of transmission events. Both CCR5-Δ32 and the much rarer CCR5 303T > A mutation (also referred to as m303 or C101X) [6,7] result in the production of truncated proteins that are not expressed on the cell membrane, thereby preventing infection. The quest for host genetic determinants of resistance did not stop with the identification of CCR5 variation, but no other human polymorphism can, so far, be consistently associated with differences in HIV-1 susceptibility [8].

The careful assessment of exposure is an integral part of studies searching for genetic determinants of resistance against HIV infection. It is, however, important to realize that infection with HIV-1 from a single exposure is a rare event [9]; therefore, it is likely that a significant fraction of individuals who were exposed, yet remained uninfected, can just be described as lucky and will not carry any resistance mutation. This complicates the realization of reliable large-scale human genetic studies of resistance and could partially explain the scarcity of such efforts, as well as the absence of positive findings [10]. A thorough description of the genetics of resistance in HIV-1-exposed sero-negative individuals is provided in Chapter 6.

HUMAN GENETIC VARIATION AND HIV CONTROL

The direct exploration of human genetic correlates of protection against acquisition has been hampered by the relative lack of well-characterized exposed yet uninfected populations. Given the extent of the pandemic and the chronic nature of HIV infection, this was not the case for the study of the genetics of HIV control; a flurry of host genetics studies used a candidate gene strategy in attempts to identify polymorphisms impacting the individual response to HIV infection in genes coding for cytokines, chemokines and chemokine receptors, or proteins involved in innate and acquired immunity [11,12]. Interesting knowledge was gained from some of those studies, notably through the careful dissection of the chemokine receptor locus on chromosome 3, containing the CCR5 and CCR2 genes. However, because of a combination of limitations, many results were unconvincing or conflicting; the sample sizes were generally small, correction for multiple testing was not always stringent, and population stratification was not taken into account, which can create false-positive associations even in populations with homogeneous self-reported ancestry [13,14].

As discussed in the introduction to this chapter, the emergence of genome-wide approaches represented a fundamental paradigm change throughout human genomics. The HIV host genetics community was relatively quick to appreciate its potential and to confront the challenges associated with the adoption of large-scale genomic technologies [15]. Chief among all factors that made genome-wide association studies possible was the existence of prospective cohorts, which collected detailed clinical data and biological material from hundreds or thousands of HIV-infected individuals over many years. After informed consent authorizing genetic testing was obtained from study participants, these cohorts proved an invaluable resource to search for human genetic determinants of HIV disease outcomes.

Genome-wide association analyses have been performed using various phenotypes, reflecting slightly different laboratory and clinical aspects of viral control and disease progression: plasma viral load (HIV-1 RNA) at set-point [14,16,17]; intracellular HIV-1 DNA [18]; exceptional capacity to control viral replication [19]; pace of CD4+ T lymphocyte decline [14]; time to clinical AIDS [20]; and rapid progressor [21] or long-term non-progressor (LTNP) status [22,23]. The precision of phenotype definition and the careful characterization of study participants represent crucial steps in study design, having the potential to seriously impact the strength of association results, as recently demonstrated empirically [24].

The main lesson from all studies is that the HLA class I region, part of the major histocompatibility complex (MHC) on chromosome 6, contains the human genetic factors that have the strongest impact on HIV control (Figure 12.1). Indeed, single nucleotide polymorphisms (SNPs) located in close proximity to the HLA-B and HLA-C genes consistently topped the lists of highly significant associations. To date, no formal meta-analysis has been performed. However, from the different studies performed on individuals of recent Western European ancestry, it is already possible to distinguish two major and independent associations with viral control in the region, corresponding to the associations with rs2395029 and rs9264942 (dbSNP IDs; see http://www.ncbi.nlm.nih.gov/projects/SNP/) identified in the first published study [16].

The rs2395029 polymorphism, located in the HCP5 gene, is in almost perfect linkage disequilibrium (LD), in whites, with the HLA-B*5701 allele. The association signal is thus at least partially attributable to the known HIV-1 restricting properties of B*5701, an allele known to play a key role in the induction of an efficient cytotoxic T lymphocyte (CTL) response. Noticeably,

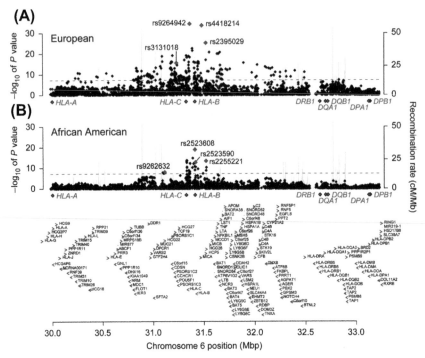

FIGURE 12.1   Regional association plot in the HLA region for (A) European and (B) African American samples from the GWAS performed by the International HIV Controllers Study. Recombination rates (in light blue) are from HapMap. The horizontal dotted line (in red) indicates genome-wide significance ($P < 5 \times 10^{-8}$). SNPs highlighted (with red diamonds) are independent markers identified through stepwise regression. The SNPs showing the strongest association with the ability to effectively control HIV-1 differ between ethnic groups, underlining the need for human population-specific analyses. The HLA region is a gene-rich region of the human genome (bottom part of the figure), making it a challenge to identify the precise causal variants responsible for the observed genetic associations. *Modified from The International HIV Controllers Study, 2010 [19].*

a very comparable result has been observed in the only genome-wide study performed in African Americans, where HLA-B*5703 was the most important determinant of viral control [17]. More recently, an in-depth analysis of the HLA region by the International HIV Controllers Consortium concluded that specific amino acids present in the peptide-binding groove of the HLA molecules summarize the variable anti-HIV potency of different HLA alleles [19].

The second associated polymorphism, rs9264942, is located in the upstream region of the HLA-C gene, 35 kb away, and has therefore often been referred to as "HLA-C-35". Although it is also in LD with HLA-B*5701, it has been shown that it has an independent association signal as well, most likely reflecting some HLA-C-related control of HIV-1. Indeed, the SNP is associated not only with clinical outcomes such as viral load and rate of CD4 T cell decline but also with mRNA and protein expression of HLA-C [16,25], suggesting that the number of molecules expressed at the surface of immune cells might play a role in the efficacy of the antiretroviral response. It seems now clear that the HLA-C-35 SNP itself plays no causal role [25,26]. Recently, Carrington and coworkers identified HLA-C-35 as a marker of variation at the binding of microRNA Hsa-miR-148a to its target site within the 3′ untranslated region of HLA-C [27]. This mechanism of post-transcriptional regulation results in relatively low surface expression of alleles that bind this microRNA and high expression of HLA-C alleles that escape.

Many additional associations were detected in the MHC (Figure 12.1). However, because of the complexity of the region, the extent of genetic variation (the MHC is the most polymorphic region in the human genome) and the long-range LD structure, it proved to be very difficult to distinguish truly independent signals using genotyping data alone. Thus, while it is now established that most human genetic factors influencing HIV disease are concentrated in the MHC and linked to HLA class I variation, an exact understanding of the underlying mechanisms is still elusive and will require careful assessment and cross-fertilization of genetic and immunological evidences. In addition, HLA class I molecules contribute to HIV-1 control not only by inducing CTL responses, but also as ligands for killer cell immunoglobulin-like receptors (KIRs), expressed at the surface of natural killer (NK) cells. KIRs regulate NK cells' activation status through inhibitory or activating signaling, and can thereby have a direct modulating effect on the innate immune response to HIV-1 infection. Specific combinations of KIR genes and HLA class I alleles have been shown to exert epistatic influences on HIV-1 infection [28]: KIR3DL1 and KIR3DS1 were discovered to be associated with better control of HIV-1 when found in patients that also have HLA-B alleles with a Bw4 specificity.

Several genome-wide studies also identified loci associated with HIV control outside of the MHC, but a single one could be replicated and can thus be confidently considered a confirmed association: heterozygosity for CCR5-Δ32, the deletion that confers resistance against infection in its homozygous form. Whether CCR5-Δ32 contributes to better HIV control by decreasing coreceptor concentration on the cell surface or by modulating additional features of the immune response remains an open question [29]. Selected genetic factors associated with functional, experimental and clinical consequences in HIV/SIV infections are shown in Table 12.1. In parallel with HLA associations identified in human studies, this table also emphasizes the role of specific MHC alleles in the control of SIV replication levels—most notably, MHC B-locus alleles Mamu-B*08 and B*17, which are associated with elite control of SIVmac infection in rhesus macaques [30,31].

A different approach to genome analysis uses *in vitro* generation of phenotypes. Loeuillet and colleagues [32] mapped a susceptibility locus on HSA8q24.3 through quantitative linkage analysis using cell lines from multi-generation families. The SNP rs2572886, which is associated with cellular susceptibility to HIV-1 in lymphoblastoid B cells and in primary T cells, is located in a region associated with regulation of the LY6 family of glycosyl-phosphatidyl-inositol (GPI)-anchored proteins. The same locus was mapped through crosses between SJL/J and BALB/cJ inbred mice as a major host factor in mouse susceptibility to adenovirus type 1 infection [33]. The Ly6 family members are attractive candidates for virus susceptibility genes because these membrane-anchored proteins are expressed on lymphoid and myeloid cells,

TABLE 12.1   Selected genetic factors associated with functional, experimental and clinical consequences in HIV/SIV infections

Gene/allele	Species	Functional consequences	Experimental and clinical consequences	References
Multiple HLA-B alleles (e.g., B27, B57, B*5802)	Human	Induction of CTL escape mutations impacting viral fitness; epistatic interaction with KIR genes	Better viral control and slower disease progression; increase in immunogenicity of T cell vaccines	14, 17, 28, 40
HLA-C -35 SNP (rs9264942)	Human	Association with variation in miRNA target site influencing HLA-C expression	Modulation of viral load and disease progression	16, 25, 27
CCR5–CCR2 locus	Human	Decrease in coreceptor expression altering viral entry; possible immunoregulatory effect	Protection from infection; better viral control and slower disease progression; development of entry antagonists for treatment	3–5, 14, 29
Mamu-A*01	Macaque	Induction of CTL escape mutations impacting viral fitness	Better viral control; risk of stratification and confounding in vaccine trials	55, 56, 59
TRIM5α alleles	Macaque	Differences in cellular restriction of incoming virus by targeting of viral capsid	Determinant of cross-species transmission, and of peak and set-point viral load; risk of stratification and confounding in vaccine trials	55, 60, 61

with proposed functions in cell adhesion and cell signaling [33]. A second approach using *in vitro* models in the study of cellular susceptibility to HIV was reported by Bol and colleagues [34]. This group infected monocyte-derived macrophages from 393 blood donors with HIV-1. Thereafter, they completed a GWAS using *in vitro* viral replication, determined using Gag p24 antigen levels, as the study phenotype. The SNP rs12483205 in DYRK1A approached genome-wide significance ($P = 2.16 \times 10^{-5}$).

Although beyond the scope of this chapter, it is important to indicate that other levels of analysis at the genome scale are increasingly being applied in HIV research. These include studies of the transcriptome of the infected individual or of specific cell subsets, proteomics and building of viral-host protein co-immunoprecipitation libraries relevant to the early innate immune responses to HIV, and large-scale functional genomics using loss-of-function (siRNA) and gain-of-function screens [35–37].

HOST GENETICS IN HIV VACCINE TRIALS

Genetic variation at the DNA level is an important contributor to every aspect of human diversity. It therefore seems reasonable to assume that host genetics will also play a role in determining immunological and clinical responses to vaccines. From early-days empiricism to more recent exploration of fundamental immunology, it is fair to say that HIV vaccine research has not devoted much attention to human genomics. However, because of the combination of unsatisfactory results on the vaccine front and rapid advances in genomic technologies, the importance of taking into account host genetic diversity in designing and testing vaccine candidates is now better appreciated (Figure 12.2); this has been outlined, for example, in the report written by the Host Genetics and Viral Diversity Working Group for the 2010 Scientific Strategic Plan of the Global HIV Vaccine Enterprise [38].

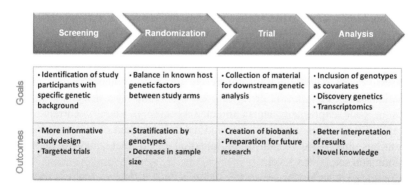

FIGURE 12.2   **Proposed applications of human genetics in vaccine trials, outlining the goals and expected outcomes for each phase of a vaccine trial.**

The first genome-wide association study focusing on a vaccine-related outcome was performed using DNA from participants in the Step trial, a phase 2b study that was designed to assess the safety and efficacy of a three-dose regimen of the Merck adenovirus serotype 5 (MRKAd5) HIV-1 gag/pol/nef vaccine, which aimed to elicit cellular immune responses [39]. Although not protective, the vaccine was highly immunogenic and induced HIV-specific T cell responses that showed considerable inter-individual variability and therefore represented an adequate phenotype for genetic exploration. The genome-wide study identified associations between a number of HLA-B alleles and the intensity of HIV-specific T cell responses, thereby demonstrating the importance of the host immunogenetic background in shaping cellular immune responses to the tested vaccine [40]. Interestingly, the HLA alleles that impacted T cell responses were already known to associate with HIV-1 control during infection (e.g., HLA-B*5701 and B*2705); a clear connection between natural viral control and vaccine response was thus confirmed. This result certainly suggests that the genetic background of vaccine trial participants has the potential to alter immunological or clinical responses to immunogens; failure to consider human genetic variation in the vaccine equation could therefore introduce serious bias in the analysis of clinical trials, while careful assessment of inter-individual differences could open up new avenues for better delineating the mechanisms of action of tested products.

Genetic investigations are also an integral part of the large effort that is underway to understand the results of the RV144 trial, which gave the first supporting evidence of any vaccine conferring some degree of protection against HIV acquisition in humans [41]. Investigators are exploring the possible impact of host genetic factors on HIV acquisition in trial participants, as well as on vaccine-induced cellular and humoral immune responses.

PRIMATE GENOME COMPARISON

This book has as one of the main emphases the identification of tools and approaches that can serve to understand differences in susceptibility to HIV and other retroviruses across primates, and to improve the animal models used in vaccine and pathogenesis research. The contribution of comparative genomics to this specific task can be summarized in the following three aspects: the identification of interspecies differences in genomic signals that can orient biological studies to specific genes or protein domains; the analysis of differences in gene expression across infected species to identify correlates of susceptibility or disease progression; and the development of systems biology approaches that place responses to infection or to vaccination at a more dynamic and integrated level.

Comparative genomics serves to catalog genetic differences across species. Evolutionary genomics defines the trajectory of genes according to the type of selective pressure that has been exerted: positive selection indicates the possibility of genetic conflicts, such as those expected from a host–pathogen interaction, and purifying or negative selection maintains the structure of the gene across species. The genes of innate immunity are characteristically less conserved than the average gene, and a subset of those genes, in particular those that are dedicated to the control of retroviruses (e.g., TRIM5α, APOBEC3G), is under strong positive selection [42]. Evolutionary data from those genes served to inform the domains and residues immediately relevant to the interaction with a given retroviral pathogen. A novel development anchored in evolutionary genomics is the possibility to reconstruct the ancestral state of proteins. Ancestral reconstruction uses recent advances in phylogenetics to infer the ancestral state of genes while taking into consideration various uncertainties about the evolutionary process [43]. In the case of TRIM5α, successful reconstruction of a 25-million-year protein allowed functional testing [44]. More recently, data on lemur TRIM5α contributed new information towards a model of TRIM5α evolution under retroviral pressure [45]. Estimation of a possible 40-million-year-old ancestral primate TRIM5α highlighted that the most striking process in TRIM5α evolution is the lineage specific expansion of variable loops v1 to v3 in the B30.2/SPRY. Variable v1 expansion characterizes hominoid and Old World monkey TRIM5α; v2 expansion is observed in some lemurs, cow TRIM5 and mouse TRIM12 and 30; while v3 expansion characterizes New World monkey TRIM5α [45].

A second level of primate genome comparison can be built using expression data. Several groups have demonstrated the different patterns of interferon response upon natural SIV infection of sooty mangabeys and African green monkeys compared with the pathogenic model of infection in rhesus macaques and Asian pigtailed macaques [46–48]. In these studies, a strong initial interferon response induced during non-pathogenic infection resolves after peak viral load. Thereafter, the non-pathogenic primate models are characterized by low levels of immune activation. More recently, Rotger and colleagues [49] investigated the minority of HIV-infected individuals that remain asymptomatic and show persistently high CD4+ T cell counts despite very high viremia for many years (viremic non-progressors, VNPs). As observed in non-pathogenic models of SIV infection, VNPs present lower expression of interferon-stimulated genes and lower levels of the monocyte-expressed LPS receptor sCD14 than human rapid progressors; they share with SIV-infected sooty mangabeys a common profile of regulation of a set of genes that includes *CASP1*, *CD38*, *LAG3*, *TNFSF13B*, *SOCS1* and *EEF1D*. VNPs, who represent 0.1 percent of patients in human cohorts, may inform our understanding of HIV pathogenesis. It is important to underscore that these cross-species analyses of transcriptome data were possible through the use of novel tools, such as Gene Set Enrichment Analysis (GSEA). GSEA tests the relative position of a collection of genes ("query gene set") within an independent, ranked dataset ("reference gene set"). GSEA is less dependent on arbitrary cut-offs such as fold change of specific *P* values, making its ability to detect an underlying process within transcriptome data potentially more sensitive than a "single-gene" approach using traditional statistics. The utilization of rank data rather than absolute intensity measurements in GSEA also affords greater flexibility to make comparisons between diverse gene-expression data (i.e., between tissues, species or array platforms [50]).

Genetic analyses are leading to more advanced functional genomics. Barreiro and colleagues [51] compared immune responses among primates by stimulating primary monocytes from humans, chimpanzees and rhesus macaques with lipopolysaccharide (LPS). They studied the ensuing time-course regulatory responses to find that Toll-like receptor responses are mostly conserved across primates, although the response associated with viral infections appeared lineage-specific. Their interpretation was that lineage-specific immune responses may help explain inter-species differences in susceptibility to infectious diseases, probably reflecting rapid host–virus mutual cycles of adaptation.

CLINICAL IMPLICATIONS

A major objective of host genomic research in HIV disease is to identify genetic factors that play a role in host–viral interaction, participate in HIV-1 pathogenesis, and have the potential to serve as novel therapeutic or vaccine targets. Beyond basic biology, however, the exploration of the human genome is also expected to pave the way toward personalization of patient care. As our understanding of the genetic basis for inter-individual differences in disease outcome and in response to therapy increases, the possibility of using this information to tailor clinical follow-up will continue to develop. A crucial point, at this stage, is to remember that results from association analyses at the population level do not immediately translate into information that is relevant at the individual level. A failure to grasp or to convey the importance of this limitation has been central to the cycles of hype and frustration observed over the past few years in the nascent field of personalized medicine. Many were too quick to transpose the paradigm of Mendelian disorders, in which single mutations are responsible for dramatic symptoms, to complex diseases, without realizing that common genetic polymorphisms often have limited influence. It is now obvious that, for most clinical outcomes, genetic information can only be meaningful when placed in a more global context, integrating demographic, environmental and social aspects.

Nonetheless, host genetic markers have the potential to be used to stratify populations based on the risk of rapid disease progression, informing decisions about when to start antiretroviral treatment: predictive scores are being developed that combine securely identified genetic determinants of HIV control and additional relevant cofactors like gender, age or non-genetic clinical correlates of disease progression [37]. Given that most of the inter-individual variability has yet to be explained at the population level, one shouldn't expect current genetic scores to be immediately applicable clinical tools. They will, however, continue to be enriched, refined and validated by more translational research, until they become an integral part of individualized patient care. One clinical application would be the identification of individuals who would not need initiation of antiretroviral treatment as recommended by current recommendations [52].

In contrast, some facets of human genetics have more immediate clinical relevance—most notably, pharmacogenetics. A paramount example is the link between HLA-B*5701 carriage and the antiretroviral drug abacavir: the demonstration that individuals carrying the B*5701 are at high risk of hyper-sensitivity reaction resulted in the adoption of guidelines recommending HLA-B*5701 testing before abacavir prescription. There are other genetic markers that could be used as predictors of the likelihood of suffering adverse effects of a drug leading to discontinuation [53]. More generally, it is now clear that differences in treatment toxicity, efficacy and pharmacokinetics are due, at least in part, to human genetic variants that affect drug metabolism, drug disposition and off-site drug targets. Translating this knowledge to the clinical world might not be straightforward because of a combination of limited familiarity with genetic analyses, the inertia of healthcare systems, and constrained budgets, but could represent a significant step forward in the quality of care.

Another setting where genetic stratification will be of increasing importance is in vaccine trials (Figure 12.2). Recent studies in primates have demonstrated the need to understand the genetic structure of the animals included in the studies. Genetic variation in TRIM5α in macaques determines, to a large extent, the outcome of infection—both peak and set-point viremia—potentially con-founding studies with a limited number of animals if the different alleles are not equally represented in all groups, or if the information is not taken into account [54,55]. The second locus that needs to be considered in the study design or interpretation is the carriage of protective HLA alleles, in particular *Mamu*-A*01 [55,56]. Examples of allelic imbalance distorting the outcome of trials has been already described [57], and it is expected that this aspect of vaccine genomics will become increasingly relevant.

CONCLUSIONS

Eric Lander coined the concept that "Within genomics, we must complete biomedicine's 'periodic table'" [58]. This is the spirit that should prevail in the stepwise collection of genomic, transcriptomic and other orders of high-content data pertinent to the analysis of the susceptibility to HIV. This concept was conveyed by the 2010 scientific strategic plan of the Global HIV Vaccine Enterprise, whose working group on host genetic and viral diversity stated that "Ideally, every human gene that impacts each mode of HIV transmission and disease outcome should be identified to improve our understanding of the mechanisms of protection" [38]. It also reinforced the notion that, for this goal to be accomplished, the investigated populations should represent human diversity, as well as cohorts enriched in individuals at the extreme of the

---

BOX 12.1

1. Genetic and genomic analyses have contributed to the understanding of the host response to HIV/SIV infection and disease progression in human and non-human primates.
2. At least 20 percent of variation in viral control at the population level is explained by known genetic polymorphisms. In the macaque model, TRIM5α and Mamu alleles explain heterogeneity in response to SIV infection.
3. Use of these data should be prioritized in the design and analysis of vaccine trials, and could be considered for clinical applications, notably decisions on "when to treat".
4. New technologies will improve the depth, the breadth and the thoroughness of analyses, expanding from the blueprint (genomic DNA) to its regulation and expression.
5. A complete description of genomic influences on HIV disease will require joint analysis of the host and viral genomes.

---

phenotypic distribution. The working group also identified as a priority, and as key to vaccination studies, the understanding of the genetic structure of non-human primate models and its impact on vaccination and infection (Box 12.1). Finally, the recommendation was made that vaccine trials should include a complete genetic characterization of study participants who become infected during the trial (vaccinated and placebo controls).

It is of critical importance to complete the understanding of the role of host DNA variation in susceptibility to infection and disease. Exome and whole genome sequencing data will soon complement the wealth of information obtained through large-scale genotyping studies, and provide a comprehensive description of the contribution of genomic DNA variation to HIV phenotypes. This step will be key to tackling the challenge of other elements of heritability: the next layers of genetic information (e.g., regulation and epigenetic markings), transcriptome and protein expression, as well as progress in the understanding of the mutual information that can be obtained from the joint analysis of the host DNA and the genome of the infecting virus.

ACKNOWLEDGEMENTS

JF is supported by a SNF Professorship grant from the Swiss National Science Foundation; AT is supported by the Swiss National Science Foundation, grant 31003A_132863.

REFERENCES

[1] Lander ES. Initial impact of the sequencing of the human genome. Nature 2011;470:187–97.
[2] Mardis ER. A decade's perspective on DNA sequencing technology. Nature 2011;470:198–203.

[3] Dean M, Carrington M, Winkler C, Huttley GA, Smith MW, Allikmets R, et al. Genetic restriction of HIV-1 infection and progression to AIDS by a deletion allele of the CKR5 structural gene. Hemophilia Growth and Development Study, Multicenter AIDS Cohort Study, Multicenter Hemophilia Cohort Study, San Francisco City Cohort, ALIVE Study. Science 1996;273:1856−62.

[4] Samson M, Libert F, Doranz BJ, Rucker J, Liesnard C, Farber CM, et al. Resistance to HIV-1 infection in caucasian individuals bearing mutant alleles of the CCR-5 chemokine receptor gene. Nature 1996;382:722−5.

[5] Liu R, Paxton WA, Choe S, Ceradini D, Martin SR, Horuk R, et al. Homozygous defect in HIV-1 coreceptor accounts for resistance of some multiply-exposed individuals to HIV-1 infection. Cell 1996;86:367−77.

[6] Blanpain C, Lee B, Tackoen M, Puffer B, Boom A, Libert F, et al. Multiple nonfunctional alleles of CCR5 are frequent in various human populations. Blood 2000;96:1638−45.

[7] Quillent C, Oberlin E, Braun J, Rousset D, Gonzalez-Canali G, Metais P, et al. HIV-1-resistance phenotype conferred by combination of two separate inherited mutations of CCR5 gene. Lancet 1998;351:14−8.

[8] Lederman MM, Alter G, Daskalakis DC, Rodriguez B, Sieg SF, Hardy G, et al. Determinants of protection among HIV-exposed seronegative persons: An overview. J Infect Dis 2010;202(Suppl 3):S333−8.

[9] Fox J, Fidler S. Sexual transmission of HIV-1. Antiviral Res 2010;85:276−85.

[10] Petrovski S, Fellay J, Shianna KV, Carpenetti N, Kumwenda J, Kamanga G, et al. Common human genetic variants and HIV-1 susceptibility: a genome-wide survey in a homogeneous African population. AIDS 2011;25:513−8.

[11] O'Brien SJ, Nelson GW. Human genes that limit AIDS. Nature Genetics 2004;36:565−74.

[12] Fellay J. Host genetics influences on HIV type-1 disease. Antivir Ther 2009;14:731−8.

[13] Campbell CD, Ogburn EL, Lunetta KL, Lyon HN, Freedman ML, Groop LC, et al. Demonstrating stratification in a European American population. Nature Genetics 2005;37:868−72.

[14] Fellay J, Ge D, Shianna KV, Colombo S, Ledergerber B, Cirulli ET, et al. Common genetic variation and the control of HIV-1 in humans. PLoS Genet 2009;5:e1000791.

[15] Telenti A, Goldstein DB. Genomics meets HIV-1. Nature Rev 2006;4:865−73.

[16] Fellay J, Shianna KV, Ge D, Colombo S, Ledergerber B, Weale M, et al. A whole-genome association study of major determinants for host control of HIV-1. Science 2007;317:944−7.

[17] Pelak K, Goldstein DB, Walley NM, Fellay J, Ge D, Shianna KV, et al. Host determinants of HIV-1 control in African Americans. J Infect Dis 2010;201:1141−9.

[18] Dalmasso C, Carpentier W, Meyer L, Rouzioux C, Goujard C, Chaix ML, et al. Distinct genetic loci control plasma HIV-RNA and cellular HIV-DNA levels in HIV-1 infection: The ANRS Genomewide Association 01 Study. PLoS ONE 2008;3:e3907.

[19] The International HIV Controllers Study. The major genetic determinants of HIV-1 control affect HLA class I peptide presentation. Science 2010;330:1551−7.

[20] Herbeck JT, Gottlieb GS, Winkler CA, Nelson GW, An P, Maust BS, et al. Multistage genome-wide association study identifies a locus at 1q41 associated with rate of HIV-1 disease progression to clinical AIDS, J Infect Dis 201:618−26.

[21] Le Clerc S, Limou S, Coulonges Cd, Carpentier W, Dina C, Taing L, et al. Genome-wide association study of a rapid progression cohort identifies new susceptibility alleles for AIDS (ANRS Genomewide Association Study 03). J Infect Dis 2009;200:1194−201.

[22] Limou S, Le Clerc S, Coulonges C, Carpentier W, Dina C, Delaneau O, et al. Genome-wide association study of an AIDS-nonprogression cohort emphasizes the role played by HLA genes (ANRS Genomewide Association Study 02). J Infect Dis 2009;199:419−26.

[23] Limou S, Coulonges C, Herbeck Joshua T, van Manen D, An P, Le Clerc S, et al. Multiple-cohort Genetic Association Study reveals CXCR6 as a new chemokine receptor involved in long-term nonprogression to AIDS. J Infect Dis 2010;202:908−15.

[24] Evangelou E, Fellay J, Colombo S, Martinez-Picado J, Obel N, Goldstein DB, et al. Impact of phenotype definition on genome-wide association signals: Empirical evaluation in HIV-1 infection. Am J Epidemiol 2011, in press.

[25] Thomas R, Apps R, Qi Y, Gao X, Male V, O'Huigin C, et al. HLA-C cell surface expression and control of HIV/AIDS correlate with a variant upstream of HLA-C. Nature Genetics 2009;41:1290−4.

[26] Ritchie AJ, Campion SL, Kopycinski J, Moodie Z, Wang ZM, Pandya K, et al. Differences in HIV-specific T cell responses between HIV-exposed and -unexposed HIV-seronegative individuals. J Virol 2011;85:3507−16.

[27] Kulkarni SS, Savan R, Qi Y, Gao X, Yuki Y, Bass SE, et al. Differential microRNA regulation of HLA-C expression and its association with HIV control. Nature 2011, in press.

[28] Carrington M, Martin MP, van Bergen J. KIR-HLA intercourse in HIV disease. Trends Microbiol 2008;16:620−7.

[29] Dolan MJ, Kulkarni H, Camargo JF, He W, Smith A, Anaya JM, et al. CCL3L1 and CCR5 influence cell-mediated immunity and affect HIV-AIDS pathogenesis via viral entry-independent mechanisms. Nat Immunol 2007;8:1324−36.

[30] Loffredo JT, Maxwell J, Qi Y, Glidden CE, Borchardt GJ, Soma T, et al. Mamu-B*08-positive macaques control simian immunodeficiency virus replication. J Virol 2007;81: 8827−32.

[31] Yant LJ, Friedrich TC, Johnson RC, May GE, Maness NJ, Enz AM, et al. The high-frequency major histocompatibility complex class I allele Mamu-B*17 is associated with control of simian immunodeficiency virus SIVmac239 replication. J Virol 2006;80:5074−7.

[32] Loeuillet C, Deutsch S, Ciuffi A, Robyr D, Taffe P, Munoz M, et al. *In vitro* whole-genome analysis identifies a susceptibility locus for HIV-1. PLoS Biol 2008;6:e32.

[33] Spindler KR, Welton AR, Lim ES, Duvvuru S, Althaus IW, Imperiale JE, et al. The major locus for mouse adenovirus susceptibility maps to genes of the hematopoietic cell surface-expressed LY6 family. J Immunol 2010;184:3055−62.

[34] Bol SM, Moerland PD, Limou S, van Remmerden Y, Coulonges C, van Manen D, et al. Genomewide Association Study identifies single nucleotide polymorphism in DYRK1A associated with replication of HIV-1 in monocyte-derived macrophages. PLoS ONE 2011;6:e17190.

[35] Bushman FD, Malani N, Fernandes J, D'Orso I, Cagney G, Diamond TL, et al. Host cell factors in HIV replication: Meta-analysis of genome-wide studies. PLoS Pathogens 2009;5:e1000437.

[36] Telenti A. HIV-1 host interactions—integration of large scale datasets. F1000 Biology Reports 2009;1:71.

[37] Fellay J, Shianna KV, Telenti A, Goldstein DB. Host genetics and HIV-1: The final phase? PLoS Pathogens 2010;6:e1001033.

[38] McMichael A, McCutchan F, for the Working Group convened by the Global HIV Vaccine Enterprise, Host Genetics and Viral Diversity (2010). Report from a Global HIV Vaccine Enterprise Working Group. Available from Nature Proceedings, <http://dx.doi.org/10.1038/npre.2010.4797.2>.

[39] Buchbinder SP, Mehrotra DV, Duerr A, Fitzgerald DW, Mogg R, Li D, et al. Efficacy assessment of a cell-mediated immunity HIV-1 vaccine (the Step Study): A

double-blind, randomised, placebo-controlled, test-of-concept trial. Lancet 2008;372: 1881−93.

[40] Fellay J, Frahm N, Shianna KV, Cirulli ET, Casimiro DR, Robertson MN, et al. Host genetic determinants of T cell responses to the MRKAd5 HIV-1 gag/pol/nef vaccine in the Step Trial. J Infect Dis 2011;203:773−9.

[41] Rerks-Ngarm S, Pitisuttithum P, Nitayaphan S, Kaewkungwal J, Chiu J, Paris R, et al. Vaccination with ALVAC and AIDSVAX to prevent HIV-1 infection in Thailand. N Engl J Med 2009;361:2209−20.

[42] Ortiz M, Guex N, Patin E, Martin O, Xenarios I, Ciuffi A, et al. Evolutionary trajectories of primate genes involved in HIV pathogenesis. Mol Biol Evol 2009;26:2865−75.

[43] Thornton JW. Resurrecting ancient genes: Experimental analysis of extinct molecules. Nat Rev Genet 2004;5:366−75.

[44] Goldschmidt V, Ciuffi A, Ortiz M, Brawand D, Munoz M, Kaessmann H, et al. Antiretroviral activity of ancestral TRIM5alpha. J Virol 2008;82:2089−96.

[45] Rahm N, Yap M, Snoeck J, Zoete V, Munoz M, Radespiel U, et al. Unique spectrum of activity of prosimian TRIM5alpha against exogenous and endogenous retroviruses. J Virol 2011;85:4173−83.

[46] Bosinger SE, Li Q, Gordon SN, Klatt NR, Duan L, Xu L, et al. Global genomic analysis reveals rapid control of a robust innate response in SIV-infected sooty mangabeys. J Clin Invest 2009;119:3556−72.

[47] Jacquelin B, Mayau V, Targat B, Liovat AS, Kunkel D, Petitjean G, et al. Nonpathogenic SIV infection of African green monkeys induces a strong but rapidly controlled type I IFN response. J Clin Invest 2009;119:3544−55.

[48] Lederer S, Favre D, Walters KA, Proll S, Kanwar B, Kasakow Z, et al. Transcriptional profiling in pathogenic and non-pathogenic SIV infections reveals significant distinctions in kinetics and tissue compartmentalization. PLoS Pathog 2009;5:e1000296.

[49] Rotger M, Dalmau J, Rauch A, McLaren P, Bosinger SE, Marttinez R, et al. Comparative transcriptome analysis of extreme phenotypes of human HIV-1 infection and sooty mangabey and rhesus macaque models of SIV infection. J Clin Invest 2011;121:2391−400.

[50] Haining WN, Wherry EJ. Integrating genomic signatures for immunologic discovery. Immunity 2010;32:152−61.

[51] Barreiro LB, Marioni JC, Blekhman R, Stephens M, Gilad Y. Functional comparison of innate immune signaling pathways in primates. PLoS Genetics 2010;6:e1001249.

[52] Thompson MA, Aberg JA, Cahn P, Montaner JS, Rizzardini G, Telenti A, et al. Antiretroviral treatment of adult HIV infection: 2010 recommendations of the International AIDS Society USA panel. J Am Med Assoc 2010;304:321−33.

[53] Lubomirov R, Colombo S, di Iulio J, Ledergerber B, Martinez R, Cavassini M, et al. Association of pharmacogenetic markers with premature discontinuation of first-line anti-HIV therapy: An observational cohort study. J Infect Dis 2011;203:246−57.

[54] Kirmaier A, Wu F, Newman RM, Hall LR, Morgan JS, O'Connor S, et al. TRIM5 suppresses cross-species transmission of a primate immunodeficiency virus and selects for emergence of resistant variants in the new species. PLoS Biol 2010;8:e1000462.

[55] Lim SY, Rogers T, Chan T, Whitney JB, Kim J, Sodroski J, et al. TRIM5alpha modulates immunodeficiency virus control in rhesus monkeys. PLoS Pathog 2010;6:e1000738.

[56] Allen TM, O'Connor DH, Jing P, Dzuris JL, Mothe BR, Vogel TU, et al. Tat-specific cytotoxic T lymphocytes select for SIV escape variants during resolution of primary viraemia. Nature 2000;407:386−90.

[57] Thompson AJ, Muir AJ, Sulkowski MS, Patel K, Tillmann HL, Clark PJ, et al. Hepatitis C trials that combine investigational agents with pegylated-interferon should be stratified by IL28B genotype. Hepatology 2010;52:2243−4.

[58] Lander ES. The new genomics: Global views of biology. Science 1996;274:536−9.

[59] Evans DT, O'Connor DH, Jing P, Dzuris JL, Sidney J, da Silva J, et al. Virus-specific cytotoxic T-lymphocyte responses select for amino-acid variation in simian immunodeficiency virus Env and Nef. Nat Med 1999;5:1270−6.

[60] Newman RM, Hall L, Connole M, Chen GL, Sato S, Yuste E, et al. Balancing selection and the evolution of functional polymorphism in Old World monkey TRIM5α. Proc Natl Acad Sci USA 2006;103:19134−9.

[61] Wilson SJ, Webb BL, Maplanka C, Newman RM, Verschoor EJ, Heeney JL, et al. Rhesus macaque TRIM5 alleles have divergent antiretroviral specificities. J Virol 2008;82:7243−7.

Conclusions

Gianfranco Pancino [1], Guido Silvestri [2,3] and Keith R. Fowke [4]

[1] INSERM and Institut Pasteur, Unité de Régulation des Infections Rétrovirales, Paris, France, [2] Department of Pathology and Laboratory Medicine, Emory University School of Medicine, Atlanta, Georgia, USA, [3] Division of Microbiology & Immunology, Yerkes National Primate Research Center, Emory University, Atlanta, Georgia, USA, [4] Laboratory of Viral Immunology, Department of Medical Microbiology, and Department of Community Health Sciences, University of Manitoba, Winnipeg, Manitoba, Canada

Readers of this book will have understood that there are three basic ways to deal with primate immunodeficiency lentivirus infections without succumbing to AIDS. The first way is to avoid infection altogether despite being intensely exposed; this is the goal achieved by the group of "HIV-exposed seronegative" (HESN) individuals. The second way is to control virus replication after being infected, which is achieved by the subset of HIV-infected individuals that are defined as "HIV controllers" (HICs). The third way is to control pathogenesis— that is, to remain with a functioning immune system, even if virus replication is not controlled. This last scenario is exemplified by the non-pathogenic SIV infections of natural hosts, such as the African green monkey (AGM) and sooty mangabey (SM), as well as a few rare HIV-infected individuals defined as "viremic non-progressors". In both HICs and natural SIV hosts a key feature of the infection is the low level of immune activation, and, at least in the case of natural SIV infections, this phenomenon appears to be evolutionarily driven by several thousand years of host—pathogen interaction, resulting in a balanced relationship between the virus and the host.

More than 15 years of studies on HESNs have demonstrated that the ways to resist infection are likely multiple. This is probably the reason why prominent mechanisms of protection against infection have not clearly arisen, except for the CCR5Δ32 variant in Caucasians. There are data supporting a role for additional genetic determinants, such as the association of HLA haplotypes, or of IRF1 polymorphisms, with the resistance to HIV-1 infection, but highly significant associations such as those found for the viral control in HICs (see below) have not been described. This may also be due to the limited size of the HESN groups studied, and to the heterogeneity of the populations. Additionally, intrinsic resistance to infection of CD4 T cells, enhanced NK cell activity, and specific immune responses, especially localized at mucosal sites, have all been implicated in the protection against infection. Environmental determinants, including antiviral factors secreted at genital sites and the mucosal microbiome, are thought to play a relevant role in the protection against viral entry and propagation. Therefore, it is plausible that some of these distinct mechanisms are needed to operate in cooperation, or in synergy, to block viral transmission or to cause abortive local infection.

HICs do get infected but succeed in containing viral replication to undetectable levels in the early phases of infection, thus avoiding excessive chronic immune activation. T cell responses, and especially cytotoxic T lymphocytes (CTLs), appear to contribute greatly to maintaining a long-lasting control of HIV infection, at least in strong responder HICs. This is underlined by the strong association of viral control with HLA alleles known to be involved in the induction of an efficient CTL response, including HLA-B57 and B27. The critical role of the genetic background in the effective immune control of HIV infection in HICs is further supported by additional associations of viral control with polymorphisms in the MHC locus, including the HLA-C-35 SNIP that modulates the surface expression of HLA-C molecules. Besides T cell responses, intrinsic mechanisms of resistance to HIV replication may contribute to viral control, since CD4 T cells and macrophages from HIC exhibit low susceptibility to HIV infection *in vitro*. Since the control of infection appears to occur in the acute/early phases of infection, the lack of data concerning these phases precludes drawing up a clear picture of the events that lead to the suppression of viral replication. A hypothetical scenario is that due to different causes, including viral restrictions in target cells, early innate immune response or, in certain cases, infection with decreased replicative fitness viruses, viral spread is rapidly knocked down. This could allow the host to mount an effective adaptive response that will keep the virus in stalemate during the chronic phase.

In contrast with HICs, specific immune responses do not play a key role in protecting SIV-infected natural hosts from disease progression. The success of controlling immune activation in African monkeys is based on the ability of the host to down-modulate innate immune responses, including type I interferon production and IFN-related gene activation, after the burst that follows acute infection. Importantly, this spares lymphoid tissue integrity and immune functions. It is still unclear how SIV-infected SMs and AGMs avoid aberrant chronic immune activation, despite having levels of virus replication comparable with those described in humans and rhesus monkeys (RMs). A large array of factors appears to contribute to the balance between viral replication and host responses, such as interactions between viral proteins, including Nef, with cell determinants involved in T cell response contributing to modulate immune activation; the downregulation of molecules required for viral entry, such as CD4 and CCR5, helping to preserve the memory T cell pool; and endowment of other lymphocyte subsets with T helper functions allowing maintenance of an efficient immune system also in the presence of SIV-induced CD4 T cell loss. Whether the absence of chronic immune activation is the result of a tolerance to the virus or is due to active mechanisms of downregulation of the initial burst of immune activation, involving Tregs or other regulatory pathways, or whether both mechanisms are involved, is matter of debate. The presence of both B and T cell responses to virus, although moderate, seems to be at odds with immune tolerance. However, the low Ab level against Gag observed in SIV-infected AGMs, as well as the TCR down-regulation induced by SIVagm or SIVsmm Nef, may support an evolution of host partial tolerance to the virus.

Given the differences in the natural history of host—virus interactions in humans and monkeys, as well as the tremendous variability of both the virus and host genes that control the immune responses, it may not be possible to build a single unifying model of protection against HIV/SIV infection and disease. However, it is noteworthy that some factors are shared by the three models discussed in this book:

1. Factors that decrease the permissiveness of target cells to HIV infection, such as downregulation of CD4 and CCR5 expression at the cell surface in African monkeys and CCR5 in HESNs, decreased numbers of activated CD4+ T cells in HESNs, or intracellular restriction mechanisms in HESNs and HICs;
2. Regulation of IFN pathways in African monkeys and in HESNs;
3. Enhanced NK cell activity in HESNs and in acute infection of SMs;
4. Associations of MHC polymorphisms with protection in HICs and HESNs (favorable MHC-associated efficient CTL responses have also been reported to control viral replication in pathogenic SIVmac infection of rhesus macaques).

Humans and non-human primates have evolved so that not all individuals mount the identical response to viral infection or exposure. The existence of rare individuals who resist infection or control viral replication without need of antiretroviral therapy constitutes proof that long-lasting remission from disease and even prevention of infection are achievable objectives. Current therapeutic approaches based on CCR5 inhibition have been inspired by results from the research on HESNs. Many vaccine studies are aimed to induce CTL responses with the same qualitative features as those found in HIC. Moreover, the induction of protective innate responses is a novel field of vaccine research. On the other hand, the apathogenic model of infection of African monkeys strongly supports therapeutic approaches aimed at reducing immune activation in HIV-infected individuals in complement to antiretroviral treatments.

Clearly, these models provide evidence that control or prevention of HIV/SIV infection is possible. Further work will define the mechanisms, and how they are to be implemented on a global scale. The hope these real-world models bring is that one day the life-costing disease of AIDS can be eliminated, and HIV transmission can be prevented altogether.

Index

Printed and bound by CPI Group (UK) Ltd, Croydon, CR0 4YY

03/10/2024

01040419-0003